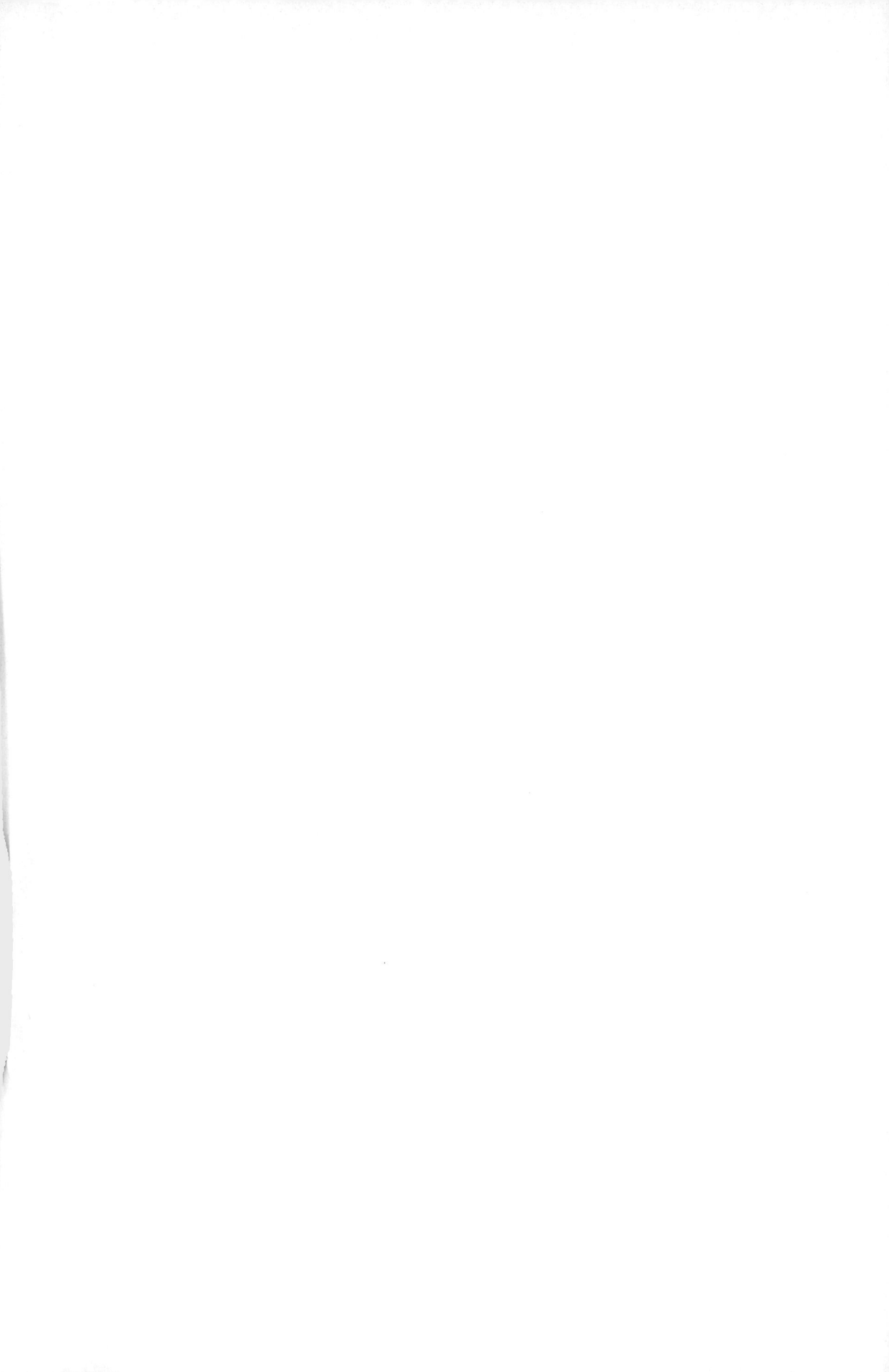

RECOVERY FROM BRAIN DAMAGE
Reflections and Directions

ADVANCES IN EXPERIMENTAL MEDICINE AND BIOLOGY

A Continuation Order Plan is available for this series. A continuation order will bring delivery of each new volume immediately upon publication. Volumes are billed only upon actual shipment. For further information please contact the publisher.

RECOVERY FROM BRAIN DAMAGE

Reflections and Directions

Edited by

F. D. Rose

Goldsmiths' College
University of London
London, United Kingdom

and

D. A. Johnson

Astley Ainslie Hospital
Edinburgh, Scotland, United Kingdom

SPRINGER SCIENCE+BUSINESS MEDIA, LLC

Library of Congress Cataloging-in-Publication Data

Recovery from brain damage : reflections and directions / edited by
F.D. Rose and D.A. Johnson.
        p.   cm. -- (Advances in experimental medicine and biology ; v.
325)
     "Proceedings of a European Brain and Behaviour Society (EBBS)
Workshop on Recovery of Function following Brain Damage, held April
11-13, 1991, at Goldsmiths' College, London, United Kingdom"--T.p.
verso.
    Includes bibliographical references and index.
    ISBN 978-0-306-44344-2   ISBN 978-1-4615-3420-4 (eBook)
    DOI 10.1007/978-1-4615-3420-4
    1. Brain damage--Patients--Rehabilitation--Congresses.   I. Rose,
David (F. David) II. Johnson, D. A., 1952-   . III. European Brain
and Behaviour Society (EBBS) Workshop on Recovery of Function
following Brain Damage (1991 : Goldsmiths' College) IV. Series.
    [DNLM: 1. Brain Injuries--rehabilitation--congresses.   W1 AD559
v.325 / WL 354 R3112 1991]
RC387.5.R38 1992
DNLM/DLC
for Library of Congress   92-35407
                                                               CIP

Proceedings of a European Brain and Behaviour Society (EBBS) Workshop
on Recovery of Function following Brain Damage, held April 11-13, 1991,
at Goldsmiths' College, London, United Kingdom

ISBN 978-0-306-44344-2

© 1992 Springer Science+Business Media New York
Originally published by Plenum Press, New York in 1992

PREFACE

The present volume is based upon the invited review lectures delivered to the European Brain and Behaviour Society's Workshop on Recovery of Function Following Brain Damage held at Goldsmiths' College, University of London, in April 1991.

Coming exactly ten years after the Society's first meeting on this subject, held at Erasmus University, Rotterdam, a major objective of the Workshop was to review progress in the intervening years. This task was begun by Professor D. G. Stein in his opening presentation. Looking ahead to possible developments in recovery research in the next decade was the subject of Professor B. Kolb's closing lecture. The intervening presentations reviewed progress made in specific areas of recovery research.

In addition to reviewing progress over the last decade we sought to achieve an additional objective in the way that the invited review lectures were organised. This was to bring together those doing basic research, usually animal research, and those whose research interests are more clinically orientated. Thus some of the lectures were "paired", one concentrating on the results of animal studies and one on clinical research findings. For example, whilst Professor A. Björklund reviewed progress in animal studies of neural implantation, Professor E. R. Hitchcock reviewed neural implantation as a treatment for Parkinson's disease patients. Similarly, in considering recovery from extensive unilateral brain damage, Professor M. W. van Hof reviewed work on hemidecorticate animals whilst Dr. F. Vargha-Khadem discussed cognitive outcome after hemispherecomy in human patients. The discussion of environmental influences on recovery followed the same pattern with Professor B. E. Will and Dr. C. Kelche reviewing the role of environmental enrichment in recovery of function following brain lesions in animals and Professor L. Diller evaluating neuropsychological rehabilitation in brain damaged humans.

The emphasis placed on strengthening the links between human and animal work represented one aspect of a final and broader objective of the Workshop. This was to discuss the organisational aspects of research on recovery of function and, particularly, the value of more systematic and widespread collaboration between those doing this type of research. Given the scale, complexity and importance of recovery research it is imperative that scientists and clinicians pay much more attention to the organisation and management of research than has traditionally been the case. Imaginative organisation and management of our activities is surely the way to fulfil the potential of recovery research in improving the outcome for those whose lives have been blighted by brain damage. At present we do not feel that this potential is being fulfilled. One session of the Workshop, out of an otherwise entirely scientific programme, was reserved for launching this discussion and was addressed by Mr. P. Colyer, Coordinator of Scientific Networks for the European Science Foundation. Some aspects of this discussion are considered in the final chapter of this volume.

The list of contributors to the present volume is not exactly the same as the list of those invited to give review lectures at the Workshop. Because of other commitments neither Professor Björklund nor Dr. J. D. Turner were able to expand their talks to form chapters. However, we are most grateful to Dr. J. D. Sinden, Dr. K. M. Marsden and Dr. H. Hodges for stepping in to contribute a very comprehensive review of the animal work on neural implantation. Other invited speakers, Professor Stein, Dr. Vargha-Khadem and Professor van Hof, have chosen to write their chapters in collaboration with others and we should like to extend our thanks to these additional contributors as well.

By the time any volume of this nature appears on a bookshelf there are many "thank you's" to be said, of course. We are most grateful to all the invited review lecturers and other contributing authors, to Mrs. Sue Weston who typed the manuscript, and to Ms. Nicola Clark, Ms. Janie Curtis and Mr. Greg Safford from Plenum Press for their advice and forebearance. We should also like to thank all those who helped us in planning and running the Workshop itself. In particular we should like to mention the other members of the Organising Committee, Professor B. A. Bell (St. George's Hospital Medical School, London), Professor J. A. Gray (Institute of Psychiatry, London), Mr. C. J. Latham (Goldsmiths' College, London), Dr. J. D. Sinden (Institute of Psychiatry, London) and Professor M. W. Van Hof (Erasmus University, Rotterdam), but also a small army of undergraduates, postgraduate students and staff from Goldsmiths' College whose enthusiasm, hard work and humour ensured the success of the Workshop. Finally we should like to thank the following organizations for their financial support for the Workshop: Bayer (UK) Ltd., Children's Head Injury Trust, Commercial Union Plc., Fisons Pharmaceuticals, Norwich Union Insurance Group, the Parkinson's Disease Society, Pearl Assurance, PPP Medical Trust Ltd., Sanofi (UK) Ltd., Scottish Widows' Fund and Life Assurance Society, Schering Berlin, the Wellcome Foundation Ltd., and the Wellcome Trust.

F.D. Rose and D.A. Johnson

CONTENTS

AN OVERVIEW OF DEVELOPMENTS IN RESEARCH ON RECOVERY FROM BRAIN INJURY

Donald G Stein and Marylou M Glasier

Brain Research Laboratory
Institute of Animal Behavior
Rutgers, the State University
Newark, New Jersey, USA

INTRODUCTION

Although there have recently been many other conferences on the subject, it was in 1981 that Professors van Hof and Mohn, under the auspices of the European Brain and Behaviour Society, organized the first major European workshop devoted exclusively to "Functional Recovery from Brain Damage." That landmark meeting, held at the Erasmus University in Rotterdam, was the first major international conference bringing together investigators from many different countries who were interested in a careful and thorough analysis of brain damage and the processes mediating behavioral recovery.

For the casual reader or for those just entering this vital and exciting area of scientific inquiry and clinical application, it is worth noting that there has been a virtual explosion of research on recovery of function in the last decade. At the Rotterdam meeting in 1981, almost everyone attending knew each other and was further acquainted with almost everyone else working on brain injury and repair. At that time there were perhaps only 50-60 investigators around the globe who were seriously committed to this kind of research. Ten years later we find that there are many international groups representing hundreds of investigators, several professional societies and a number of journals dedicated primarily to research on recovery of function following central nervous system (CNS) damage[a].

---

[a] Professional groups such as the Neurotrauma Society, National Head Injury Foundation; journals focusing on recovery from brain and spinal cord injury including (but not limited to): Restorative Neurology and Neuroscience, Journal of Neurotrauma, Brain Injury Rehabilitation, and Experimental Neurology.

Recovery from Brain Damage, Edited by F.D. Rose and
D.A. Johnson, Plenum Press, New York, 1992

1

The first volume[85] of the EBBS conference proceedings provided a good representation of the ideas about recovery mechanisms that were prevalent just a decade ago. In a time span of only ten years, however, recovery research has greatly changed. The difference becomes evident in a comparison of the kinds of papers reported in the van Hof and Mohn book with some 1991 topics in neurotrauma research. In the 1981 meeting, 65% of the papers focused on behavioral and performance deficits following brain damage, in order to examine the prevailing views about structure/function relationships in the central nervous system. About 20% of the papers were concerned with anatomical substrates of neuronal plasticity in developing animals, while only 15% reported on pharmacological interventions designed to treat CNS damage. As an example of the change in focus in recovery research, in 1981 only one author briefly mentioned the possibility of using fetal brain tissue transplants as potential treatment for CNS injury and one speculated that glial cells might have an important role to play in injury-induced brain plasticity. In 1990 alone there were hundreds of articles on neural grafting into the damaged CNS and a growing recognition that glia play a key role in the mediation of both normal and pathological brain functions.

In the last several years, symposia and publications have addressed myriad concerns with respect to recovery after brain damage. Topics reported range from multidimensional aspects of neural transplantation, such as genetically engineered cells, immunological problems and delivery systems to EEG analysis in disease states[b] and neurotransmitter response to injury[28,94]. At the first International Neurotrauma Symposium, held in 1991, molecular aspects of neurotrauma research were addressed, including growth, inhibitory, guidance and protective factors in CNS injury and repair, glial response, and the role of calcium and free radicals in injury response.

In looking over the books and proceedings of Recovery meetings over the last 10 years, there has been a major shift away from behavioral work and towards a much more molecular approach in which analysis of allied behaviour seems to play little, if any role. For example, at the 1991 International Neurotrauma Society meeting whose theme was CNS injury and repair, only 6% of the papers presented reported any data at all related to behavioral/functional assessment despite the primary emphasis on "recovery of function." Thus, even a cursory glance at the literature of the last decade will reveal that the major thrust of recovery research has moved away from the more descriptive and holistic behavioral analyses to a much greater emphasis on molecular biology and pharmacology - especially in the area of drug discovery and clinical development. This shift to an emphasis on molecular biology has provided a much better understanding of the physiological mechanisms underlying potential treatments designed to facilitate recovery after CNS damage; however, the complete picture will only emerge when cellular models are combined with the examination and evaluation of behaviour.

---

[b] For examples of these and related issues, see the abstracts and selected papers of the 3rd International Symposium on Neural Transplantation in the special issue of *Restorative Neurology and Neuroscience*. Vol. 1, No. 2, January 1990 and Vol. 82 of *Progress in Brain Research*, entitled "Neural Transplantation: From Molecular Basis to Clinical Applications," S.G. Dunnett and S.-J. Richards, editors, Amsterdam, Elsevier, 1990. Also see *Annals of the New York Academy of Sciences* (Volume 457, 1990), entitled "Windows on the Brain, Neuropsychology's Technological Frontiers."

RECOVERY RESEARCH AND THE CONCEPT OF LOCALIZATION OF FUNCTION

What has accounted for the shift in focus to molecular mechanisms, detached from their accompanying behavioral results? Several factors are implicated, some of which are practical, while others are philosophical. On a practical level, there has been a growing awareness that traumatic brain (and spinal cord) injury represent a very serious medical problem. Recently, Dr. Murray Goldstein[37], the Director of the National Institute of Neurological Disorders and Stroke (USA) wrote that:

> Mortality from traumatic brain injury over the past 12 years has exceeded the cumulative number of American battle deaths in all wars since the founding of our country. The enormity of the problem, often referred to as the silent epidemic, becomes even clearer when we realize that the total number of head injuries is conservatively estimated at over 2 million each year. The overall economic cost to society approaches $25 billion each year. (page 327)

Given the high cost of treatment for brain injury, attention has settled on means of effective initial treatment. Such a focus does not necessarily reflect the time-span of recovery processes. With few exceptions, physicians are concerned with immediate treatment and immediate results, as opposed to long-term follow up of patient progress. Such an argument also applies to laboratory research with animal models, as necessary behavioral assessment of recovery processes is more time consuming and costly.

With patient-oriented, head injury associations gaining impetus and increased success in lobbying for more government support for research and treatment, funds for neurotrauma, stroke and recovery have become more available. Pharmaceutical companies and bioventure capitalists have also begun to recognize that the market for new drugs to treat CNS injury in all its forms (including degenerative disorders such as Parkinsonism, Alzheimer's disease, Huntington's Chorea, etc.) could be quite significant, and so more private funding has become available as well. Since researchers will "go where the money is," and with many neurologists and neurosurgeons beginning to see the potential for a lucrative practice in treating brain damage, recovery research has now become both respectable and mainstream. The shift in emphasis from behavioral to molecular research has been reinforced by the fact that most physicians and biomedical researchers have, in recent years, followed the most recent prevalent view, and thus have typically shown little interest in the analysis of behaviour as an important scientific discipline. In the case of genetic disorders, such as Huntington's Chorea, the molecular bases could be deemed to be overwhelmingly critical. However, for other types of CNS injury, such as stroke or other brain trauma, the necessity remains to evaluate the known molecular alterations with correlative behavioral changes.

A second major causative factor in the continuation of the shift has been one of a philosophical nature. There has been a change in paradigmatic thinking about nervous system organization on the part of biomedical researchers. The initial work on recovery of function was not done with a therapeutic purpose in mind. For the most part, early research on recovery following brain damage was seen primarily as a tool used by experimental psychologists to examine and test the prevailing theories of cerebral organization which stressed localization of function, the assigning to each brain region a specific behavioral role[57,60,63]. Most proponents of strict localization theory argued that the particular impairments produced by lesions to circumscribed brain regions demonstrated localization of function (e.g. cerebral hemispheric control of speech and related aphasias after injury) related to the brain's cytoarchitecture.

Concomitantly, it was easy to think that, if behavioral functions were highly localized, the destruction of the areas controlling the behaviour would lead to permanent and irreversible deficits - the prognosis for recovery then being extremely poor.

In contrast, more holistically oriented psychologists (e.g. Karl Lashley and his students) suggested that localization of impairments following brain damage did not imply localization of function but rather, localization of symptoms[47]. Non-localizationists argued that behavioral sparing or recovery of function following brain lesions should be taken as a demonstration that assignment of complex behaviours to discrete brain "centers" was not helpful for understanding how the central nervous system actually "works" as a complex, integrated and dynamic system.

For the most part, this latter "systems approach" to brain function was initially ignored in favour of much more reductionistic thinking about brain functions. Why? First, individuals with brain damage typically showed very severe and permanent impairments - and prognosis for recovery was virtually nil. Second, cytoarchitectural research was the driving force behind most neuroscience in this century and it made intuitive sense to think that for each type of distinctive neuroarchitectonics, there had to be distinctive functions to "go with" the structures. This view was further reinforced by improvements in laboratory technology which permitted and encouraged fine-grained analyses of neuronal activities. Some examples of this approach can be seen in electrophysiological recording studies popular in the 60's and 70's in which the purported specific involvement of a single neuron in one specific activity gave rise to speculation about the existence of highly complex "perceptual" decision-making cells controlling the organism's behaviour, such as pontifical cells or grandmother cells. Third, there were no consistent treatments for brain injury and until only the last few years, none were even contemplated, further enforcing a limited view of CNS plasticity and of any potential for functional recovery.

Until very recently, many neurologists and neuropsychologists involved with head injury showed little interest in recovery of function as a subdiscipline of their field. With respect to head injury, their main tasks were first to stabilize the patient and then to diagnose and localize the deficits caused by stroke or trauma, a perspective entirely in keeping with localization doctrine,(e.g., see 53). Any therapy or treatment for recovery of function was left to psychiatrists and rehabilitation workers who "might" be able to help patients cope more effectively with their permanent disabilities.

In the early 1970's, the field of neuroscience began to develop rapidly as a separate discipline. Rather than emerging out of experimental psychology, the newly formed programs in neuroscience usually were located in anatomy or cell biology departments in medical schools where the emphasis was much more biological. As anatomy is basically a descriptive science, hypothesis testing so common in psychology departments gave way to the demonstration and perfection of exquisite map-making, tract-tracing and chemical assay techniques. Indeed, the most widely read textbook of neuroscience, by Kandel, Schwartz and Jessel[50] claims that:

> ... all behaviour, including higher mental functioning (affective as well as cognitive), can be localized to specific regions or constellations of regions within the brain. Descriptive neuroanatomy provides us with a functional guide to local sites within the brain that correspond to specific behaviours. (page 15)

This rigid localization perspective has influenced a whole generation of researchers to think of recovery and plasticity as not much more than a curious anomaly - especially in adult organisms. Now, thanks to the last decade of research clearly demonstrating brain plasticity as related to potential for recovery, lesion analysis is being viewed from a different perspective - even by those who are rather firmly committed to the localization paradigm. For example, Damasio and Damasio[19], working within parcellation theory encompassing the aforementioned "constellations of regions," write that:

> ... brain tissue contains numerous systems, composed of networks that are made up of functional regions interconnected by feedforward and feedback projections. (page 12)

This perspective also leads them to conclude that:

> ... complex psychological activities are not viewed as the result of the operation of a single area or even a single functional region, but rather as the consequence of concerted activity in networks made up of multiple regions. (page 13)

While the increasing awareness of "complexity" in brain activities is heartening, many current notions still imply a strictly fixed system, in which injury is reflected solely in subsequent loss of part of the connected areas and such behaviour as is purported to be associated with the damaged part. The inclusion of concerted activity or an overall localization of connected regions, often utilizing metaphors taken from the computer engineering field, does not adequately explain the mechanisms of extensive cortical reorganization after injury, such as are seen in primates after sensory deafferentation[72], the variable functional effect of lesion size on degree of recovery[46], or the serial lesion effect, in which slow-growing lesions are associated with less severe deficits than lesions occurring rapidly[27]. A complex interconnected localized system also does not explain known alterations in rodent cortical somatosensory maps, which appear dependent on such factors as genetics and experience[87], nor does it fit well with what are commonly referred to clinically as "unexpected recoveries."

During the 1970's and 80's, armed with much new technology (e.g. CAT-scan, SPECT, PET, MRI and immunocytochemistry), the emphasis on describing and mapping the structure of the nervous system grew understandably stronger. The study of behaviour as an important dependent variable in localizing injury and in understanding CNS function became less important.

Thus, while molecular neuroscience was becoming more refined and sophisticated, those concerned with describing behavioral recovery were losing ground because they could do little more than speculate about the biochemical and/or anatomical substrates accounting for their observations. Without "real" physiological events capable of direct manipulation, biologists could argue that the observed "recovery" was not recovery at all, but simply a series of "tricks" or new strategies used by the brain-damaged subject to replace the behaviours that were permanently lost following CNS injury.

In brief, prior to the structural demonstration of injury-induced neuronal plasticity in the late 1960's[73], most explanations of functional recovery, when they were provided, were primarily speculative or phenomenological. For example, when recovery of function after brain damage was observed, investigators suggested that "spontaneous reorganization" had occurred in which other brain areas "took over" the functions of the injured tissue (see references 26,27 for detailed reviews of this and other related issues). Phenomenological concepts of spontaneous reorganization, denervation supersensitivity, and removal of "inhibition" (diaschisis) were difficult to test empirically and even more difficult to relate to specific and known physiological events. Therefore, with the growing emphasis on structure and biochemistry, investigators turned to examining questions that were easier to quantify, were less capricious and variable and lent themselves to more direct determination of structural mechanisms mediating nervous activity. The frustration with the analysis of behaviour is best summed up in the popular neuropharmacology text of Cooper, Bloom and Roth[17], where they state that:

... at the molecular level, an explanation of the action of a drug is often possible, at the cellular level, an explanation is sometimes possible, but at a behavioral level, our ignorance is abysmal. (page 4)

Fortunately, with the considerable strides which occurred in functional neuroanatomy in the late 1960's and early 1970's, the view that the adult central nervous pathways were fixed and immutable began to change. As new techniques for measuring the functional activity of neurons in situ became available, the potential for relating behavioral "plasticity" following brain damage to specific, physiological mechanisms seemed like a more attainable goal. With the advent of new and more sensitive metabolic markers and staining techniques, researchers were able to show that, in response to limited deafferentation of CNS areas, nerve fibers could sprout new terminal branches to replace those that were lost as a result of the injury[38,51,61,73]. It was noted that partially damaged nerve fibers could produce additional nerve terminals to replace those that were destroyed, or that intact fibers in the vicinity of the injury could generate new terminal branches that would reafferent brain areas deprived of their "normal" inputs following damage.

What made these findings particularly exciting and important was that injury-induced regenerative (neuroplastic) phenomena were observed in adult mammals and seemed, in general, to obey principles of organization, growth and guidance found in the nervous systems during development. For the first time, researchers now had some specific and understandable structural mechanisms that could be employed to account for the functional recovery observed when the adult brain was injured.

SOME IMPORTANT MILESTONES IN RESEARCH ON RECOVERY FROM BRAIN DAMAGE

Once a physiological basis for neural plasticity had been established, it then became logical to ask how the specific structure and function of adult neurons could be directly controlled and modified. The implications for such potential modification quickly became apparent to basic researchers and clinicians alike. If the "plasticity" of adult neurons could be understood and controlled, perhaps it would be possible to develop specific treatments to enhance neural growth when and where it was needed. Perhaps it would also be possible to block the neuronal loss that accompanies a variety of degenerative, central nervous system disorders when that goal was a primary consideration.

The answer to these questions continues to be provided by new and exciting developments in molecular biology and neurochemistry. With respect to the development of a pharmacology of recovery, the major advances over the last decade have come in the form of a much broader understanding of the mechanics and genetics of metabolism and chemical activity in neurons and glial cells. Whereas a decade ago, most research focused on defining the up- or down-regulation of neurotransmitters released by pre-synaptic terminals, more current efforts have been directed to discovering and characterizing a large array of new, endogenous substances which modulate neuronal and glial activity under normal and pathological conditions. As the new receptors on neurons and glia were identified, it became increasingly clear that neurotransmitters were not the only controlling factors influencing how the cells perform under normal and pathological conditions. Other classes of molecules called neuromodulators or neurohormones[17] were recognized as playing an important role in determining how the nervous system could be so "modifiable" and responsive to environmental conditions.

With respect to the development of a specific pharmacology of recovery from brain damage over the last decade, there were several fundamentally important areas of research that had significant impact. First, it was confirmed that amino acids involved in CNS metabolism also might serve as neurotransmitters in their own right. In fact, Cooper, Boom and Roth[17] argue that:

> ... from a quantitative standpoint, the amino acids are probably the major neurotransmitters in the mammalian CNS, while the better-known transmitters ... (acetylcholine, norepinephrine, dopamine, histamine and 5-hydroxytryptamine) probably account for transmission at only a small percentage of central synaptic sites. (page 124)

Investigators soon found that the amino acid neurotransmitters are not just important for regulation and control of neurotransmission under normal conditions. It was also determined that traumatic brain injury often results in the excessive release of excitatory amino acids such as glutamate[8,68,70,79]. The term "excessive" is used because, in higher amounts, the same substances necessary for neural transmission become capable of causing neural degeneration, in an effect mediated by actions of NMDA receptors[22,71]. This secondary cell loss could be more detrimental to the patient than the initial injury itself. In particular, ischemia or hypoglycaemia produce a "glutamate cascade" (also seen as a delayed or secondary effect after traumatic brain injury) resulting in an excess of calcium ions entering into vulnerable neurons, with resultant cell death (for details of the process, see the excellent reviews in references 78, 95).

Once the pathways for the excitotoxic effects had been determined at the beginning of the decade, it then became feasible to develop specific compounds which could be used to antagonize and block the excitotoxic cascade of events leading to cell death and thus possibly prevent the loss of behavioral functions allied with the damage. The noncompetitive glutamate (NMDA) receptor antagonists, which are able to penetrate the blood brain barrier, act by blocking the receptor-gated calcium channel. For example, the NMDA receptor antagonists MK-801 and CGS 19755 (cis-4-(phosphonomethyl)-2-piperidine-carboxylic acid) appear to diminish a number of ischemic-related negative effects in rat and gerbil models. In the rat model[66], reductions were seen in cerebral edema and tissue sodium, along with a protective effect on the intracellular free magnesium concentrations. In the gerbil model, a decrease in hippocampal[11] and striatal[89] necrosis was observed, along with a reduction in behavioral hypermotility[11]. In one study[89], it was suggested that the effect of agents such as MK-801 may be temperature dependent and inversely related to the extent of the injury. Nimodipine and verapimil, which also block calcium channels, have been reported to produce diminished acidosis after ischemic injury[40].

In a similar category, recognition of the destructive effects of ions and their toxic by-products, such as free radicals, was a major step in the understanding of deleterious events occurring after brain injury, and created concrete possibilities for treatment (for review, see reference 32). Use of antioxidants, such as alpha-tocopherol, with in vivo animal models of ischemic brain damage, has shown that increases in plasma alpha-tocoperol levels are associated with a protective effect on membrane phospholipids against free radical attack[93].

There is a growing literature demonstrating that there are agents capable of blocking a number of "negative" processes which occur after brain injury[24,32,82,95]. Blocking some of the secondary consequences of brain injury may be as important to the recovery process(es) as providing neurotransmitter replacement or other forms of pharmacotherapy later in the course of treatment[24,36].

The second step of importance in understanding the mechanisms of recovery came with the discovery that, in response to damage, the brain itself secretes complex proteins and peptides which are capable of stimulating the repair of damaged neurons[5,18,55]. Such substances are usually called "neurotrophic factors" because when they are extracted from the brain and placed into culture dishes containing neurons, they keep the cells from dying and actually promote growth of new processes called neurites. In vivo, trophic factors serve to guide regenerating or sprouting terminals to their appropriate target areas in the brain[3,41,54]. Trophic factors appear to have their highest concentrations at or near sites of injury, and they reach their peak after about 10 and 15 days post-injury, for adult and aged animals, respectively, thereafter declining in concentration and activity[18].

Some researchers have argued that injury-induced activation of certain glial cells, called astrocytes, functions importantly in the production of neurotrophic factors after CNS trauma[29]. This hypothesis has resulted in a whole new look at the "beneficial" role of glia in promoting brain injury recovery. Glial expression of trophic factors, such as nerve growth factor (NGF), had been shown several decades ago[6,86]. Whitaker-Azmitia proposed a two-stage response of glia to injury[90], in which the initial effects of reactive astrocytes are beneficial, giving way to the later formation of the glial scar. It has been recently suggested that glia participate in a cascade of events, involving microglial activation of astrocytes through production of interleukin-l, with subsequent astrocytic expression and release of NGF, which itself is then primary in cholinergic sprouting responses[23,29]. The relationship of these proposed time-dependent events to observed behavioral responses after injury remains to be explored.

With each type or class of new substance being discovered and investigated, another important realization began to emerge which had important consequences for recovery research. As the mechanisms of action for different receptors, excitatory amino acids, neuromodulators, transmitter agonists and antagonists, trophic factors, guidance factors and regulating factors were being developed, it became evident that brain injury itself is not a monolithic event. This means that when damage occurs it triggers a complex cascade of processes that take place over potentially very long periods of time (days, weeks, months and perhaps even years) and produce changes throughout the entire nervous system which are not just limited to the injury site alone[22,32,72,83,84,95].

As they learned more about the complexity of the injury/recovery process, investigators began to focus upon the different stages of the process to determine which specific agents might be most effective in blocking neuronal loss and functional impairments and when they needed to be administered. Thus, a substance appropriate for treatment early in the injury process might actually be counterproductive or ineffective later on. For example, the potential for survival of striatal transplants into injured rat cortical tissue was found to coincide with periods of peak endogenous trophic factor expression[70]. Conversely, some treatments which could be beneficial later in the course of therapy could be detrimental when given early on. For example, administration of diazepam (an indirect GABAergic agonist) for several weeks beginning immediately after injury in the rat caused an enhancement of secondary neural degeneration after selected brain lesions[77]. After unilateral injury to the anterior-medial region of the neocortex in rats, normal recovery was seen within one week. Administration of diazepam immediately after injury, continued for three weeks, effectively prevented behavioral recovery for the length of the experiment, which continued to over nine weeks after cessation of diazepam treatment[76]. Thus, during this last decade, we learned that proper treatments require more complex tailoring to the individual needs of the subject - and must consider the type of injury, when and where it occurs and its time course and duration before and during treatment.

It is not possible to discuss trends and developments in research on recovery of function without also mentioning the tremendous wave of experiments using fetal brain tissue grafts to enhance recovery from CNS injury (for reviews, see 9, 14). Although the use of embryonic brain tissue grafts has a long history (for details, see 10), the major developments in this area began in the 1980's. The attraction of this method lies in its initial simplicity. Embryonic brain cells can be harvested in solid pieces or in suspensions and then placed directly into the host's zone of injury. Both solid blocks of fetal tissue and cell suspensions will survive in host brain[13,67]. Although any connections established do not replicate normal cytoarchitecture, the cells will proliferate and grow in size. Within the last five years it is safe to say that hundreds of studies have been published in which the neuroanatomy and neurochemistry of the graft-host interactions have been examined. Approximately 10% of the published papers report on the behavioral consequences of the grafts. For the most part, in animal models, embryonic brain tissue grafts have been successful in reducing (but not completely eliminating) sensory, motor and cognitive deficits caused by traumatic injury to the adult brain. For example, we were able to demonstrate that implants of fetal frontal cortex into bilaterally injured medial-frontal cortex, in rats, significantly reduced the number of trials necessary to reach the established learning criteria in a spatial alternation task using a T-maze[56]. Transplant research captured the public's attention when neurosurgeons attempted to use portions of a patient's own adrenal medulla (the cells produce low levels of dopamine) to reduce some of the symptoms associated with Parkinson's Disease. Later, Scandinavian and Mexican physicians[4,64] used human fetal tissue in an attempt to ameliorate the rigidity seen in the later stages of this disorder. Although the results have been very mixed[33,64], attempts to use grafts as potential therapy have continued. In the United States, there is considerable controversy over the use of fetal tissue research in general and, in particular, against the use of aborted fetuses for the purposes of obtaining tissue for any treatment conditions.

As a result of this adverse publicity and the current lack of government support for fetal research, investigators have turned to the use of non-neural and/or genetically engineered cells that can be raised and modified in culture to produce some of the missing substances needed by the injured or diseased brain[13,16]. Such research necessarily employs the latest techniques in molecular biology and attracts considerable interest in the biotechnology community because of the commercial potential of developing patentable cells for therapeutic use. Altered cells, capable of replacement of neurotransmitters, trophic factors, or hormones, could be particularly useful in disease states where specific neural degeneration has led to a critical lack of a specific agent. Recently, fibroblast 3T3 cells, genetically modified to express human tyrosine hydrosylase (which converts tyrosine to L-DOPA), were grafted into rats in which the dopamine neurons had been damaged unilaterally by selective toxin[45]. The modified cells secreted DOPA into the surrounding striatal tissue, after which the host tissue effected the decarboxylation of DOPA, yielding dopamine. Rats treated in this way showed a mean significant reduction in apomorphine-induced rotation, a behavioral deficit normally shown with this lesion.

Although genetically engineered cells avoid some of the problems posed in finding suitable fetal tissue, there is still the risk of tumerigenicity and the possibility of immune rejection of tissue placed into the compromised (damaged) brain. Investigators are also seeking ways to encapsulate specific substances needed for repair. For example, NGF slowly released from a polymer matrix has been shown to prevent the loss of choline acetyltransferase activity in septum and diagonal band regions which occurs after unilateral fimbria fornix lesion in the rat[44].

The techniques mentioned above are not yet available for clinical use and they still pose more of a risk than any systemic administration of pharmacological agents. Nonetheless, this work represents an exciting marriage between biotechnology and basic neuroscience. Even though there are considerable clinical problems to face, the use of grafts and supplemental substances as research tools may aid in development of a much better understanding of how the damaged brain attempts to repair itself, what signals are necessary to initiate the process, and what determines the growth and guidance of immature cells placed into the damaged adult brain.

This very brief overview of the last 10 years of "milestones" and the events leading up to them demonstrates that recovery of function research has certainly come of age as an important subspecialty of neuroscience and restorative neurology. Certainly, another writer might focus on a different set of parameters he or she would think critical to the field. Whatever those parameters would be, it is certainly the case that we now have a much better understanding of the mechanisms causing loss of brain tissue, both from primary and secondary insults, and a better idea of what some of the mechanisms might be that facilitate brain injury repair.

Despite very important progress in our understanding of brain damage, there are still significant gaps in our knowledge, which will be reviewed briefly in this last section. Here, we need to examine some of the constructs and basic hypotheses (spoken and unspoken) that guide current thinking. Some of these constructs may be leading us down false paths that could deter progress in delivering treatments to those who need it.

PERSISTING PROBLEMS IN RESEARCH ON RECOVERY FROM BRAIN DAMAGE

I. Defining "recovery of function"

One area which still seems to pose a problem for researchers revolves around the question of what is the most appropriate definition of "functional recovery"? Should recovery be defined primarily in terms of the specific, physiological/morphological changes taking place after injury? Are there different "levels" of recovery ... can there be physiological recovery without behavioral recovery, or vice versa? How do we use the definition to develop appropriate instruments to test and measure recovery? Unfortunately, no simple answer to any of these questions is currently available and it would seem that there are as many definitions as there are groups working on the problem. Almli and Finger[1] have examined the various descriptions by researchers and clinicians which have been given to "functional (behavioral) recovery," such as:

1. ... resumption of normal life even though there may be minor neurological and psychological deficits."[49]

2. ... a return to normal or near normal levels of performance following initially disruptive effects of an injury to the nervous system."[58]

3. ... when persistent behavioral deficits are reduced by special training or by pharmacological, surgical or other independent manipulations."[12]

4. ... impairments in behavioral or physiological functions that abate as time since injury increases"[65]

5. ... the post-lesion reinstatement of the specific behaviours [behavioral isomorphism] that were disrupted by the brain injury."[59] (bracket insert ours)

As can be seen from the different definitions provided in the above quotes, defining "recovery" is much more difficult than identifying chemical reactions, or obtaining photographic images of selectively stained neurons in the process of growth or regeneration. As a result of this confusion, there is both controversy and criticism of the research and clinical practice in this field. With respect to the latter, the lack of precise and agreed upon definitions of what constitutes "functional recovery" have important medical and social implications.

In the first place, who should decide on what constitutes adequate functional recovery? The patient's physician? The nursing staff? Social workers? Family members? Employer? Insurance and workman's compensation representatives? Each group could very well have its own standards and criteria for recovery based on different needs. The emergency medical staff, for example, might define recovery in terms of the patient requiring less intensive care during his or her hospital stay. Social work staff might define recovery in terms of the patient becoming more manageable and being able to use social skills. Family members might be concerned with the patient being able to participate more fully in activities of daily life, while employers and insurance representatives might apply criteria concerned with whether the patient can return to work and perform his or her job in a satisfactory manner. Each definition makes sense and is neither right nor wrong, and each has important medical, economic and social implications (e.g. how serious is the initial impairment [which would determine how recovery is assessed]; when should therapy or treatment begin; what type of therapy needs to be given and for how long; where should the patient go for treatment; how much will it cost...?). Definitions of recovery also become crucially important when litigation is involved in the case of CNS injury, as each side calls on its own "experts" to determine the patient's status and need for further treatment and/or compensation.

Patients who suffer concussion injuries often appear to "return to normal" rather quickly, but they may report a range of affective disturbances ranging from tiredness to inability to concentrate. Even in cases of less severe head injury, the issue of defining full recovery can become very important. According to Diller[21]:

> Recent work on the neuropsychology of emotion ... suggests that some affective disturbances in people with brain damage may have a neurological basis. (page 7)

Personal relationships as well job performance may often suffer but the patients, assumed to be "normal" and "fully recovered," may be accused by family, health providers and employers of "malingering." Whether they are seen to be malingering or truly impaired may very well depend upon the definition(s) used to determine what is full, functional recovery and upon the sensitivity and suitability of the neuropsychological tests utilized.

In the laboratory the problem is similar - what tests are used to assess recovery from brain injury and what are the criteria for recovery on those tests? Different researchers tend to be idiosyncratic in their uses of behavioral testing, such that each laboratory tends to develop its ways of using the "same task" to measure a given behaviour, or individual laboratories use tasks that they think are more "sensitive" to detecting impairments and recovery than someone else's. When working with laboratory animals, very subtle differences in parameters such as (a) how the animals are handled and housed; (b) size of the behavioral testing equipment; (c) feeding schedules; (d) the experimenter's experience and comfort in handling and testing; (e) strain and gender of the test subjects; (f) surgical procedures used to create brain injury; (g) post-injury treatment schedules (amount, duration, route of administration), are among the more important factors in determining the extent and quality of the recovery that would vary from one laboratory (and one experiment) to another.

Without some degree of standardization and agreement as to what is being measured when one uses the term "recovery of function," it becomes rather difficult to determine the effectiveness of a new treatment. Often, too, the extent of testing (i.e. the number of different tasks employed) will play an important role in the assessment of recovery. In laboratory models of recovery from brain injury, it is not surprising to find that the same, specific treatments may enhance recovery on some tasks, have no effect on others, and on still others, the treatment might actually prove to be disruptive (i.e. be worse than no treatment at all)! For example, Casamenti and co-workers[15], using a rat model with lesion of the cholinergic forebrain nuclei and ganglioside GMl treatment, were able to show an improvement, with treatment, in acquisition of active avoidance behaviour. However, passive avoidance responses were not improved.

In many pharmacological studies only very simple and rapidly determined "behaviours" are used to assess the effects of treatments on recovery, such as: reduced mortality from the injury, general levels of activity and/or reflexes, response to noxious stimulation, pole climbing, avoidance of shock or balancing on a narrow runway. Although under such circumstances, recovery of simple behaviours might be observed after treatment, there might be no effect on more complex behaviours needed by the organism to function in a more complex, "real world" situation.

To assess cognitive and perceptual recovery after injury, some investigators use simple mazes, such as the T-maze, to evaluate performance while others require animals to solve more difficult kinds of learning tasks. Depending upon the task difficulty and the criteria used in the behavioral assessments, the investigator can record success or failure, recovery or permanent impairment. As a result of these inconsistencies, efforts may be unnecessarily duplicated because researchers cannot agree on consistent definitions of recovery and appropriate tasks to use. Investigators in spinal cord recovery research met recently to see if they could develop definitions of recovery and appropriate behavioral tasks that would be used as acceptable standards in their field, indicating increased recognition of the importance of this problem to progress in treatment[35].

II. In trying to promote functional recovery, is there any reason to distinguish between restitution and substitution of function?

A number of years ago, when research on functional recovery was still primarily concerned with behaviour, Laurence and Stein[58] drew attention to the question of whether recovery from brain damage represented a true restitution of function or whether the "treatments" permitted the organism to substitute new behaviours for those lost as a result of the initial injury. Put another way, one could ask whether any treatment to promote recovery of function works simply by helping the subject to learn "tricks" to adapt to its new sensory, motor, and cognitive alterations[34]. Under such circumstances, it could be argued that there really is no true restitution of function and that some treatments simply permit the organism to develop alternative strategies to replace those that were lost (for a more detailed look at vicariation theory, see 80). In fact, LeVere[59] proposed that such response substitution might actually serve to block "true" recovery of function in terms of affecting the optimal reorganization of central nervous system pathways.

This question has been addressed in two related studies reporting similar results. First, Gentile, et al[30] and more recently Slavin, et al[81] examined this problem in rats with bilateral injuries of the sensory-motor cortex who were examined on beam-walking behaviour before and after the brain lesions. The rats were trained to perform the task before the injury and when they had learned to traverse the beam in only a few seconds, their performance was filmed with a high-speed camera and the data subjected to a frame-by-frame analysis of their hind-limb gait. In the Gentile, et al experiments, no post-injury treatments were provided; however, the rats received bilateral, one-stage or unilateral, 2-stage cortical removals with a 30 day interval between the first and second surgery. In the Slavin, et al experiments, the rats were given one-stage operations, which were followed by (a) grafting of fetal brain cells into the zone of injury, (b) injections of GMl ganglioside (a drug previously shown to facilitate recovery from brain damage[75], or (c) combinations of ganglioside and fetal brain tissue grafts.

Normal, intact rats learn to traverse the beam for water reward within a very few days and make very few errors (such as foot-faults, falling off the beam, loss of balance, etc). Rats with bilateral removals of sensory-motor cortex show an initial, post-operative deficit (foot-faults, falling off the beam, increased running times, etc), but within one week their performance rapidly improves and for all intents and purposes, the animals' running behaviour "looks normal." When subjected to cinematographic gait analysis, a different picture emerges. In the Gentile, et al study[30], the investigators found both substitution and restitution of function, dependent on the type of surgery given to the rats. To the naked eye, it would appear that the one-stage animals ran perfectly well on the balance beam but, when their hind limb gait was carefully analyzed, they showed a highly aberrant pattern of gait that looked completely different from that of normal animals. The rats with two-stage (serial) lesions (which created the same extent of injury and loss of thalamo-cortical fibers) had hind-limb gait patterns virtually identical to that observed in intact rats. Here, the type of surgery (one- or two-stage) played a role in determining whether the "recovery" could be attributed to restitution (i.e. post-traumatic behaviour was identical to pre-operative state) or substitution (recovery occurred but was manifested by a different pattern of behaviour than that seen in the normal state).

In the Slavin, et al study[81], animals with bilateral, single- stage lesions of motor cortex were also able recover, but the gait patterns were significantly different from those that had no treatments, or that had received combinations of fetal brain tissue grafts and ganglioside treatments to promote recovery. In other words, while all animals, including those with lesions alone, showed some "recovery" on the beam-walking task, the specific treatments resulted in different gait patterns (or behavioral strategies) of recovery.

We believe that these findings are of more than just theoretical importance for those involved in rehabilitation and recovery of function in a clinical setting. Therapists need to recognize that underlying any program of rehabilitation, be it pharmacological, behavioral or some combination of both, is neuronal reorganization. Such reorganization occurs not just at the site of the injury itself but even in brain regions that are quite remote from the damaged area[20,72,77] - and it can occur quite rapidly and with important implications for therapy and training.

In a series of elegant experiments, Jenkins et al[48], using adult, non-human primates, were able to show that "the neocortex of adult mammals has the capacity for functional reorganization, even under normal, non-pathological conditions." By recording the receptive fields of neurons in the somatosensory cortex (i.e. the hand is stimulated and single-neuron recordings in the cortex are taken to reveal which cells are activated by the tactile stimulation), Jenkins and colleagues were able to show that cortical lesions can produce a dramatic reorganization of these fields and also of cortical-thalamic interactions within a very short period of time after the injury. This means basically that cortical and thalamic areas previously not involved in specific hand digits and pad representations began to respond to tactile stimulation within hours after the removal of the primary fields. Perhaps more importantly, simple, tactile training in normal animals also had the effect of extensively altering the cortical maps. Similar results have recently been reported (i.e. massive cortical reorganization following peripheral deafferentation in adult monkeys by Pons and co-workers[72]), thus demonstrating that extensive changes in the adult cortex can occur as a result of experience, be it learned or traumatic!

Why do we mention this work in the context of therapy for brain injury? When taken together with the work of Gentile, et al and Slavin, et al, it becomes evident that therapists should begin to consider whether "rote" or standardized rehabilitation strategies may be having effects on cerebral reorganization that could be detrimental to functional recovery. Thus, "negative plasticity" could be induced by requiring the patient to use behavioral strategies that might inhibit the unmasking of new, more appropriate pathways and thus block subsequent optimum reorganization in critical CNS areas.

In this context, Jenkins and co-workers[48] also reported observing very significant individual differences in the location and size of cortical receptive fields in normal adult primates. These workers suggest that the individual differences may be determined by a combination of genetic and environmental influences. In planning rehabilitation strategies, such individual differences in cerebral organization need to be given serious consideration in attending to individual differences in response to therapies.

That there is growing concern over these issues among rehabilitation specialists can be seen in the following quote taken from Held[42], who wrote:

> Because of the current pressures, in the United States at least, for cost containment, it is critical that therapists carry out clinical research studies to demonstrate the effectiveness of therapeutic approaches. We can no longer afford to simply become a disciple of any particular approach, believing blindly that our way is the best way. ... We are currently being forced into interventions "to get the patient out" that are supposedly cost effective. However, <u>are we training compensatory strategies that will prevent true recovery</u> [underline ours], thus lengthening the time and increasing the level of care that the patient will need in the long run? (page 174)

As the mapping of cortical reorganization in patients would be difficult, time-consuming, and expensive, what are some practical steps to be taken to assure that routine or standard "therapy" does not prove to be more detrimental than doing nothing at all? While awaiting the development of non-invasive, new testing protocols available in a rehabilitation setting, perhaps the following suggestions might be considered.

1. Therapists (behavioral or neurological) should begin to recognize that any treatments provided will have multilevel effects - especially in a complex system undergoing injury-induced reorganization. This means that small changes in one part of the system can have widespread effects throughout the entire system - the whole patient is being treated and not just the damaged brain "part." At the practical level this implies that "standard" doses of drugs or "routine" behavioral manipulations should, whenever possible, be considered in the context of developing highly specific programs tailored to the individual case history and medical, social and environmental context of the patient.

2. Cerebral reorganization begins early after injury and is part of a complex cascade of biochemical and morphological events that may continue for months or even years after the initial injury. Pharmacological and behavioral treatments should be designed to meet the physiological conditions of the specific stage of the injury. This means that there may be precise "windows of opportunity" for different types of pharmacologic agents during which they are more likely to be effective, while at other time periods they may be ineffective or even harmful[36]. For example, the same NMDA antagonists which promote sparing after ischemic brain damage produce detrimental effects at a later time in the recovery period in rats with unilateral lesions of the sensorimotor cortex[7]. This effect is thought to occur through blockage of long-term potentiation, which has been proposed as one mechanism whereby "relearning" after injury may take place[36]. Careful and systematic evaluation of proper dose levels, treatment duration and time for initiation of treatment after injury must be performed in both the clinical and laboratory setting (for specific details and review, see 36,95), in order to increase the probability of functional recovery.

3. The post-traumatic environment of the patient may be important in determining functional outcome. Environment can shape the scope and extent of functional recovery from brain injury and directly affects neuronal reorganization[25,27,43,52,92]. The sterile and deprived environments of many nursing homes and convalescent centers, especially for the elderly patient with brain damage (e.g. in the state of California, 65% of nursing home patients are either physically or chemically restrained[c]) may actually produce or exacerbate some of the behavioral impairments that the therapist is seeking to avoid, much as impoverished, deprived conditions have been shown to dramatically affect the intelligence and capabilities of deprived children[42].

4. Research on how much time should be devoted to rehabilitation or other forms of post-injury "therapy" is another area that needs careful investigation. Norman Geschwind[31] felt that most clinicians not only did not pay sufficient attention to "seeking the right maneuvers" to elicit recovery, they also did not give enough attention to the time necessary for the processes leading to recovery to become manifest. Referring to the aphasias, He said that:

> Most neurologists are gloomy about the prognosis of severe adult aphasias after a few weeks and pessimism is reinforced by a lack of prolonged follow-up in most cases. I have, however, seen patients severely aphasic for over one year, who then made excellent recovery. One patient returned to work as a salesman, the other as a psychiatrist. Furthermore, there are patients who continue to improve over many years, for example, the patient whose aphasia is still quite evident six years after onset, cleared up substantially by 18 years. (page 3)

We take Geschwind's observations to suggest that perhaps we are not doing enough to provide long-term therapy and rehabilitation to patients whose progress through the spectrum of recovery may be arduous and long. There is no principle of neuronal organization that demands that functional recovery occur immediately or not at all. As Held[42] pointed out, the decision to withhold or terminate either pharmacological treatments or rehabilitation therapy is probably based more on economic (i.e. it would cost too much to continue) and social factors (let's get on to something with a more rapid, personal pay-off; i.e. seeing a quick recovery) than it is on purely physiologic grounds; i.e. what we know about how the nervous system actually works.

The time-course of recovery can also be taken to mean that the therapy itself may need to change as the CNS endogenous response to the trauma progresses. As the underlying physical substrates change over time, so should the therapy. Thus, for example, in the earliest stages of CNS injury, it may eventually prove appropriate to give drugs which block edema, reduce free radical formation and reduce excitotoxicity (e.g. methylprednisolone, NMDA receptor antagonists, alpha-tocopherol), then shortly follow this regimen with neurotrophic factors that could enhance neural sparing or reduce neuronal loss by repairing damaged membranes (e.g. gangliosides, brain-derived trophic factors).

5. At present, there is virtually no systematic research on the outcome of rehabilitation "therapies for brain dysfunctions." Carefully controlled outcome studies must be done to determine if patients are truly benefitting from the specific duration and types of therapy that they are receiving. This means that objective and agreed-upon criteria for recovery must be developed and applied in systematic fashion, so that investigators can compare inter-institutional data and results.

---

[c] For further information on this issue, see *The New York Times'* editorial entitled "Unshackle Nursing Home Patients," in the April 8, 1991 issue, page A14.

CONCLUSIONS

As the subsequent chapters in this volume will show, great strides in understanding the nature and scope of recovery from brain damage have been made, although much more still remains to be discovered. One area very much in need of attention is whether there are gender differences in recovery from brain damage and whether different courses and types of therapy might be needed for males and females. There are virtually no clinical studies in this area despite research showing that the hormonal status of females at the time of brain injury can play a role in determining severity of deficit[2], sex-related differences occur in response to injury[62,88] and males and females respond differently to treatment[39].

Another area needing study concerns the "more is better syndrome." In other words, we tend to think that producing new, neuronal growth, or stimulating the development of new pathways in response to brain damage is the best solution to prompt and complete recovery. However, there is research demonstrating that such growth may be, in reality, detrimental to the recovery process[74,83,91]. Research focusing upon when neuronal "replacement" is beneficial and when it might be detrimental is in its infancy and this is why caution should be exercised before trophic, growth--promoting substances are administered or the grafting of embryonic brain tissue or cell replacement into damaged brains is considered as the best way to promote recovery of function in all stages of a particular disorder.

One of the reasons that the recovery research is so exciting, from both an experimental and clinical perspective, is that there are so many questions and so many possibilities available for those wishing to become involved. Given the speed with which new discoveries are being made in molecular biology and the growing interest of pharmaceutical companies in developing new treatments for brain and spinal cord trauma, the next EBBS recovery meeting a decade hence should prove to be most exhilarating.

REFERENCES

1. Almli, C.R., and Finger, S., 1988, Toward a definition of recovery of function, in *Brain Injury and Recovery: Theoretical and Controversial Issues*, S. Finger, T.E. LeVere, C.R. Almli and D.G. Stein., eds., pp. 1-14, Plenum Press, New York.

2. Attella, M.J., Nattinville, A., and Stein, D.G., 1987, Hormonal state affects recovery from frontal cortex lesions in adult female rats, *Behav. Neural. Biol.*, **48**, 352-367.

3. Auburger, G.R., Heumann, R., Hellweg, S., Korsching, S., and Thoenen, H., 1987, Developmental changes of nerve growth factor and its mRNA in the rat hippocampus: Comparison with choline acetyltransferase, *Develop. Biol.*, **120**, 322-328.

4. Backlund, E-O., Granberg, P-O., and Hamberger, B., 1985, Transplantation of adrenal medullary tissue to striatum in Parkinsonism. First clinical trials, *J. Neurosurg.*, **62**, 169-173.

5. Barde, Y-A., 1989, Trophic factors and neuronal survival: Review, *Neuron*, **2**, 1525-1534.

6. Barde, Y-A., Lindsay, R.M., Monard, D., and Thoenen, H., 1978, New factor released by cultured glioma cells supporting survival and growth of sensory neurons, *Nature*, **273**, 818.

7. Barth, T.M., Grant, M.L., and Schallert, T., 1990, Effects of MK-801 on recovery from sensorimotor cortex lesions, *Stroke*, **21** (*Supplement III*) III 153-III 157.

8. Benveniste, H., Drejer, J., Schousboe, A., and Diemer, N.H., 1984, Elevation of the extracellular concentrations of glutamate and aspartate in rat hippocampus during transient cerebral ischemia monitored by intracerebral microdialysis, *J. Neurochem.*, **43**, 1369-1374.

9. Bjorklund, A. and Gage, F.H., 1985, Neural grafting in animal models of neurodegenerative diseases, *Ann. N. Y. Acad. Sci.*, **457**, 53-81.

10. Bjorklund, A., and Stenevi, U., 1985, Intracerebral neural grafting: A historical perspective, in *Neural Grafting in the Mammalian CNS*, A. Bjorklund and U. Stenevi, eds., pp. 3-14, Elsevier, New York.

11. Boast, C.A., Gerhardt, S.C., Pastor, G., Lehmann, J., Etienne, P.E., and Liebman, J.M., 1988, The N-methyl-D-aspartate antagonists CGS 19755 and CPP reduce ischemic brain damage in gerbils, *Brain Res.*, **442**, 345-348.

12. Braun, J.J., 1978, Time and recovery from brain damage, in *Recovery from Brain Damage: Research and Theory*, S. Finger, ed., pp.165-197, Plenum, New York.

13. Bredesen, D.E., Hisanaga, K., and Sharp, F.R., 1990, Neural transplantation using temperature-sensitive immortalized neural cells: A preliminary report, *Ann. Neurol.*, **27**, 205-207.

14. Buzsaki, G., and Gage, F.H., 1988, Mechanisms of action of neural grafts in the limbic system, *Can. J. Neurol. Sci.*, **15**, 99-105.

15. Casamenti, F., Bracco, L., Bartolini, L., and Pepeu, G., 1985, Effects of ganglioside treatment in rats with a lesion of the cholinergic forebrain nuclei, *Brain Res.*, **338**, 45-52.

16. Chen, L.S., Ray, J., Fisher, L.J., Kawaja, M.D., Schinstine, M., Kang, U.J., and Gage, F.H., 1991, Cellular replacement therapy for neurologic disorders: Potential of genetically engineered cells, *J. of Cell. Biochem.*, **45**, 252-257.

17. Cooper, J.R., Bloom, F.E., and Roth, R.H., 1986, *The Biochemical Basis of Neuropharmacology*, Oxford University Press, New York.

18. Cotman, C.W., and Nieto-Sampedro, M., 1985, Progress in facilitating the recovery of function after central nervous system trauma, *Ann. N. Y. Acad. Sci.*, **457**, 83-104.

19. Damasio, H., and Damasio, A.R., 1989, *Lesion Analysis in Neuropsychology*, University Press, New York.

20. Dietrich, W.D., Alonso, 0., Busto, R., Watson, B.D., Loor, Y., and Ginsberg, M.D., 1990, Influence of amphetamine treatment on somatosensory function of the normal and infarcted rat brain, *Stroke, (Supplement III)* **21** III 147-III 150.

21. Diller, L., 1987, Neuropsychological rehabilitation, in *Neuropsychological Rehabilitation*, M.J. Meier, A.L. Benton and L. Diller, eds., pp. 3-17, The Guildford Press, New York.

22. Faden, A.I., Demediuk, P., Panter, S.S., and Vink, R., 1989, The role of excitatory amino acids and NMDA receptors in traumatic brain injury, *Science*, **244**, 799-800.

23. Fagan, A.M., and Gage, F.H., 1990, Cholinergic sprouting in the hippocampus: A proposed role for IL-l, *Exp. Neurol.*, **110**, 105-120 .

24. Feeney, D.M., and Sutton, R.L., 1987, Pharmacotherapy for recovery of function after brain injury, *CRC Critical Reviews in Neurobiology*, **3**, 135-197 .

25. Finger, S., 1978, Environmental attenuation of brain lesion symptoms, in *Recovery from Brain Damage: Research and Theory*, S. Finger, ed., pp. 297-325, Plenum, New York.

26. Finger, S., LeVere, T.E., Almli, C.R., and Stein, D.G., eds., 1988, *Brain Injury and Recovery: Theoretical and Controversial Issues*, Plenum Press, New York.

27. Finger, S., and Stein, D.G., 1982, Fast- versus slow-growing lesions and behavioral recovery, in *Brain Damage and Recovery: Research and Clinical Perspectives*, pp. 1513-173, Academic Press, New York.

28. Fischer, W., and Bjorklund, A., 1991, Loss of AChE- and NGFr-labeling precedes neuronal death of axotomized septal-diagonal band neurons: Reversal by intraventricular NGF infusion, *Exp. Neurol.*, 113, 93-108.

29. Gage, F.H., Olejniczak, P., and Armstrong, D.M., 1988, Astrocytes are important for sprouting in the septohippocampal circuit, *Exp. Neurol.*, 102, 2-13.

30. Gentile, A.M., Green, S., Neiburgs, A., Schmelzer, W., and Stein, D.G., 1978, Disruption and recovery of locomotor and manipulatory behavior following cortical lesions in rats, *Behav. Biol.*, 22, 417-455.

31. Geschwind, N., 1985, Mechanisms of change after brain lesions, *Ann. N. Y. Acad. Sci.*, 457, 1-11.

32. Ginsberg, M.D., Watson, B.D., Buston, R., Yoshida, S., Prado, R., Hakayama, H., Ikeda, M., Dietrich, W.D. and Globus, M.Y., 1988, Peroxidative damage to cell membranes following cerebral ischemia: A cause of ischemic brain injury? *Neurochem. Path.*, 9, 171-193 .

33. Goetz, C.G., Olanow, C.W., and Koller, W.C., 1989, Multicenter study of autologous adrenal medullary transplantation to the corpus striatum in patients with advanced Parkinson's Disease, *New Eng. J. Med.*, 320, 337-341.

34. Goldberger, M.E., 1974, Recovery of movement after CNS lesions in monkeys, in *Plasticity and Recovery of Function in the Central Nervous System*, D.G. Stein, J.J. Rosen and N. Butters, eds., pp. 265-337, Academic Press, New York.

35. Goldberger, M.E., Bregman, B.S., Vierck, C.J. Jr., and Brown, M., 1990, Criteria for assessing recovery of function after spinal cord injury: Behavioral methods, *Exp. Neurol.*, 107, 113-117.

36. Goldstein, L.B., 1990, Pharmacology of recovery after stroke, *Stroke*, 21 (*Supplement III*) III 139-III 142.

37. Goldstein, M., 1990, Traumatic brain injury: A silent epidemic. *Ann. Neurol.*, 27, 327.

38. Goodman, D.C., Bogdasarian, R.S., and Horel, J.A., 1973, Axonal sprouting of ipsilateral optic tract following opposite eye removal, *Brain, Behav. Evol.*, 8, 27-50.

39. Gould, E., Westlind-Danielsson, A., Frankfurt, M., and Mc-Ewen, B., 1990, Sex differences and thyroid hormone sensitivity of hippocampal pyramidal cells, *J. Neurosci.*, 10, 996-1003.

40. Hakim, A.M., 1986, Cerebral acidosis in focal ischemia: II. Nimodipine and verapamil normalize cerebral pH following middle cerebral artery occlusion in the rat, *J. Cerebral Blood Flow and Metabolism*, 6, 676-683.

41. Hefti, F., Hartikka, J., and Knusel, B., 1989, Function of neurotrophic factors in the adult and aging brain and their possible use in the treatment of neurodegenerative diseases, *Neurobiology of Aging*, 10, 515-533.

42. Held, J.M., 1987, Recovery of function after brain damage: Theoretical implications for therapeutic intervention, in *Movement Science: Foundations for Physical Therapy in Rehabilitation*, J.H. Carr, R.B.

Shepherd, J. Gordon, A.M. Gentile and J.M. Held, eds., pp. 155-157, Aspen Publishers, Inc., Rockville, M.D.

43. Held, J.M., Gordon, J., and Gentile, A.M., 1985, Environmental influences on locomotor recovery following cortical lesions in rats, *Behav. Neurosci.*, **99**, 678-690.

44. Hoffman, D., Wahlberg, L., and Aebischer, P., 1990, NGF released from a polymer matrix prevents loss of ChAT expression in basal forebrain neurons following a fimbria-fornix lesion, *Exp. Neurol.*, **110**, 39-44.

45. Horellou, P., Brundin, P., Kalen, P., Mallet, J., and Bjorklund, A., 1990, In vivo release of DOPA and dopamine from genetically engineered cells grafted to the denervated rat striatum, *Neuron*, **5**, 393-402.

46. Irle, E., 1987, Lesion size and recovery of function: Some new perspectives, *Brain Res. Rev.*, **12**, 307-320.

47. Jackson, J.H., 1898, Relations of different divisions of the central nervous system to one another and to parts of the body. Lancet, (Reprinted in J. Taylor, ed., [1958]). *Selected Writings of John Hughlings Jackson*, Basic Books, New York.

48. Jenkins, W.M., Merzenich, M.M., and Reconzone, G., 1990, Neocortical representational dynamics in adult primates: Implications for neuropsychology, *Neuropsychologia*, **28**, 573-584.

49. Jennett, B., and Bond, M., 1975, Assessment of outcome after severe brain damage, *Lancet*, **1**, 480-484.

50. Kandel, E.R., Schwartz, J.H., and Jessell, T.M., 1991, *Principles of Neural Science* (3rd edition), Elsevier, New York.

51. Katzman, R., Bjorklund, A., Owman, C., Stenevi, U., and West, K., 1971, Evidence for regeneration axon sprouting of central catecholamine neurons in the rat mesencephalon following electrolytic lesions, *Brain Res.*, **25**, 579-596.

52. Kelche, C., Dalrymple-Alford, J.C., and Will, B., 1988, Housing conditions modulate the effects of intracerebral grafts in rats with brain lesions, *Behav. Brain Res.*, **28**, 287-295.

53. Kertesz, A., 1988, Recovery from stroke, in *Pharmacological Approaches to the Treatment of Brain and Spinal Cord Injury*, D.G. Stein and B.A. Sabel, eds., pp. 361-376, Plenum Press, New York.

54. Korsching, S., 1986, The role of nerve growth factor in the CNS, *Trends in Neurol. Sci.*, **9**, 570-573.

55. Kromer, L.F., and Cornbrooks, C.J., 1987, Identification of trophic factors and transplanted cellular environments that promote CNS axonal regeneration, *Ann. N. Y. Acad. Sci.*, **495**, 207-225.

56. Labbe, R., Firl Jr., A., Mufson, E.J. and Stein, D.G., 1983, Fetal brain transplants: Reduction of cognitive deficits in rats with frontal cortex lesions, *Science*, **221**, 470-472.

57. Lashley, K.S., 1964, originally published 1929, *Brain Mechanisms and Intelligence*, Hafner Publishing Company, New York.

58. Laurence, S., and Stein, D.G., 1978, Recovery after brain damage and the concept of localization of function, in *Recovery from Brain Damage: Research and Theory*, S. Finger, ed., pp. 369-407, Plenum, New York.

59. LeVere, T. E., 1980, Recovery of function after brain damage: A theory of the behavioral deficit, *Physiol. Psychol.*, **8**, 297-308 .

60. Lindsley, D.B., Schreiner, L.H., Knowles, W.B., and Magoun, H.W., 1949, Behavioral and EEG changes following chronic brain stem lesion in the cat, *Electroenceph. Clin. Neurophys.*, **1**, 455-473.

61. Loesche, J., and Steward, 0., 1977, Behavioral correlates of denervation and reinnervation of the hippocampal formation of the rat: Recovery of alternation performances following unilateral entorhinal cortex lesions, *Brain Res. Bull.*, **2**, 31-39.

62. Loy, R., and Milner, T.A., 1990, Sexual dimorphism in extent of axonal sprouting in rat hippocampus, *Science*, **208**, 1282-1284 .

63. Luria, A.R., 1963, *Restoration of Function after Brain Injury*, The Macmillan Company, New York.

64. Madrazo, I., Drucker-Colin, R., and Diaz, V., 1987, Open microsurgical autograft of adrenal medulla to the right caudate nucleus in two patients with intractable Parkinson's Disease, *New Eng. J. Med.*, **318**, 51.

65. Marshall, J.F., 1985, Neural plasticity and recovery of function after brain injury, *Int. Rev. Neurobiol.*, **26**, 201-247 .

66. McIntosh, T.K., Vink, R., Soares, H., Hayes, R., and Simon, R., 1990, Effect of non-competitive blockade of N-methyl-D-aspartate receptors on the neurochemical sequelae of experimental brain injury, *J. Neurochem.*, **55**, 1170-1179 .

67. McLoon, L.K., Mcloon, S.C., Chang, F.-L.F., Steedman, J.G., and Lund, R.D., 1985, Visual system transplanted to the brain of rats, in *Neural Grafting in the Mammalian CNS*, A. Bjorklund and U. Stenevi, eds., pp. 267-283, Elsevier, New York.

68. Meldrum, B., 1985, Possible therapeutic applications of antagonists of excitatory amino acid neurotransmitters, *Clinical Science*, **68**, 113-122 .

69. Nieto-Sampedro, M., 1988, Growth factor induction and order of events in CNS repair, in *Pharmacological Approaches to the Treatment of Brain and Spinal Cord Injury*, D.G. Stein and B.A. Sabel, eds., pp. 309-332, Plenum Press, New York.

70. Nieto-Sampedro, M., Manthrope, M., Barbin, G., Varon, S., and Cotman, C.W., 1983, Injury-induced neuronotrophic activity in adult rat brain: Correlation with survival of delayed implants in the wound cavity, *J. Neurosci.*, **3**, 2219-2229 .

71. Olney, J.W., 1978, Neurotoxicity of excitatory amino acids, in *Kainate as a Tool in Neurobiology*, E.G. McGeer, J.W. Olney and P.L. McGeer, eds., pp. 95-121, Raven Press. New York.

72. Pons, R.P., Garraghty, P.E., Ommaya, A.K., Kaas, J.H., Taub, E., and Mishkin, M., 1991, Massive cortical reorganization after sensory deafferentation in adult macaques, *Science*, **252**, 1857-1860.

73. Raisman, G., 1969, Neuronal plasticity in the septal nuclei of the adult rat, *Brain Res.*, **14**, 25-48.

74. Ramirez, J.J., Fass-Holmes, B., Karpiak, S.E., Harshbarger, R., Zengel, D., Wright, P., and Valbuena, M., 1991, Enhanced recovery of learned alternation in ganglioside-treated rats after unilateral entorhinal lesions, *Behav. Brain Res.*, **43**, 99-101.

75. Sabel, B.A., Slavin, M.D., and Stein, D.G., 1984, GMI ganglioside treatment facilitates behavioral recovery from bilateral brain damage, *Science*, **225**, 340-342.

76. Schallert, T., Hernandez, T.D., and Barth, T.M., 1986, Recovery of function after brain damage: Severe and chronic disruption by diazepam, *Brain Res.*, **379**, 104-111.

77. Schallert, T., Jones, R.A., and Lindner, M.D., 1990, Multilevel transneuronal degeneration after brain damage: Behavioral events and effects of anticonvulsant gamma-aminobutyric acid-related drugs, *Stroke*, **21** (*Supplement III*) III 143-III 146.

78. Siesjo, B.K., and Bengtsson, F., 1989, Review: Calcium fluxes, calcium antagonists, and calcium-related pathology in brain ischemia, hypoglycemia, and spreading depression: A unifying hypothesis, *J. Cerebral Blood Flow and Metabolism*, **9**, 127-140.

79. Simon, R.P., Swan, J.H., Griffiths, T. and Meldrum, B.S., 1984, Blockade of N-methyl-D-aspartate receptors may protect against ischemic damage in the brain, *Science*, **226**, 850-852.

80. Slavin, M.D., Laurence, S., and Stein, D.G., 1988, Another look at vicariation, in *Brain Injury and Recovery: Theoretical and Controversial Issues*, S. Finger, T.E. LeVere, C.R. Almli and D.G. Stein, eds., pp. 165-179, Plenum Press, New York.

81. Slavin, M.D., Held, J.M., Basso, D.M., Lesensky, S., Curran, E., Gentile, A.M., and Stein, D.G., 1988, Fetal brain tissue transplants and recovery of locomotion following damage to the sensorimotor cortex in rats, in *Transplantation Into the Mammalian CNS*, D.M. Gash and J.R. Sladek Jr., eds., pp. 33-38, Elsevier, New York.

82. Stein, D.G., and Sabel, B.A., 1988, *Pharmacological Approaches to the Treatment of Brain and Spinal Cord Injury*, Plenum Press, New York.

83. Steward, 0., 1989, Reorganization of neuronal connections following CNS trauma: Principles and experimental paradigms, *J. Neurotrauma*, **6**, 99-143.

84. Teasdale, G., 1991, The treatment of head trauma: Implications for the future, *J.Neurotrauma*, **8** (*Supplement I*) S 53- S-58.

85. van Hof, M.W. and Mohn, G., eds., 1981, *Functional Recovery from Brain Damage*, Elsevier/North-Holland Biomedical Press, New York.

86. Varon, S., Raiborn, C.W., and Norr, S., 1974, Association of antibody to nerve growth factor with ganglionic non-neurons (glia) and consequent interference with their neuron-supportive action, *Exp. Cell Res.*, **88**, 247-256.

87. Wall, J.T., 1988, Variable organization in cortical maps of the skin as an indication of the lifelong adaptive capacities of circuits in the mammalian brain, *Trends in Neurosci.*, **11**, 549-557.

88. Wan-Hua, A.Y., 1982, Sex difference in the regeneration of the hypoglossal nerve, *Brain Res.*, **238**, 404-406.

89. Warner, M.A., Neill, K.H., Nadler, J.V., and Crain, B.J., 1991, Regionally selective effects of NMDA receptor antagonists against ischemic brain damage in the gerbil, *J. Cerebral Blood Flow and Metabolism*, **11**, 600-610.

90. Whitaker-Azmitia, P.M., Ramirez, A., Noreika, L., Gannon, P.J., and Azmitia, E.C., 1987, Onset and duration of astrocytic response to cells transplanted into the adult mammalian brain, *Annals. N. Y. Acad. Sci.*, **495**, 10-23.

91. Whitson, J.S., Glabe, C.G., Shintani, E., Abcar, A., and Cotman, C.W., 1990, B-amyloid protein promotes neuritic branching in hippocampal cultures, *Neurosci. Lett.*, **110**, 319-324.

92. Will, B.E., Rosenzweig, M.R., Bennett, E.L., Hebert, M. and Morimoto, H., 1977, Relatively brief environmental enrichment aids recovery of learning capacity and alters brain measures after postweaning brain lesions in rats, *J. Comp. Physiol. Psychol.*, **91**, 33-50.

93. Yoshida, S., Busto, R., Santiso, M., and Ginsberg, M.D., 1984, Brain lipid peroxidation induced by postischemic reoxygenation in vitro: Effect of vitamin E, *J. Cerebral Blood Flow and Metabolism*, **4**, 466-469.

94. Zhou, F.C., Bledsoe, S. and Murphy, J., 1991, Serotonergic sprouting is induced by dopamine-lesion in substantia nigra of adult rat brain, *Brain Res.*, **556**, 108-116.

95. Zivin, J.A., and Choi, D.W., 1991, Stroke therapy, *Sci. Amer.*, **265**, 56-63.

RECOVERY OF FUNCTION: NUTRITIONAL FACTORS

J W T Dickerson

School of Biological Sciences
University of Surrey
Guildford, England

INTRODUCTION

This volume is concerned with recovery from damage to a specific organ, the brain. Since damage to the brain may occur at any age, it would seem pertinent to discuss briefly the growth, development and metabolic characteristics of this organ, particularly in relation to the effects of nutrition upon it. I will then discuss the effects of injury on the body's metabolism and the effects of brain damage specifically. This discussion forms a necessary background to understanding the importance of nutrition in the recovery process. Finally, I will discuss nutritional requirements, food administration and long-term follow-up.

BRAIN DEVELOPMENT

Unlike most other organs in the body, the brain has a single growth spurt with only limited possibility for regeneration. The brain accounts for 13% of the body weight of a full-term baby, and at birth has reached its peak rate of growth[9]. The brain continues to grow, albeit at a decreasing rate, and achieves 90% of its adult size by 6 years and almost adult size by 12 years.

The different parts of the brain grow and develop at different rates. The surface area is increased by the development of convolutional patterns[3]. Early growth of the brain is by cell multiplication followed by cell enlargement[27]. The exact timing of the cessation of cellular multiplication in the human brain has not been determined, but the bulk of neuronal multiplication in the cerebral hemispheres occurs before about 18 weeks gestation. Multiplication of various types of glial cells continues. Oligodendroglial cells have been of most interest from a nutritional viewpoint since the membranes of these cells are converted into the myelin sheath. The process of myelination occurs in cycles differing in their age relationships in different parts of the brain[39]. This process is reduced by nutritional deprivation due to a reduction in oligodendroglial multiplication. Though neuronal multiplication in the cerebrum may cease before birth, the linking of the neurones by the dendrites and the development of synapses continues after birth and this process of dendritic arborization is affected considerably by both nutritional and sensory deprivation[13]. In fact, there is evidence from studies in rats[28] that delayed synaptic development induced by under-nutrition can be prevented by sensory stimulation. In addition to nutrition and sensory stimulation, brain growth and development are affected by hormonal balance. These variables are interdependent and may be altered after brain damage, and disturb complex relationships affecting the management of the head injured child.

Cerebral blood flow reaches a peak at different times in different regions and is proportional to the speed of regional maturation; areas with a high density of white matter show the highest blood flow at peak myelination; and blood flow is proportional to metabolic rate. Cerebral blood flow and oxygen consumption are maximal at 6 years of age when the brain has achieved about 90% of its adult size. At this age the brain consumes about 60 ml oxygen/min/brain which represents about 50% of the basal metabolic rate; in adults the corresponding value is 20 - 30%.

The brain contains very little glycogen and neutral fat and hence is dependent on a continuous supply of fuel entering the organ. Glucose is the major fuel and in an adult is utilised at the rate of 0.3 - 1.0 mmol/kg/min with more than 90% of the glucose metabolised via glycolysis. The brain of a newborn baby can readily use ketones. The uptake and utilisation of ketones by the adult brain is dependent on their circulating concentrations and their passage through the blood-brain barrier. Ketones act as a brain fuel in conditions of starvation and ketone production after injury (ketone adaption) can be an important factor in survival.

Dietary carbohydrate causes the release of insulin from the pancreas. Insulin plays an important role in the control of the plasma glucose concentration. It also affects protein synthesis by regulating the uptake of neutral amino acids into muscle. This effect has been shown to be important in the regulation of the synthesis of the neurotransmitter, 5-hydroxytryptamine (5-HT) or serotonin. 5-HT is synthesised in the synapses of serotoninergic neurones from the amino acid, tryptophan. Tryptophan is a neutral amino acid which competes with other large neutral amino acids (tyrosine, phenylalanine, leucine, isoleucine and valine) for a common mechanism for passage across the blood brain barrier into the brain[15]. Thus, the synthesis of 5-HT is regulated by the supply of tryptophan, an essential amino acid, and also by dietary carbohydrate. Present evidence suggests that these relationships relate to individuals of all ages. Other examples of dietary precursors of neurotransmitters are phenylalanine and tyrosine as precursors of noradrenaline and dopamine, and lecithin and choline as precursors of acetylcholine. Moreover, certain amino acids themselves act as neurotransmitters.

The pathways of energy, protein and lipid metabolism involve a number of enzymes which require vitamins as cofactors including thiamin, niacin, pyridoxin, vitamin B12, folic acid and vitamin C. A number of minerals including magnesium, zinc and manganese are important nutrients acting as co-factors for enzymes.

METABOLIC RESPONSE TO TRAUMA

The classical studies on fracture patients[8] led to the identification of three phases in the metabolic response to injury - the 'ebb', 'flow' and 'anabolic' or 'convalescent' phases. The 'ebb' phase occurs immediately and is characterised primarily by an increase in catecholamine secretion. The magnitude of the increases in blood concentrations of epinephrin and norepinephrin depend on the severity of the injury, being least for minor and moderate trauma, higher when sepsis supervenes and highest following cardiac arrest (Table 1). In burn injury, values are similar to those following severe trauma. During this phase the metabolic rate falls and patients may die if there is massive blood loss not compensated for by transfusion, or if sepsis occurs. This phase lasts no longer than 6-18 hours even after severe injury. The 'flow' phase, sometimes erroneously called the 'catabolic' phase, varies in length and may last up to 8 weeks or even more. It is characterised by an increase in metabolic rate, breakdown of protein (predominantly from skeletal muscle) with increased ureagenesis and excretion of nitrogen. Some of the amino acids released are used in the liver to synthesise acute phase reactant proteins, other amino acids are deaminated in the muscle and with the carbon fragments, e.g. pyruvate, are transported to the liver via the 'alanine shuttle'. There the carbon moiety is resynthesized via pyruvate to glucose. It is this process of gluconeogensis, stimulated by cortisol and glucagon, which is thought to be responsible for the hyperglycaemia, the so-called 'diabetes of trauma' which follows injury[23].

Table 1. Plasma concentrations of catecholamines in trauma and stress. (Mean values in µmol per litre - Modified from Frayn[16])

Group	Epinephrin	Norepinephrin
Controls	0.4	2.1
Acutely injured		
Minor and moderate injury	1.0	3.4
Severe injury	13.0	13.0
Septic shock	6.5	17.0
Cardiac patients		
Acute infarction	1.6	7.5
Cardiac arrest	29.0	40.0

Cortisol is released from the adrenal in response to ACTH which is regarded as one of the three 'trauma' or 'stress' hormones. The other hormones in this group are prolactin and vasopressin. The functions of prolactin are obscure. Increased secretion of vasopressin occurs in response to an increase in the osmolality of the extracelluar fluid and a fall in blood volume or blood pressure. Vasopressin is also secreted in response to emotional trauma. In contrast, ACTH is released in response to all noxious stimuli. In respect of the effects of brain injury it is perhaps important to recognise that ACTH is formed in the adenohypophysis in response to 'corticotrophin releasing factor' (CRF). CRF is produced in the hypothalamus. It is now generally agreed[4] that CRF consists of several components which act synergistically. These include a 41 residue CRF, vasopressin and epinephrin.

Neural mechanisms control the release of CRF. Excitatory and inhibitory nervous pathways originating from other parts of the CNS are involved. These come from several parts of the brain. Studies in laboratory animals show that the amygdala, hippocampus, thalamus and others are involved. There is some evidence that cholinergic neurons have a stimulatory effect. The role of serotinergic neurones is less well understood. GABA (Gamma amino butyric acid) -ergic neurones appear to exert a tonic inhibitory influence over the hypothalamic secretion of CRF. Catecholaminergic neurones are also concerned but their effects differ from species to species. Opioid substances may play a role but the physiological importance of opioid receptors in regulating CRF remains to be established. In man, opiate drugs and opioid peptides inhibit the release of ACTH and related peptides. Measurements of plasma and urinary cortisol levels in opiate addicts suggests that the function of the hypothalamic-pituitary-adrenal axis is impaired by prolonged exposure to opiate drugs[4].

The largest energy reserves in the body are in the neutral triglycerides found in adipose tissue. Lipoprotein lipases are activated by the catecholamines resulting in breakdown of triglycerides and release of free fatty acids and glycerol into the blood stream. The glycerol moiety participates in gluconeogensis in the liver. The free fatty acids are either used to produce energy in peripheral tissue or converted into ketone bodies, acetoacetate and β-hydroxybutyrate, in the liver. These ketone bodies can be used as an energy substrate for many tissues, including, as we have seen, the brain. Hyperketonaemia may be linked with prognosis in undernourished surgical patients[38]. Oxidation of fat can provide 70 - 80% of the energy required after injury.

Following injury there are also changes in water and electrolyte metabolism consequent upon increased production of aldosterone and ADH so that oliguria, or anuria, occur with retention of sodium.

CYTOKINES

The hormonal changes described above provide the means of facilitating, coordinating and controlling the metabolic actions of cytokines[17]. Cytokines are a diverse range of polypeptides produced in response to inflammatory stimuli. Cytokines are produced by phagocytic immune cells, T and B lymphocytes, fibroblasts and various endothelial cells. Besides being produced by inflammation, cytokines are also produced by trauma, cancer, sepsis and as a result of chronic inflammatory diseases. Of considerable possible importance in relation to patents with head injuries, is the fact that cytokines, besides enhancing the production of hormones which cause the breakdown of proteins, lipolysis and changes involved in the metabolic response to injury, also lead to the production of fever, anorexia and eventually to a reduction in the production of cytokines. CRF may be important in all three of these activities. In the production of fever, circulating cytokines may act on an area of the hypothalamus called the organum vasculorum laminae terminalis (OVLT). Prostaglandins are subsequently produced from endothelial cells of the OVLT, and either directly stimulate the temperature-sensitive neurons nearby that may induce fever, or stimulate production of neurotransmitters which act in the same way. CRF can induce fever when given intracerebrovascularly[33]. CRF may also be involved in the anorexia produced by cytokines, although the precise mechanism remains to be determined. It has been suggested that cytokines may act directly on the appetite centres via an effect on glucose sensitive neurons in the lateral hypothalamus[30].

THE METABOLIC RESPONSE IN BRAIN-INJURED PATIENTS

Increased ventricular activity of the cytokine, interleukin 1 (IL-1), has been reported in head-injured patients[24]. This report, coupled with the finding that intracerebroventricular adminstration of IL-1 in experimental animals produces a much more profound metabolic response compared with intravenous or intraperitoneal administration of the same dose of IL-1[1,36] suggests that small amounts of strategically located IL-1 in the brain of head-injured patients might also cause a profound systemic metabolic response in man[40]. These workers studied the acute-phase response in 25 patients from admission up to 21 days post injury. The patients were divided into two groups according to the Glasgow Coma Scale (GCS) to determine if the severity of injury influenced the response. Patients with GCS scores of 4 or less (severely injured) were compared with those with scores of 8 or greater (moderately severe). Measurement of acute phase proteins (α -1 acid glycoprotein, caeruloplasmin and C-reactive protein) and of serum copper, zinc and serum albumin showed that both groups of patients had a profound acute-phase response which lasted for the duration of the study period. Other studies have similarly suggested that altered metabolic status in brain-injured patients lasts for an extended period of time. One study[19] suggested that hypermetabolism may persist for up to 1 year after brain injury. However, it may be that not all aspects of the metabolic response are affected for the same length of time. Thus, Deutschman et al[10], on the basis of measurement of nitrogen excretion and plasma amino acid profiles, suggested that brain-trauma patients have a short period of altered metabolic response of approximately 1 week duration.

An earlier report[6] had indicated that in a majority of head-injured patients there was difficulty in achieving nitrogen balance. In this study of 14 steroid-treated comatose patients it was found that the resting metabolic energy expenditure (RMEE) as a percentage of that expected in an individual of equivalent age, sex and body surface area varied from 79 to 190% with a mean of 138% +/- 37%. The mean nitrogen excretion, measured for 135 patient-days was 20.2 +/- 6.4 gm/d. The mean contribution of protein to the energy expenditure was 23.9% with values over 25% for 6 patients. In non-injured normal individuals protein contributes 10-15% of the energy. In the seven patients in whom a positive nitrogen balance was achieved over any 3-day period it was necessary to administer 161% to 240% of RMEE with externally administered formula. The authors commented that the metabolic response in their patients was similar to that reported for patients with burns of 20% to 40% of the body surface. A failure to meet the hypermetabolic response in brain injured patients is likely to precipitate malnutrition with attendant risks of infection and death[2]. Risk of infection may be increased also by changes in vitamin and trace elements, particularly zinc, status. Wound healing increases the need for vitamin C which, besides playing a major role in the hydroxylation of proline to form hydroxyproline for collagen synthesis, plays a role in the synthesis of the neurotransmitters norepinephrin and dopamine. Vitamin C is also important for the maintenance of immuno-competence. Vitamin A is essential in creating the cross-links between collagen fibrils and thus for the maturation of collagen fibres. Plasma retinol levels are controlled only in part by dietary vitamin A. A major factor affecting plasma retinol concentration is the hepatic synthesis of the specific carrier protein, retinol binding protein (RBP). This protein has a short half-life and its synthesis is therefore dependent on nutritional status. Synthesis of RBP also depends on zinc nutriture and thus may be seriously affected by the depletion of body zinc which has been reported[25] to occur in severely head-injured adults. In addition, both vitamin A and zinc status affect immunocompetence.

The autonomic status of severely head-injured patients is similar to that of surface burns patients, with hypertension, tachycardia, hyperthermia and wasting of body mass even when food intake appears to be adequate[5]. Hypermetabolic intensity is related to an hyperadrenergic state. This is manifest as increased nutritional requirements and by a hyperdynamic cardiovascular state with increased oxygen delivery to tissues[6]. Serum and urinary catecholamine levels appear to increase in relation to injury severity[7] and are implicated as a major component in post-traumatic hypermetabolism, also as co-factors with steroids[10]. Hyperadrenergic states may arise from increased muscular tone, since paralysis and sedation may reduce RMEE in some patients, suggesting activity level as a contributory factor. Normovolaemia is of primary importance to early recovery, as volume depletion impairs the supply of oxygen, energy and nutrients to damaged organs and so increases the mortality rate. Similarly, as oxygen consumption increases in proportion to catecholamine elevation, the combination of hypermetabolism and inadequate delivery of oxygen is destructive. The hypermetabolic process should resolve as the patients' neurological and general stress condition improves, although a history of other disease or of inadequate nutrition may hinder early recovery.

GLUCOSE INTOLERANCE

Reference has been made to the fact that trauma is followed by an increase in blood glucose concentration. Hyperglycaemia may be a function of increased glucose production by gluconeogensis rather than reduced glucose utilisation. A relative insensitivity to both insulin and glucose may also arise. Insulin deficiency or insensitivity promotes protein breakdown and skeletal muscle in particular is wasted. Each gram of a negative nitrogen balance is equivalent to the loss of almost 30 gm of skeletal muscle. Incidently, it is largely this muscle wasting, with consequent muscle weakness, which is responsible for the often long period of recovery after injury.

The brain normally uses glucose as a source of energy but can use alternative substrates including the ketone bodies β-hydroxybutyrate and acetoacetate, short chain fatty acids, lactate and pyruvate[20]. During periods of hypoxia/ischaemia increased availability of glucose for metabolism via the anaerobic pathways may result in additional neuronal damage while increased availability of non-glucose substrates such as ketone bodies may have protective effects[21]. Robertson et al[31] reported a study of the effect of intravenous glucose on the availability of other substrates. Patients deemed eligible for the investigation were randomly assigned to receive glucose or saline. All received 12g nitrogen per day as amino acids and appropriate electrolytes and vitamins. The results are summarised in Table 2. Caloric intake was higher and negative nitrogen balance marginally lower in patients receiving glucose. Arterial glucose concentrations were similar in both groups. However, insulin concentrations were significantly lower and the concentrations of β-hydroxybutyrate, acetoacetate, glycerol and free fatty acids higher in patients who received saline. It is clear that administration of glucose to patients during the first 5 days following injury suppressed the availability of alternative energy substrates. Pertinent to our present discussions was the observation that patients who made a good recovery had arterial glucose concentration of 5.52 μmol/ml, vegetative patients 6.79 μmol/ml and those who died 7.11 μml/ml. Corresponding arterial lactate concentrations were 0.55, 0.71 and 0.81 mol/ml. Although the lack of ketogensis in response to hypocaloric intake may be only a reflection of the severity of injury, hypoketonaemia may also contribute to ischaemic lactic acidosis. A number of clinical studies of head injured patients have demonstrated the relationship between hyperglycaemia and neurological outcome, with non-ketotic hyperglycaemic hyperosmolar coma almost always predicting a poor outcome (e.g. 26,29).

In addition to the general metabolic responses to injury, areas of focal injury may cause specific and long-term changes in nutritional status and behaviour. Rolls[32] showed that severe bitemporal damage in the monkey may result in both food and non-food items being placed in the mouth. Pica is sometimes a problem in individuals with mental subnormality and in patients with head injury visual discriminative learning difficulties may lead to difficulty in forming correct associations between stimulus (food item) and reinforcement. Orbitofrontal injury may alter food preferences with failure to control inappropriate feeding responses.

Table 2. Effect of glucose administration on protein-sparing and availability of energy substrates on days 3 to 5 after head injury (Modified from Robertson et al[31])

	Glucose	Saline
Nitrogen intake (g/d)	10.6	10.5
Calorie intake (Kcal/d)	643	271
Nitrogen balance (g/d)	-3.7	-5.0
Cumulative N balance (g/5d)	-21.5	-25.6
Arterial concentrations (per ml)		
Glucose (µmol)	6.65	6.40
Insulin (µU)	14.8	10.3*
ß-Hydroxybutyrate (µmol)	0.06	0.78**
Acetoacetate (µmol)	0.02	0.06**
Glycerol (µmol)	0.09	0.12*
Free fatty acids (µmol)	0.09	0.11*
Cerebral availability (µmol/g/min)		
Glucose	3.04	2.71
ß-Hydroxybutyrate	0.03	0.45
Acetoacetate	0.01	0.03
Glycerol	0.04	0.05
Free fatty acids	0.04	0.05

Values for saline-treated patients significantly different from glucose-treated patients shown * when $P < 0.05$; ** when $P < 0.01$.

Moreover, treatment in some patients may have nutritional consequences. This is so even in non-injured patients with diseases of the CNS. Thus management of a patient with a tumour given dexamethasone may become difficult due to appetite changes and consequent obesity.

NUTRITION DURING TREATMENT AND RECOVERY

The nutrition of children with head injury has been discussed elsewhere[12]. Salient and additional points including the management of adults will be discussed here.

Patients with brain injuries are often critically ill. As we have seen, their post-injury metabolic condition is somewhat similar to that of a patient with burns to 20% to 40% of their body surface[6]. The intensity of the metabolic responses may vary widely from one patient to another. RMEE may be increased to 190% of the non-injured values, hypermetabolism and hypercatabolism may last for an extended period and, in a proportion of patients, positive nitrogen-balance be difficult to achieve. Furthermore, glucose, the brain's normal energy source, may not be the best fuel to provide during the immediate post-injury period[31]. Further matters which should be considered are the need to provide optimum conditions for the transport of precursors of neurotransmitters into the brain[15] and the effects of drugs on nutrient requirements[11]. For the moderately and severely injured patients it seems that assessment of nutritional requirements, and possibly the construction of tailor-made diets, will be an important part of total patient management. Failure to do this may jeopardise recovery of normal function. It cannot be over-emphasised that patients are not 'fed' by giving 5% dextrose solutions. It is to be hoped that there is now better understanding of this than when Clifton and colleagues[6] wrote:

> "Another choice of feeding would have been adminstration of 5% dextrose... This would provide approximately 500 kcal/day, and represents the level of nutrition which many comatose head-injured patients have received in the acute phase of their treatment."

They added:

> "Preliminary data in patients fed at this level have shown that both RMEE and nitrogen excretion were markedly elevated in some patients."

Research into the nutrition of head-injured patients is not without difficulty. Randomisation of patients may not be totally satisfactory because of the complex interplay of factors that affect clinical outcome. Ethical considerations have to be taken into account so that any control feeding must be adequate with respect to known nutrients. Having a control group given 5% dextrose solution would be unethical! Moreover assessment of outcome and benefit to the patient may yield equivocal results due to the inadequacies of the techniques used rather than be an indication of minimal or no benefit. Thus, in the study by Hadley and colleagues[18] there is no indication that the greater average daily nitrogen intakes and smaller nitrogen losses resulting from giving TPN within 48 hrs and over 14 days actually benefitted the patient. In the study by Robertson and colleagues[31] giving glucose rather than saline increased the caloric intake and tended to reduce the negative nitrogen balance but practically switched off the production of ketones with possible ill effects to the brain.

At the present time it seems necessary to assess each patient individually. If the gastrointestinal tract is functional it should be used giving feeds via a fine-bore tube if necessary. These enteral feeds may be needed to supplement oral feeding. Young et al[41] recommended that enteral feeding should not be started until bowel sounds are active and gastric residual volumes are less than 100 ml /hr. It may be better to pass the fine bore (1-2mm diameter) tube past the pyloric sphincter into the duodenum or jejunum. A pump should be used so that the flow can be maintained at the desired rate. Careful recording on a flow chart is essential so that the amounts prescribed are actually given.

Total parenteral nutrition (TPN) may be necessary before enteral feeding can be used or may be a necessary adjunct to enteral feeding. It is essential to prevent overload of amino acids or energy, particularly glucose. Mixtures may need to be different initially, when there is a need to promote ketogenesis, from what is optimum later. If TPN is given careful attention should be paid to monitoring[22]. This is better done by specially trained nurses. A recent study[37] has drawn attention to the need to keep careful sequential records of the management of patients receiving TPN if serious underfeeding is to be avoided and risk of infection kept to a minimum.

REHABILITATION

It is not sufficient to provide appropriate nutrition only during the acute phase after injury. Children face the stressful stages of physical, cognitive and educational rehabilitation. Inadequate nutrition may delay these processes. Poor food choice can easily result in inadequate intakes of vitamins and minerals. These difficulties may be exacerbated in patients who have difficulty feeding themselves or in sucking, biting, chewing or swallowing foods. Other factors may be parental difficulties in controlling children's behaviour. Overeating may increase at 2 year follow-up in some head-injured children[34]. Obesity consequent upon inactivity and/or overeating may result in social ridicule by peers thus adding to psychological disturbance. Dietetic follow-up in the community is essential to continuing nutritional well-being and to maximal recovery in brain-injured patients.

As with recovery of muscle function, so too with the brain, stimulation and use play an important role. For the child whose brain has been damaged by head-injury there are perhaps lessons to be learnt, and encouragement to be derived, from the results of appropriate persistent stimulation in brain injured children[14]. Strength and control can be given to spastic limbs, some sight to blind eyes, some hearing to the deaf and some speech to those who hitherto have made only incoherent sounds. These results have been, and are achieved as the result of commitment and perseverance by parents and carers. In the long-term recovery of patients with brain injuries it may be that nutrition and stimulation will together hold the key.

REFERENCES

1. Bailey, P. T., Abeles, F. B., Hauer, E. C. and Mapes, C. A., 1976, Intracerebroventricular administration of leukocytic endogenous mediators (LEM) in the rat, *Proc. Soc. Exp. Biol. Med.*, **153**, 419-423.
2. Becker, D. P., Miller, J. D., Ward, J. D. Greenberg, R.P., Young, H.F. and Sakalas, R., 1977, The outcome from severe head injury with early diagnosis and intensive management, *J. Neurosurg.*, **47**, 491-502.
3. Berry, M., 1982, The developoment of the human nervous system, in *Brain and Behavioural Development*, J. W. T. Dickerson, and H. McGurk, eds., pp 6-47. University of Surrey Press.
4. Buckingham, J. C., 1985, Hypothalamo-pituitary responses to trauma, *Brit. Med. Bull.*, **41**, 203-211.
5. Clifton, G. L. and Robertson, C. S., 1986, Metabolic response to severe head injury, in *Neurotrauma: Treatment, Rehabilitation and Related Issues*, M.E. Miner and K.A. Wagner eds., pp. 73-88, Butterworths, Boston.
6. Clifton, G. L., Robertson, C. S., Grossman, R. G., Hodge, S., Foltz, R., 1984, and Garza, C., The metabolic response in severe head injury, *J. Neurosurg.*, **60**, 687-696.
7. Clifton, G. L., Ziegler, M. G. and Grossman, R. G., 1981, Circulating catecholamines and sympathetic activity after head injury, *Neurosurgery*, **8**, 10-13.
8. Cuthbertson, D. P., 1930, The disturbance of metabolism produced by bony and non-bony injury with notes on certain abnormal conditions of bone, *Biochem. J.*, **24**, 1244-1263.
9. Davison, A. N. and Dobbing, J., 1966, Myelination as a vulnerable period in brain development, *Brit. Med. Bull.*, **22**, 40-44.
10. Deutschman, C. S., Konstatinidis, F. N., Raup, S, and Cerra, F. B., 1987, Physiological and metabolic responses to isolated closed head injury. II Effects of steroids on metabolism potentiation of protein wasting and abnormalities of substrate utilisation, *J. Neurosurg.*, **66**, 388-395.
11. Dickerson, J. W. T., 1988, The inter-relationships of nutrition and drugs, in *Nutrition in the Clinical Management of Disease (2nd Ed.)* J.W.T. Dickerson, and H. A. Lee eds., pp. 392-421. Arnold, London.
12. Dickerson, J. W. T., Johnson, D. A. and MacLean, A., 1989, Food for thought.

A Role for nutrition in recovery, in *Children's Head Injury - Who Cares?* D. A. Johnson, D. Uttley, and M. Wyke, eds., pp. 55-70. Taylor Francis, London.

13. Dickerson, J.W.T., Merat, A., and Yusuf, H.K.M., 1982, Effects of malnutrition on brain growth and development, in *Brain and Behavioural Development,* J. W. T. Dickerson, and H. McGurk, eds., pp. 73-108, University of Surrey Press.

14. Dickerson, J. W. T., Tingle, P., Barrington, P. and Pennock, J. K., 1987, Development of brain injured children, *J. Roy. Soc. Health.*, **107**, 115-123.

15. Fernstrom, J. D. and Wurtman, R. J, 1971, Brain serotonin content: increase following ingestion of a carbohydrate diet, *Science*, **174**, 1023-1025.

16. Frayn, K.N., 1986, Hormonal control of metabolism in trauma and sepsis, *Clin. Endocrinology*, **24**, 577-599.

17. Grimble, R. F., 1990, Nutrition and cytokine action, *Nutr. Res. Revs.*, **3**, 193-210.

18. Hadley, M. N., Graham, T. W., Harrington, T., Schiller, W. R., McDermott, N. K.and Posillico, D. B., 1986, Nutritional support and neurotrauma: a critical review of early nutrition in 45 acute head injury patients, *Neurosurgery*, **19**, 367-373.

19. Haider, W., Benzer, H., Krystof, G., Lackner, F., Mayrhoffer, O., Steinberleithner, K., Irsigler, K., Korn, A., Schlick, W., Binder, H. and Gerstenbrand, F., 1975, Urinary catecholamines in excretion and thryoid hormone blood level in the course of severe acute brain damage, *Europ. J. Intensive Care Med.*, **1**, 115-123.

20. Hawkins, R. A. and Mans, A. M., 1981, Intermediary metabolism of carbohydrates and other fuels, in *Handbook of Neurochemistry Vol. 3.* A. Lajtha, ed., pp. 259-294, Plenum Press, London.

21. Kirsch, J. K. and D'Alecy, L. G., 1984, Hypoxia induces preferential ketone body utilisation in rat brain slices, *Stroke*, **15**, 319-323.

22. Lee, H. A., 1988, Parenteral nutrition, in *Nutrition in the Clinical Management of Disease (2nd Ed.)*, J. W. T. Dickerson, and H. A. Lee eds., pp. 496-511, Arnold, London.

23. Long, C. L., Spencer, J. L., Kinney, J. M. and Geiger, J. W., 1971, Carbohydrate metabolism in man: Effect of elective operations and major injury, *J. Appl. Physiol.*, **31**, 110-116.

24. McClain, C. J., Cohen, D., Ott, L., Dinarello, C. A. and Young, B., 1987, Ventricular fluid interleukin-1 activity in patients with head injury, *J. Lab. Clin. Med.*, **110**, 48-54.

25. McClain, C. J., Twyman, D. L., Ott, L. G., Rapp, R. P., Tibbs, P. A., Norton, J.A., Kasarkis, E. J., Dempsey, R. J. and Young, B., 1986, Serum and urine zinc response in head injury patients, *J. Neurosurg.*, **64**, 224-230.

26. Merguerian, P. A., Perel, A., Wald, U, et al, 1981, Persistent non-ketotic hyperglycaemia as a grave prognostic sign in head-injured patients, *Crit. Care Med.*, **9**, 838-840.

27. Morgan, B.L.G. and Dickerson, J.W.T., 1982, Effects of hormonal and other factors on growth and development, in *Brain and Behavioural Development,* J. W. T. Dickerson and H. McGurk, eds., pp. 6-47, University of Surrey Press.

28. Morgan, B. L. G. and Winick, M., 1980, Effects of environmental stimulation on brain N-acetylneuraminic acid content and behaviour, *J. Nutr.*, **110**, 425-432.

29. Park, B. E., Meacham, W. E. and Netsky, M. G., 1976, Nonketotic hyperglycemic hyperosmolar coma. Report of neurosurigcal cases with

a review of mechanisms and treatment, *J. Neurosurg.*, **44,** 409-417.

30. Plata-Salaman, C. R., Oomura, Y and Kai, 1988, Y. Tumor necrosis factor and interleukin Iβ ; suppression of food intake by direct action in the central nervous system, *Brain Res.*, **448,** 106-114.

31. Robertson, C. S., Goodman, J. C., Narayan, R. K., Contant, C. F. and Grossman, R. G., 1991, The effect of glucose administration on carbohydrate metabolism after head injury, *J. Neurosurg.*, **74,** 43-50.

32. Rolls, E. T., 1985, The neurophysiology of feeding, in *Psychopharmacology of Food*, M. Sandler and T. Silverstone, eds., pp. 1-16, Oxford University Press, Oxford.

33. Rothwell, N.J., 1989, CRF is involved in the pyrogenic and thermogenic effects of interleukin 1β in the rat, *Am. J. Physiol.*, **256,** E111-115.

34. Rutter, M., Chadwick, O. and Shaffer, D., 1984, Head Injury, in *Developmental Neuropsychiatry*, M. Rutter, ed., pp. 1-16, Churchill Livingstone, Edinburgh.

35. Sinclair, D., 1978, *Human Growth After Birth (3rd Ed.)*, Oxford University Press, London.

36. Thurchik, J. B. and Bornstein, D. L., 1980, Role of the central nervous system in acute phase responses to leukocytic pyrogen, *Infect. Immun.*, 30, 439-444.

37. Turner, J. PhD Thesis, 1992, University of Surrey.

38. Wright, P. D. and Rich, A. J., 1981, Ketosis and nitrogen excretion in undernourished surgical patients, *Acta Chirurg. Scand.*, Suppl. 503, 41-48.

39. Yakovlev, P. I. and Lecours, A. R., 1967, The myelogenetic cycles of regional maturation of the brain, in *Regional development of the Brain in Early Life,* A. Minowski, ed., pp. 3-65, Blackwell, Oxford.

40. Young, B., Ott, L., Beard, D., Dempsey, R. J., Tibbs, P. A. and McClain, C.J., 1988, The acute phase response of the brain-injured patient, *J. Neurosurg.*, **69,** 375-380.

41. Young, B., Ott, L., Rapp, R. and Norton, J., 1987, The patient with critical neurological diseases, *Critical Care Clinics,* **3,** 217-233.

NEURAL TRANSPLANTATION AND RECOVERY OF FUNCTION:

ANIMAL STUDIES

John D Sinden, Kathryn M Marsden and Helen Hodges

Department of Psychology
Institute of Psychiatry
London, England

AN OVERVIEW

Historical Background

Experiments on the transplantation of brain tissue in mammalian species began as early as the end of the nineteenth century[133]. In spite of a long scientific past and some excellent demonstrations prior to 1940 that grafted neonatal[30] and embryonic[82] central nervous system (CNS) tissue could under certain circumstances survive and differentiate in the host brain, little scientific interest in neural transplantation arose for several decades. The modern era commenced only in the mid-seventies, when two critical observations created a new *zeitgeist* by showing that neural transplants possessed the potential for a greater understanding of development and plasticity within the CNS, functional interrelationships between neural systems and, of most importance to this review, the capacity to repair damaged neuronal circuits and functional systems.

While the early reports showed that developing neural tissue would survive in its new environment, Lund and Hauschka[87] were first to demonstrate the potential of studies of graft-host neuronal integration. They showed that fetal retinas grafted to neonatal rat tectum would develop outgrowing axons and make synaptic connections on host neurons. At the same time, Stenevi et al.[128] were able to demonstrate potential for functional activity within neural transplants, by showing that fetal central and peripheral monoaminergic neurons retained their catecholamine histofluorescence following transplantation to adult hosts. Taken together, these studies provided the essential foundation for studies of the effects of grafted neurons within lesioned host brain, and suggested that grafted cells may provide hormonal or neurotransmitter (perhaps via synapses) innervation of denervated sites within the host brain, and that such neurochemical or, under some circumstances, circuit reconstruction, may have functional, including behavioral, advantage. An extension of this hypothesis was that grafted neurons could replace neurons or neuronal systems lost in neurodegenerative disease or more acute brain damage, hence providing radical new possibilities for surgical intervention to produce functional recovery in humans.

Recovery from Brain Damage, Edited by F.D. Rose and
D.A. Johnson, Plenum Press, New York, 1992

The early experiments of the modern era also importantly established a set of neural transplantation techniques that were to permit reliable and consistent viability of grafted pieces of dissected fetal brain or of cell suspensions derived from these dissections[15,16]. Since that time, these techniques have remained the basis for neural transplant work in all species and all laboratories.

Transplants, Neurotransmitters and Neurodegeneration

Contemporaneous with the modern developments in neural transplant research, the first valid behavioural models of human neurodegenerative diseases were being developed. Earlier work had clearly shown that in humans, degeneration of the substantia nigra pars compacta dopamine (DA) projections to the striatum (caudate nucleus and putamen) is responsible for most of the motor dysfunction of Parkinson's disease, and that systemic administration of L-DOPA, the DA precursor, could partially alleviate many of these symptoms[64]. In animals, the bilateral destruction of this small number (less than 40,000 in the rat) of DA-secreting cells results in a profound behavioural syndrome of adipsia, aphagia, bradykinesia, catalepsy and sensorimotor neglect, similar to human Parkinsonism[136,137]. The unilateral destruction of the nigro-striatal DA pathway with the selective neurotoxin 6-hydroxydopamine (6-OHDA) and subsequent challenges with DA agonists[138] provided a convenient and easily quantifiable index of motor asymmetry which provided a useful model for the first study of the close relation between transplant-induced recovery of both neurochemical and behavioral function[104].

The initial, consistent successes in demonstrating significant normalisation in turning behavior following either solid ventral mesencephalon grafts to the lateral ventricle[45,104] or into a prepared cortical lesion cavity overlying dorsal striatum[33], or as a dissociated cell suspension graft directly injected into striatal parenchyma[14], encouraged clinicians to attempt trials of catecholamine-rich grafts in Parkinsonian patients using adrenal medulla autografts as early as 1982[9]. Recovery in motor asymmetries in rats following transplants of fetal substantia nigra, or of catecholamine-rich adrenal medulla tissue (the tissue chosen for practical and ethical reasons in the early human studies) was always associated with recovery in biochemical and histochemical markers for dopamine in striatum (see ref. 44 for review of these early studies). In spite of early reports of dramatic clinical success with adrenal medulla grafting procedures[88], the subsequent failures have sharpened the need for more basic animal research on transplant mechanisms, and particularly the need to assess preclinical effectiveness in primates.

These demonstrations of transplant-induced recovery in motor performance in animals following striatal dopamine depletion suggested that a similar 'neuropharmacological' transplant strategy might produce successful functional recovery in other damaged neurochemical systems. Although the neural bases for cognitive processes such as attention and memory are not nearly as clearly mapped out as they are for motor performance, this approach was soon applied to deficits in cognitive function following septo-hippocampal damage. Fimbria-fornix lesions, which destroy the major cholinergic, noradrenergic and serotonergic inputs to the hippocampus and produce a distinctive pattern of spatial learning and memory deficits in the rat[101], have provided the most frequently studied experimental model for transplant-induced recovery of cognitive function. Low et al.[86] and Dunnett et al.[36] were first to investigate the effects of fetal septal transplants some seven months post-grafting on recovery in radial maze and T-maze rewarded alternation respectively. The transplants were placed in or near the denervated hippocampus and contained *inter alia* the primordial cholinergic cell bodies that normally innervate the hippocampal formation. In the first of these studies[86], an improvement in radial maze performance was not seen in the grafted, fornix-lesioned rats unless administration of the acetylcholinesterase (AChE) inhibitor, physostigmine, was made concurrently with behavioral testing. Improvements in T-maze rewarded alternation, however, were seen without AChE inhibition following septal grafts, but not control grafts of the noradrenergic locus coeruleus primordia[36]. Taken together, these experiments indicated that at least partial behavioral recovery on these spatial cognitive tasks was dependent on recovery in hippocampal cholinergic function produced by grafts of septal tissue that had grown *in situ* to be sufficiently mature to provide a near-normal AChE relamination[13].

As with growth of research into dopaminergic motor mechanisms and graft-induced recovery, so interest grew in the role of the ascending forebrain cholinergic projection system[57] (FCPS) in the cognitive decline characteristic of aging and, at the extreme, senile dementia associated with Alzheimer's disease[11]. Pharmacological strategies for enhancement of cholinergic function in aged and demented subjects were also explored[29]. Although the symptoms of Alzheimer's disease are wide-ranging, with a progressive deterioration in language, visual-spatial skills and judgement[91], a prominent early sign is impairment in memory, especially working or short-term memory[93]. Post-mortem, the damage to the Alzheimer brain is equally wide-ranging[134], being characterized by the presence of neurofibrillary tangles in neurons of the cortex, hippocampus and amygdala and extracellular deposits of ß-amyloid containing plaques in cerebral parenchyma and around blood vessels[21]. However, the best post-mortem neurochemical correlate of the degree of dementia measured in life was the extent of loss of cholinergic markers in the FCPS, in both the areas containing the neuronal cell bodies, namely the nucleus basalis of Meynert and the medial septal area and nucleus of the diagonal band[142], as well as the cholinergic terminals of these neurons, namely in neocortex, the hippocampal formation and amygdala[19,105]. This was but one strand in a network of evidence implicating forebrain cholinergic systems in cognitive function and decline. Other evidence came from the deleterious effects of cholinergic antagonists, and beneficial effects of agonists, on cognitive function in both animals and humans[25]. If reinstatement of the modulatory role of the cholinergic input to the terminal regions of the damaged FCPS could be achieved by neural grafts, then the associated cognitive deficits might also be potentially amenable to transplant-induced recovery[50].

Recovery of function following transplants of fetal cholinergic-rich brain tissue has been extensively investigated in two experimental models of the cognitive decline in aging and dementia. The first of these models was based on a large set of data that showed excitotoxic lesions of the rat homologue of the nucleus basalis of Meynert in the human (nucleus basalis magnocellularis - NBM) produced a wide-ranging set of cognitive deficits consistent with those seen in human dementia (see refs. 28, 107 and 120 for reviews). Dunnett et al.[38] demonstrated that following large unilateral ibotenic acid lesions of the NBM, deficits in passive avoidance retention and spatial navigation in the Morris water maze were improved by intracortical cell suspension grafts of fetal basal forebrain, but not control fetal hippocampal tissue, partial behavioral recovery being paralleled by recovery in cortical cholinergic markers, especially in levels of the enzyme responsible for acetylcholine synthesis, choline acetyltransferase (ChAT).

Acute lesion methods, however, do not adequately model the slow and chronic neurodegenerative processes that characterize the pathogenesis of human dementias. Like aged humans, aged rats (about 2 years) show sensory, motor and cognitive deficits. Unlike humans, aged rats do not normally develop plaques and tangles, although declining activities in a number of neurotransmitter systems are similarly observed, with most interest focused on depletions in cholinergic, dopaminergic and noradrenergic function. Gage et al.[50,51] studying aged rats identified sub-populations that were impaired in either motor coordination (balance beam) or tests or cognitive function, assessed by spatial navigation in the water maze; the former deficits improved after transplants of suspensions containing dopamine neurons into the striatum, but not of cholinergic neurons into hippocampal formation; whereas improved water maze performance followed the implantation of cholinergic- but not the dopamine-rich suspensions. After prior fimbria-fornix lesions, cholinergic-rich grafts extensively reinnervated the hippocampus, but there were no gross differences in the density or pattern of AChE innervation in rats that showed behavioral recovery compared to those that did not[50]. A later replication of the positive effects of septal grafts on water maze performance of aged rats[49], however, demonstrated that the improvements seen in grafted rats could be blocked by administration of atropine, providing indirect support for the view that the transplants subserved their functional effects by a cholinergic mechanism, although non-transplant mechanisms could not be ruled out.

These studies support the hypothesis that cholinergic dysfunction underlies at least part of the cognitive decline characteristic of normal aging, and suggest that fetal neural transplants are capable of reversing this decline through replacement by grafted functional neurochemical systems with a considerable degree of specificity. An alternative experimental approach to the graft-induced recovery of cognitive function following a chronic process of neurodegeneration arose from the observation[7] in post-mortem Korsakoff brains of a loss of NBM and medial septal area cells of a similar order to the losses seen in Alzheimer brains. This observation suggested that the memory and other cognitive impairments that characterize both Korsakoff's syndrome and alcoholic dementia[85] might be due to impairment in cholinergic function.

A large experimental literature has demonstrated both cognitive impairments and depletions in cholinergic neurochemical markers in animals given chronic alcohol (see references in ref. 5). The specificity of this correlation is, however, in doubt, given that chronic alcohol also produces falls in markers for several other neurochemical systems (references in ref. 5). Thus, in a study of the cognitive and neurochemical effects of varying durations of exposure to chronic ethanol ingestion, Arendt et al.[5] found an equally strong relationship between, on the one hand, the extent of impairment in both spatial and non-spatial working and reference memory in the radial maze and, on the other, falls in markers for cholinergic, 5-hydroxytryptamine, noradrenaline and dopamine neurons throughout the forebrain. A noteworthy feature in this study[5,6] was the lack of damage to diencephalic areas (mamillary bodies and anterior thalamus) which has usually been associated with memory loss in humans with Korsakoff's syndrome[140]. This finding supports other evidence[83] that the thiamine deficiency associated with alcoholism is a major contributory factor to the diencephalic lesions seen in the Korsakoff brain and that alcohol alone may not play a causal role in the memory dysfunction which is characteristic of this syndrome. Moreover following seven months of alcohol consumption by rats, cholinergic-rich, but not -poor (i.e. fetal hippocampal), transplants into neocortex or hippocampal formation each significantly ameliorated the alcohol-induced deficits in spatial and non-spatial working and reference memory. Importantly, transplants into both sites in the same animal had additive effects, indicating that the two branches of the FCPS act as a unitary system diffusely modulating the local circuitry within the cortex and hippocampal formation responsible for specific cognitive processing[5,6].

In dementing diseases in humans, it remains unclear whether damage to the FCPS may in fact be secondary to the pathology of the cortex and hippocampus. One report has suggested that neuronal plaques may be seen after NBM lesions in the rat[4], but a recent study has suggested this was a histological artifact[131]. There is a recent report of increased levels of ß-amyloid precursor protein (ß-APP) mRNA in local astrocytes following neurotoxic lesions in the hippocampus[116], but the life-span of the rat may be too short for full-blown Alzheimer-like pathology to develop. Of great future importance are the new transgenic mouse models; in one of these the terminal fragment of human ß-APP has been linked to a neuron-specific promoter, Thy-1, and presence of full Alzheimer-like neuropathology occurs by eight months of age[66].* Such models will provide enormous scope for testing the role of the FCPS and cognitive function in the transgenic animals[152] as well as assessing a variety of therapeutic (including transplant) strategies.

Transplants and Recovery of Damaged Neuronal Circuits

The above discussion has concentrated on a selection of important data demonstrating that transplants of fetal cell populations can exert positive functional effects within damaged brains by placing appropriate neurochemically-specific cells in denervated, but otherwise intact, targets of the damaged neurotransmitter system. The considerable success of this approach encouraged researchers early on to attempt the more ambitious goal of restoring damaged local circuits themselves. Experiments on recovery under such circumstances were based on the hypotheses that grafted neurons may freely interchange axonal and synaptic connections with the host brain, and that with homotypic grafts (i.e. when the fetal donor tissue is placed into the same location in the host CNS as it occupied in the donor CNS), the pattern of interconnectivity may resemble that seen in normal brain. Evidence for at least the first of these, namely limited graft-host anatomical and electrophysiological interconnectivity in adult host rats, has been demonstrated in homotypic cortex[54,122,123,154], striatum[144,145,146] and hippocampal formation[41,94,135,155]. Evidence for the importance of graft-host interconnections and the extent to which these need to restore normal patterns of innervation for successful recovery of function will be considered in more detail below.

The first experiments on circuit reconstruction and recovery of behavioral function in adults were carried out in rats with lesions in perhaps the most complex of circuitry, namely association neocortex. Frontal cortex lesions in both rats and primates produce no overt sensory or motor dysfunction, but cause deficits in a wide range of delayed response tasks[76]. Labbe et al.[79] showed that a bilateral aspiration lesion of medial frontal cortex in the rat produced sustained deficits in performance of a T-maze delayed alternation task. Remarkably, transplantation of solid pieces of late foetal (E20 - 21) frontal cortex into the lesion cavity significantly reduced deficits in learning the task compared to rats with lesions alone, although none of the animals with transplants performed as well as intact controls. The behavioural training was begun only a few days following transplantation, before any possible neuronal circuit integration was likely to have occurred, hence the results were interpreted in terms of graft-induced induction of the release of trophic substances (see below), rather than any rewiring of the neural elements responsible for the behavioural function.

Confirmatory evidence of the non-specific trophic explanation of these results has come from work by the same group on recovery after visual cortex damage[127]. Large bilateral aspiration lesions of occipital cortex were made in adult rats and two groups were given late fetal solid transplants of either occipital cortex or frontal cortex tissue. On a simple black-white brightness discrimination problem - which rats with this lesion would eventually be able to learn - the rats with homotypic occipital grafts showed no improvement, whereas the rate of learning of the group with heterotypic frontal cortex grafts was enhanced relative to the lesion alone group. On a more difficult pattern discrimination problem, where no recovery in lesioned rats is normally seen, neither cortical graft enhanced performance. Hence the heterotypic frontal cortex grafts facilitated a limited recovery process by a non-specific process, whereas

---

* The report of Alzheimer-like neuropathology in their transgenic mice has very recently been retracted by Kawabata et al., 1992, *Nature*, **356**, 265.

the homotypic occipital grafts, which would be expected to be more successful in reinstating normal functional circuitry, were unable to produce any recovery in these tasks.

It could be argued that cortical circuitry (other than perhaps in primary sensory or motor cortex regions) is too complex to expect that sufficient graft-induced reconstruction would ever occur to restore cognitive function. Moreover, cortical circuitry is too poorly understood to permit experimental determination of the necessary anatomical and physiological conditions for restoration of cognitive function. Anatomical and physiological evidence for circuit reconstruction has been investigated in lesioned neuronal systems, especially in cerebellum, striatum or hippocampus, whose organization is more accessible to experimental study. Evidence for recovery in behavioral deficits induced by homotypic grafts within the latter two systems, and whether recovery depends on circuit restoration or non-specific neurochemical or trophic mechanisms, will be considered later in this review. However, in the cerebellum, there is excellent evidence for the capacity of the adult brain to incorporate grafted neurons and for those grafted neurons to then migrate and organize to restore point-to-point circuitry.

Sotelo and colleagues[124,125] have extensively studied grafts of E12 isogeneic C57BL fetal cerebellar primordia to the Purkinje-cell-degeneration (*pcd*) mutant of this strain of mouse. In this mutant, progressive death of cerebellar Purkinje cells occurs between postnatal days 17 and 45, leading to ataxia. Following either solid or cell suspension grafts, Purkinje cells migrate for some distance in all directions from the graft site and occupy the host molecular layer, in a position slightly displaced from that occupied in the ontogenetic arrangement of Purkinje cells. A single graft will occupy only 5 - 17% of the total volume of the mutant molecular layer. As yet no attempt has been reported to establish a sufficient number of grafts to achieve recovery of the mutant animal's gait. This cellular invasion of the host cerebellum from the graft is restricted to Purkinje cells only, and will not occur unless the host Purkinje layer is degenerated. The migrated graft cells will form essentially normal dendritic trees throughout the host molecular layer and receive normal synaptic connectivity from host climbing fibres. Axonal connections from grafted Purkinje neurons to the host deep nucleus, however, occur very infrequently, due to the relative proximity of cerebellar deep nucleus neurons in the graft remnant itself. Since the transplant itself contains all types of cerebellar neurons in close proximity, there is a stronger likelihood that grafted neurons will 'talk to themselves' rather than to the host. However, if migrated graft-derived Purkinje cells are closer to the host deep nucleus than to the graft remnant and the outgrowing axons can avoid the graft-related glial scar, complete circuit integration of the grafted cells is possible. This also suggests that if a pure line of, for example, late-developing cerebellar stem cells[108] which may differentiate into Purkinje neurons, could be grafted and show the same pattern of migration, then a high proportion of these cells may innervate the host without their projections being disturbed by graft-associated targets and glial barriers.

MECHANISMS OF TRANSPLANT-INDUCED RECOVERY OF FUNCTION

So far we have considered some landmark studies of brain transplantation and recovery of function and loosely ascribed the processes by which recovery occurs in these experiments to one of three major mechanisms, which, in increasing order of neuronal complexity, are: (1) Stimulation of host brain recovery processes by the secretion of growth factors or other non-specific supportive molecules from the graft itself or from host brain due to the at least temporary presence of the graft; (2) secretion by the ectopically placed graft of neurotransmitters (or their precursors) with either diffuse paracrine or endocrine effects or synaptic release on host brain; (3) synaptic integration of the graft into the host brain, restoring damaged local circuitry via two-way interconnections. (For a detailed illustration of these and other related possible transplant mechanisms, see ref. 52). These different mechanisms are not mutually exclusive, and more than one may play additive or interactive roles in a particular case; furthermore, as has been shown above, different combinations of brain damage, type and site of transplant may well recruit different mechanisms. In addition, the behavioural deficits and tasks used to assess behavioural recovery and the post-graft interval may also covary with these other factors. Therefore the variety of ways in which experimental choices between these different mechanisms can be made is very complex. However, determining the mode of action of any transplanted cells that produce behavioral recovery for a given form of brain damage is essential to refining neural grafting procedures in order to produce a maximum of efficacy with a minimum of adverse side effects. Much current research in neural transplantation is directed towards this overall aim, driven by the clinical success that could be achieved if significant breakthroughs are made. In the remainder of this chapter, we review progress in the application of neural transplantation techniques to the amelioration of behavioral function, examining the extent to which neural transplants fit the above mechanisms of action as a basis for developing appropriate research strategies.

Trophic Mechanisms and Recovery of Function

Nerve growth factor (NGF) has a critical role in both neuron survival and the promotion of neurite outgrowth during development[139]. Although originally believed to be targeted only to peripheral sensory and sympathetic neurons, it is now clear that NGF has an important role in the developing and adult brain. NGF mediates its neurotrophic effects by interacting with specific NGF receptors, and in the CNS the FCPS is particularly targeted. Basal forebrain cholinergic neurons have NGF receptors and the terminal areas of these neurons, hippocampus and cortex, contain the highest levels of NGF mRNA in brain[55]. It has been shown that the administration of exogenous NGF is able to promote the growth of cholinergic cells and to prevent their death after axotomy[139]. Neurotrophic factors will also increase as a temporary response to brain lesions, and can thereby increase the growth rate and eventual mass of neural transplants[98]. NGF also appears to have related *tropic* action, it will attract the growth of developing or regenerating axons, or encourage the sprouting of undamaged fibres[17].

A number of other trophic factors have recently been identified, including brain derived neurotrophic factor (BDNF), fibroblast growth factors (FGFs) and ciliary growth factor[132], whose activities differ from NGF largely in terms of the types of neurons for which they have greater supportive affinity. Basic FGF, for example, has been shown to prevent loss of nigrostriatal dopamine neurons after exposure to the dopaminergic toxin, MPTP[102], and BDNF[65,75], but not NGF, has been shown to enhance *in vitro* survival and dopamine uptake of cultured nigro-striatal cells. Given the range of protective and tropic effects that trophic factors have on a variety of neuronal systems, it is tempting to suggest that at least some neural transplants may exert their positive effects on behavioral recovery by the secretion of growth factor molecules that directly or indirectly support the function of damaged neurons in a lesioned or degenerating system. One line of indirect evidence to suggest that this is the case comes from recent work on implants of cell lines genetically engineered to produce recombinant NGF[40,113]. Studies to date have used transfected autologous fibroblast cell lines which are amitotic and will survive in brain parenchyma at a constant size for up to 8 weeks[67], where, it is argued, they act in an unregulated, constitutive manner to focally secrete NGF, i.e. as "biological minipumps"[48]. Implants of these NGF-producing cell lines have been shown to provide substantial trophic support to cholinergic neurons by, for example, dramatically enhancing survival of medial septal neurons following fimbria-fornix axotomy[113]. The implanted cells also encourage AChE-positive fibres to grow towards them, indicating the NGF-secreting cells will induce tropic actions on cholinergic terminals[40]. NGF-secreting cells implanted in striatum will induce cholinergic axons from host NBM to abnormally sprout and penetrate the graft milieu[68]. As yet there are no reports of recovery of behavioral function with NGF cell line grafts. This is surprising since some years ago it was shown that in memory-impaired aged rats, prolonged intracerebroventricular (icv) infusion of NGF partly reversed the atrophy of cholinergic cell bodies in the FCPS and improved performance on a spatial memory task[42].

There is as yet no direct evidence that transplants which derive from fetal brain continue to secrete growth factors with an appropriate time course able to account for the sometimes permanent behavioural recovery; a lacuna that will no doubt soon be filled. Trophic effects due to the associated surgical trauma are likely to be maximal within the first few days of transplantation[98]. There are few reports of a detailed time course of behavioural change after transplantation. Among these, some are consistent with a short-term trophic effect of this kind[37,77,79], but in others behavioral improvement is not seen until 7-9 weeks after transplantation[5,59,69]. As far as we are aware there is no evidence that fetal grafts made *after* experimental lesions have substantial *neurotrophic* actions; e.g. fetal basal forebrain transplants that restore cholinergic markers in the hippocampus are unable to protect against cholinergic cell loss in the medial septum after axotomy. Striatal grafts however, are able to protect against *subsequent* striatal excitotoxic lesions, provided the lesions are made during the time window (up to 10 days) when grafting procedures exert their maximal trophic actions[103]. It remains unknown whether or to what extent a longer-term *neurotropic* action of graft-derived growth factors on sprouting of host terminal fibres may contribute to what is assumed to be outgrowth from fetal grafts.

Nevertheless, there is a large body of indirect evidence for some role for trophic factors in fetal transplant-induced behavioural recovery. A number of early studies in Stein's laboratory showed that recovery from the behavioural effects of cortical lesions was seen too early after grafting to be explained by new connections forming between graft and host[79,127] (see above). These findings have been replicated and extended in other laboratories. Dunnett et al.[37] showed that rats with frontal cortical aspiration lesions and subsequent homotypic transplants showed improvement in T-maze alternation learning one week post-transplant, but were significantly impaired with respect to their lesion alone counterparts when tested 6 months later. Similarly, Kolb et al.[77] trained rats after comparable lesions and transplants to find a hidden platform in the water maze either immediately or one month after transplant surgery. Again, the early training group showed improved learning, whereas the one month training group was significantly worse, compared to the lesion alone groups. The authors postulated that the eventual formation of graft-host connections may disrupt performance "by adding noise to the system"[77].

That the early recovery seen in these experiments on cortical transplants was clearly of a non-specific nature was unequivocally demonstrated by Kesslak et al.[70]. These authors argued that since *in vitro* evidence had shown that microglia could support growth of neurons[96] - a trophic mechanism later recognized to be through release of NGF by astrocytes[153] - it was possible that glial implants might produce recovery in similar tasks. They showed that recovery of T-maze alternation was as effective with an implant of purified (neuron free) astrocyte culture, or gelfoam soaked with a lesion wound extract, as it was with transplants of frontal cortex[70]. This non-specific effect may, however, not always generalize to rats with lesions in the hippocampal formation. This same group has shown that following kainic acid lesions of hippocampus, recovery in T-maze alternation occurred after fetal hippocampal grafts, but not after astrocyte culture implants[71]. In another study, large aspiration lesions of the hippocampus induced deficits in a series of spatial maze tasks[73]. Grafts of fetal hippocampus improved performance of the lesioned rats, but little evidence of normal hippocampal cytoarchitecture or connectivity could be seen in the transplants. The authors argued that the recovery may have been due to the development of trophic bridges linking regions of undamaged brain[73]. Similarly, after a large hippocampal lesion, deficits in a differential reinforcement of low rates of response (DRL) task were partially ameliorated by fetal hippocampal grafts[150]. Little evidence of graft-host connectivity could be demonstrated, hence the authors interpreted the positive effects in terms of trophic processes.

In an important early commentary on mechanisms of graft action, LeVere and LeVere[84] argued that if some trophic action had promoted host recovery, then removal of an established transplant should not interfere with the corresponding behavioural recovery. Woodruff et al.[149] have shown that surgical aspiration of the transplants effective in improving DRL performance did not eliminate the behavioral recovery, supporting their argument for a trophic mechanism. However, one must be cautious about interpreting the effects of a second major surgical procedure without data from more appropriate surgical controls than were used in this experiment. Moreover, while surgical removal is relatively easy with solid grafts located on the brain surface, it is much harder for cell suspension grafts implanted deep in the brain. Techniques to provoke immunological rejection of cross-species or cross-inbred strain grafts which may more selectively and non-invasively achieve this are currently being explored[22] (see below).

Using a more selective form of hippocampal formation damage, namely focal loss of dentate gyrus granule cells by colchicine injections, Barone et al.[10] have recently studied the effects of E17-18 fetal hippocampal cell suspension transplants and 4 weeks of continuous icv NGF infusion (both separately and combined) on spatial learning and memory in the water maze, with two different post-treatment intervals. Beginning six weeks post-lesion (and 4 weeks post-transplant and/or at the end of the NGF infusions), the lesion impairment was substantially ameliorated by the NGF infusions, but not by the fetal grafts; the combined NGF-graft group gave intermediate results. At 12 weeks post-lesion, however, neither the NGF nor transplant treatments improved spatial learning. The authors could draw few conclusions about the possibility of graft-induced hippocampal circuit restoration, since the whole fetal hippocampal grafts contained mostly neurons whose size and shape resembled pyramidal cells and few organized granule cell clusters. The data, however, do suggest that the presumably trophic action of NGF is quite independent of any effects of the fetal grafts in behavioural recovery.

The evidence that a large component of transplant-induced recovery of function is due to trophic factor secretion is, given the data reviewed above, somewhat mixed. What is clear is that trophic factors, in particular NGF, delivered exogenously and possibly also through transfected cell line grafts, have powerful, if temporary, positive effects on behavioral recovery from a number of kinds of brain damage. What remains very unclear is the extent to which fetal grafts may operate via the same mechanisms. Furthermore, some of the data reviewed above which has tested animals at different post-transplant intervals, suggests that the trophic properties and the 'neuronal integration' properties (i.e., transmitter release and/or graft-host connectivity) of transplants may operate not cooperatively, but antagonistically in many functional systems.

In our laboratory we have attempted to unravel the multiplicity of local neurochemical changes at the site of transplants that may mediate behavioral effects in transplant experiments[141]. Using dissected samples of frontal cortex from a subset of rats with ibotenic acid lesions of medial septum and NBM that produce long-lasting impairments in both spatial and non-spatial reference and working memory in the radial arm maze[5,59], we examined what protein changes occurred in the presence of transplants of fetal basal forebrain that produced long-term behavioural recovery versus transplants of fetal hippocampus that were behaviorally ineffective. Recovery in ChAT activity from the fetal grafts in the frontal cortex accounted for most of the variance in behavioural recovery in these experiments and this will be discussed in the next section. However, fetal transplants consist of many cell types and neurotransmitters. After 2-dimensional electrophoresis 33 proteins were reliably identified on each sample gel and measured by image analysis. The normalized values were related to type of transplant group (cholinergic-rich versus -poor) and individually correlated with performance on the radial maze. Of the 33 proteins, 7 showed differences which depended on type of transplant and/or were correlated with behaviour. Only one identified protein was elevated in cholinergic-rich compared to cholinergic-poor transplants in frontal cortex tissue and was positively correlated with behaviour. This protein, glial fibrillary acidic protein, is a glial marker, mostly of astrocytes. On the other hand, some non-specific neuronal cytoskeletal proteins and neuron specific enolase were negatively correlated with radial maze performance, but did not differ between transplant groups[141]. These data suggest that, even when measured 12 months post-lesion and seven months post-transplant, the trophic support provided by cholinergic-rich transplant-related glia may aid cognitive recovery, whereas proliferation of some neural elements may inhibit the recovery process.

Neurotransmitter Release and Recovery of Function

There is now a large body of evidence (some of it reviewed in the Overview above) demonstrating that transplants derived from fetal dopaminergic, noradrenergic, serotonergic and cholinergic cell body regions, as appropriate, can reinnervate denervated target regions of the brain and thereby restore many behavioural deficits resulting from the denervating lesions. Comprehensive recent reviews of these data are published elsewhere[31,32,57,72], so detailed descriptions of many of these findings will not be repeated here. However, a number of important questions remain about the nature of the graft-derived neurotransmitter release which is necessary to promote successful behavioural recovery.

One issue concerns whether or not graft-derived neurotransmitter replacement requires a regulated system to produce functional effects because anatomical integration may be seen as a prerequisite for normalized physiological function. Ectopically placed fetal grafts that restore behavioral function following 6-OHDA lesions to the nigrostriatal pathway or following fimbria-fornix lesions show not only specific recovery of neurochemical markers and axonal reinnervation of the denervated target areas, but also (from electron microscopy evidence) synaptic contacts between the graft-derived fibres and vacated host target neurons[23,47]. Tyrosine hydroxylase-positive (TH) neurons and their dendrites in fetal substantia nigra grafts have been shown to receive normal synaptic inputs, possibly from host striatal afferents. However, many synaptic connections seen within the grafts are aberrant graft-derived TH-positive ones[18]. Nevertheless, dopaminergic neurons in these grafts appear to have normal electrophysiological properties and transmitter release on target neurons, responding to local applications of DA (presumably through autoreceptors) and disinhibiting the previously denervated striatal neurons[130]. In fimbria-fornix-lesioned hippocampus, fetal tissue derived from a variety of different cholinergic-rich sources, namely septum, NBM, striatum, brain stem and spinal cord have different degrees of survival and ChAT-positive afferent innervation. Only septal-derived cholinergic neurons showed vigorous axonal innervation and provided near-normal synaptic contacts with the denervated target, demonstrating a high degree of specificity of 'organotype' integration in grafted cholinergic neurons[24]. *In vivo* dialysis studies in freely moving rats have shown that KCl-stimulated acetylcholine release in fimbria-fornix lesioned hippocampus is normalized after both solid septal grafts (in the lesion cavity) and cell suspension grafts placed in hippocampal parenchyma. The transmitter release was increased by behavioural activation through handling or by electrical stimulation of the lateral habenula, in a similar fashion to intact rats[99]. It would be interesting to know whether grafts derived from other cholinergic-rich fetal regions produced the same type of functional neurotransmitter integration.

The presence of highly specific one- or two-way synaptic integration of ectopic fetal grafts in target regions which have been deprived of their distal, transmitter-specific projection systems, raises the question of whether such auto- and/or host regulation of the grafted neurons provides a regenerated system potentially capable of normal functional capacities. Alternatively, neuronal regulation in grafts may be redundant to the range of graft-induced recovery phenomena that have been studied. One way to address this question is to consider what kinds of constraints on recovery of behavioural function have been identified.

Dunnett et al.[39] showed that DA-rich fetal grafts innervating the denervated rat caudate-putamen which normalized motor asymmetries and simple sensorimotor function, did not produce recovery in a skilled forelimb reaching task. They argued that in the absence of normal host-derived feedback circuit integration, ectopic grafts are unable to restore skilled motor behavior. Similarly, we have shown that deficits in complex conditional memory tasks (win-shift/lose-stay and win-stay/lose-shift) produced by ibotenate lesions of the NBM, were not improved by transplants of fetal basal forebrain cell suspensions into neocortex, but deficits in acquisition and retention of step-through passive avoidance were improved in the same rats[117]. Intuitively, the task-specificity of recovery, such that tasks which may require greater levels of feedback control do not show recovery, is probably due to the lack of opportunity for ectopically placed grafts to participate in normal neural circuit controls. However, failures of recovery in complex tasks with both DA- and cholinergic-rich ectopic transplants in rats may be partly due to the relative lack of anatomical specificity of both striatum and the basal forebrain nuclei in this species. In primates, for example, the striatum is clearly divided into caudate and putamen components and the basal forebrain cholinergic nuclei are more clearly differentiated within substantia innominata and ventral globus pallidus than in rodents[2]. Although equivalent transplant research in primates is hindered by the relative unavailability of fetal material, recent work with marmosets has shown that transplants of fetal DA-rich cell suspensions into caudate nucleus but not into putamen restore motor abnormalities, whereas the reverse pattern of implant sites seems to be responsible for recovery in skilled forelimb use[3,109]. This suggests that where the opportunity exists for more accurate graft placement, and therefore improved likelihood of input-output integration of ectopic graft neurons, then more specific or comprehensive behavioral recovery can be obtained.

The few primate studies of ibotenate lesions to the NBM have shown that the loss of cholinergic afferents to cortex produced deficits in the learning of object recognition tasks. The deficits were exacerbated by cholinergic antagonists and improved by cholinergic agonists[1,110]. Interpretations of experiments on cognitive deficits induced by NBM lesions in rats, however, are complicated by the lack of neurochemical specificity of the excitotoxic lesion technique. Indeed, some reports (reviewed in ref. 34) suggest that the cholinergic dysfunction caused by NBM lesions is unrelated to the accompanying learning and memory impairment, since injections of quisqualate or AMPA appeared to produce more selective damage within the NBM region and a greater fall in neocortical ChAT levels than did ibotenate. However, only the latter toxin impaired performance on operant conditional discrimination or water maze spatial memory tasks[112]. These authors[34] have thus argued that the deficits following loss of cholinergic input to the cortex are essentially non-cognitive in nature, involving sensorimotor neglect[38] and attention to lateralized stimuli[111].

Our own research has concentrated on the unitary nature of the FCPS in modulating cognitive function, based on three major converging lines of evidence from two models of forebrain cholinergic depletion: (i) the similar and additive disruptive effects of ibotenate lesions to the NBM or medial septum on memory in the radial arm maze[5], and recently also demonstrated in object discrimination learning tasks with primates[1]; (ii) the effects of chronic alcohol consumption on markers of cholinergic function in both branches of the FCPS with deficits in radial maze performance similar to those of FCPS lesions[5,61]; and (iii) the additive recovery of memory function following fetal basal forebrain transplants into cortex, hippocampus or both areas[5,6,59]. We have recently shown that not only ibotenate, but also quisqualate and AMPA lesions produce equivalent radial maze impairments when NBM and medial septal area are lesioned at the same time (ref. 62 and unpublished data), providing further support for the functional unity of the two branches of the FCPS in cognitive function[57].

The deficits in spatial and non-spatial reference and working memory in the radial maze produced by combined ibotenate lesions of the NBM and medial septal area were partially reversed by the systemic injection of the cholinergic agonists, nicotine and arecoline[60], with effects on working memory performance being very pronounced. Subsequent transplants of E15 cholinergic-rich, fetal basal forebrain, but not cholinergic-poor E17 hippocampal cell suspensions into cortex and/or hippocampus produced recovery in all four measures of memory function, with the greatest recovery seen in working memory performance[59] (Fig 1 a and b). The time course of recovery, with positive effects manifest several weeks after grafting, was suggestive of the need for development of the grafts and innervation of host tissue, rather than early non-specific trophic actions. Although recovery was good in the groups with implants in either cortex or hippocampus, the combined placement grafts produced greater benefit.

The requirement that transplants which are effective by replacing damaged afferents must have contact with their normal targets was shown by the inability of cholinergic-rich grafts placed in the lesioned basal forebrain to improve radial maze performance (Fig 1 c and d) in spite of excellent survival of the transplanted cells. Except for slow-developing human neuroblasts[143], fetal grafts are unable to extend long axons to innervate distal targets in adult rats.

Given that administration of cholinergic agonist drugs apparently produced similar recovery to the cholinergic-rich terminal grafts, it might be suggested that the grafts were acting in a simple fashion as unregulated drug-delivery cells. However, the grafted rats that showed near normal behavioral performance on the radial maze did not show the same responses to cholinergic agonists and antagonists as did the unlesioned rats[60]. The recovered grafted animals, for example, showed more substantial deficits following scopolamine administration than normal rats. Paradoxically, nicotine, which had a null effect in the unlesioned rats and improved the performance of lesioned rats, increased dramatically the number of errors on the maze in the recovered transplanted rats. These interactions between drug and graft condition suggest that a complex autoregulatory system may have operated to control transmitter release from the fetal grafts[60].

One further way to investigate the importance of graft regulation in behavioral recovery is to examine the functional effects of several types of graft which are capable of effectively delivering neurotransmitters but which are likely to be regulated differently. A number of cell lines have been assessed for their capacity to restore behavioral function, all of which lack the regulatory controls that are an important feature of homotypic fetal grafts. These cells include: (i) peripheral nervous tissue, particularly from adrenal medulla; and (ii) fibroblast or neuroblastoma cell lines, some of which have been transfected to express transmitter precursors. Research on adrenal cells has been stimulated by the search for a non-fetal alternative transplant sources for Parkinsonian patients; whereas the fibroblasts and neuroblastoma cells can determine the extent to which a pure cell product, uncontaminated by the heterogeneity of cell types and products in fetal dissections, can influence function.

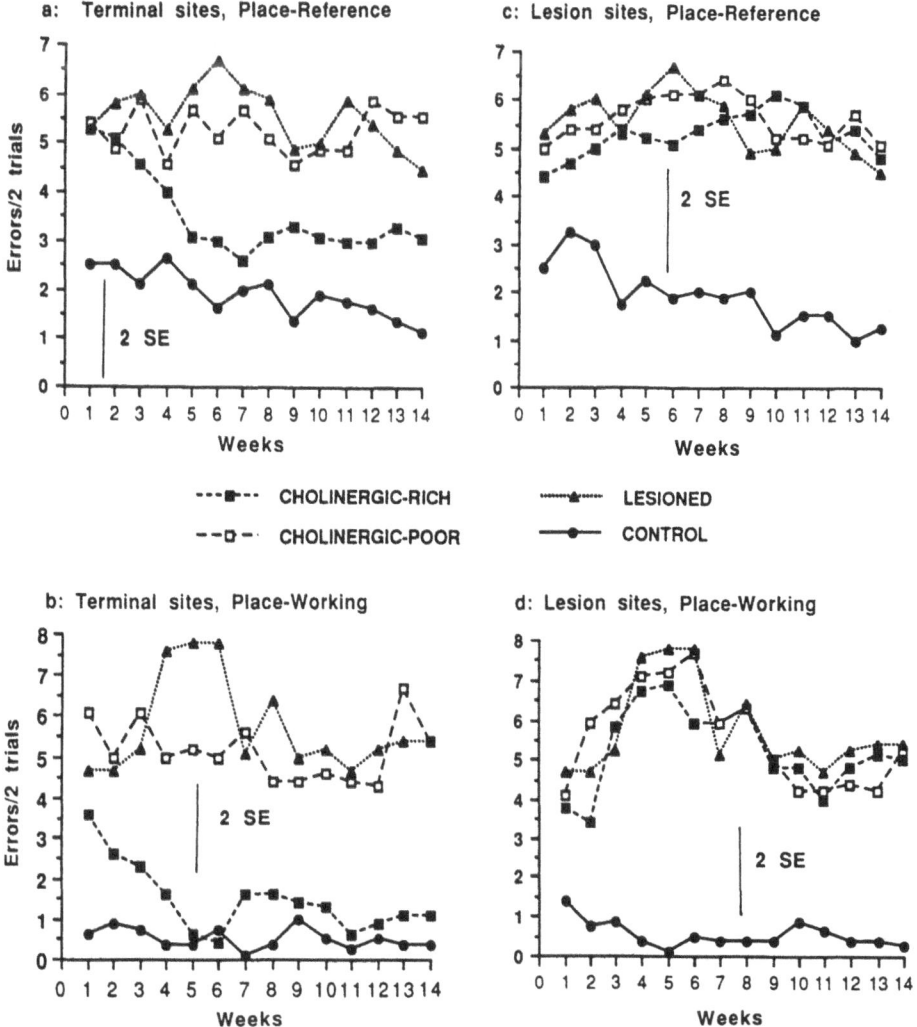

Figure 1. Effects of fetal grafts into terminal areas and excitotoxin-induced lesion sites of the forebrain cholinergic projection system. Mean number of reference (a,c) and working (b,d) memory errors in the place task in the radial arm maze are presented for 14 weeks of post-graft testing. Rats with cholinergic-rich, but not equally thriving cholinergic-poor, transplants into both cortex and hippocampus (a,b) showed recovery in both types of memory. When the grafts were placed into the lesioned basal forebrain sites (c,d), neither transplant was effective. Adapted from Hodges et al.[59]

Adrenal chromaffin cells produce and secrete catecholamines[74]. These cells, even when taken from mature animals, can undergo a partial morphological transformation, including development of neuron-like processes, either when grown in tissue culture or transplanted to the anterior chamber of the eye[100]. The extent of the transformation towards a neuronal phenotype is affected by the presence of growth factors such as NGF[129].

The chromaffin cells in adrenal medulla grafts, identified by immunoreactivity for chromagranin A, TH, and dopamine ß-hydroxylase, have been shown to demonstrate short processes which, unlike fetal substantia nigra grafts, did not appear to enter into the host brain or develop synapses[46]. Graft survival in ventricles is limited and even poorer in striatal parenchyma. Furthermore, there is no clear relationship between the number of surviving transplanted chromaffin cells and the extent of recovery of motor abnormalities[46]. It has been suggested that adrenal grafts exert a trophic or tropic effect resulting in sprouting of residual DA fibres toward the site of the graft[106], possibly induced by basic fibroblast growth factor, which is produced by the adrenal medulla[102]. However, there is no conclusive evidence to determine whether the trophic action is a specific feature of the cells or more related to non-specific damage by the response of macrophages/microglia and astrocytes following surgical procedures and tissue implantation[58]. It therefore seems unlikely that adrenal medulla cells are as effective as fetal neurons for both dopamine release and recovery from Parkinsonian motor abnormalities.

Fibroblast cell lines have been transfected with a retroviral vector containing cDNA for tyrosine hydroxylase and implanted in rats with unilateral nigrostriatal dopamine lesions[43]. These cells produced L-dopa *in vitro* which, if synthesis also occurred *in vivo*, would then be converted to dopamine by dopa decarboxylase still present in the denervated striatum. Compared to control BGal-transfected fibroblasts, the rats showed a significant reduction in motor asymmetry, although the recovery declined over the eight weeks of testing. A further study employing *in vivo* dialysis of transgenic fibroblast grafted striatum demonstrated increased levels of DA around the graft which correlated with reductions in motor asymmetry[63]. It remains to be determined whether the cells have a more permanent ability to reduce rotational behaviour than has so far been demonstrated before it can be convincingly argued that these unregulated grafts are as effective as fetal DA-rich transplants.

Neuroblastoma cell lines, which are embryologically related to neurons[8] and are thus likely to permit expression of neuron-specific traits, may provide a better alternative to fibroblasts for transplantation. Several studies have employed cultured immortal neuroblastoma cell lines as donor material. These studies demonstrated that implants of the human LAN-2 or IMR-32 cell lines with cholinergic features *in vitro*, when rendered amitotic with chemical agents[53,78], survived for up to 12 weeks *in vivo*. Implants into hippocampus of the LAN-2 amitotic neuroblastoma cell lines produced limited recovery in a T-maze alternation task following septal lesions in rats[78].

In our laboratory we have examined recovery in cognitive function following lesions of the FCPS by comparing implants of differentiated neuroblastoma cell lines with putative cholinergic features to grafts of fetal basal forebrain, with the aim of determining by what properties these unregulated cell grafts may operate. In our first study[69], IMR-32 cells were first differentiated in culture with dibutyryl cyclic adenosine monophosphate and prostaglandin E_1 and then implanted into the hippocampus of rats with fimbria-fornix lesions. Comparison groups were either unlesioned or given lesions plus E15 basal forebrain or sham transplants. Performance on a T-maze rewarded alternation task was assessed for 3 months post-transplant. Improvement in the fetal group began several weeks post-transplant and reached a level mid-way between the performance of the lesion alone and intact groups. The IMR-32 group also showed recovery with a similar time-course to that of the fetal group; however, because some rats were excluded because they developed tumours, the recovery just failed to reach statistical significance. Like a previous report using LAN-2 cells[78], no evidence of recovery in cholinergic markers was seen in the IMR-32 group, nor could any IMR-32 cells be positively identified *post mortem*.

Further transplant studies with differentiated neuroblastoma cells depended on clear evidence for their continued survival. Hence we labelled differentiated IMR-32 cells in culture with fluorescent latex microspheres to visualize both cell bodies and processes in culture. Prior treatment with mitomycin C and bromodeoxyuridine prevented their reversion to tumours. After survival times up to 12 weeks post-implant, the labelled cells could be clearly identified as dispersed elements within the grafted cortex and hippocampus, and ultrastructurally resembled their *in vitro* appearance[90]. In rats with ibotenate lesions of NBM and medial septal area, deficits in radial arm maze performance were improved by grafts of both IMR-32 and NS20Y cells, the latter being a mouse-derived neuroblastoma cell line which expressed high levels of ChAT activity in culture[89]. At the end of testing, performance of the neuroblastoma graft groups was not significantly different from that of the unlesioned controls (Fig 2 a and b). Moreover, the time course of recovery was similar to that of fetal basal forebrain grafts (data not shown), suggesting a similar mechanism of graft-induced recovery.

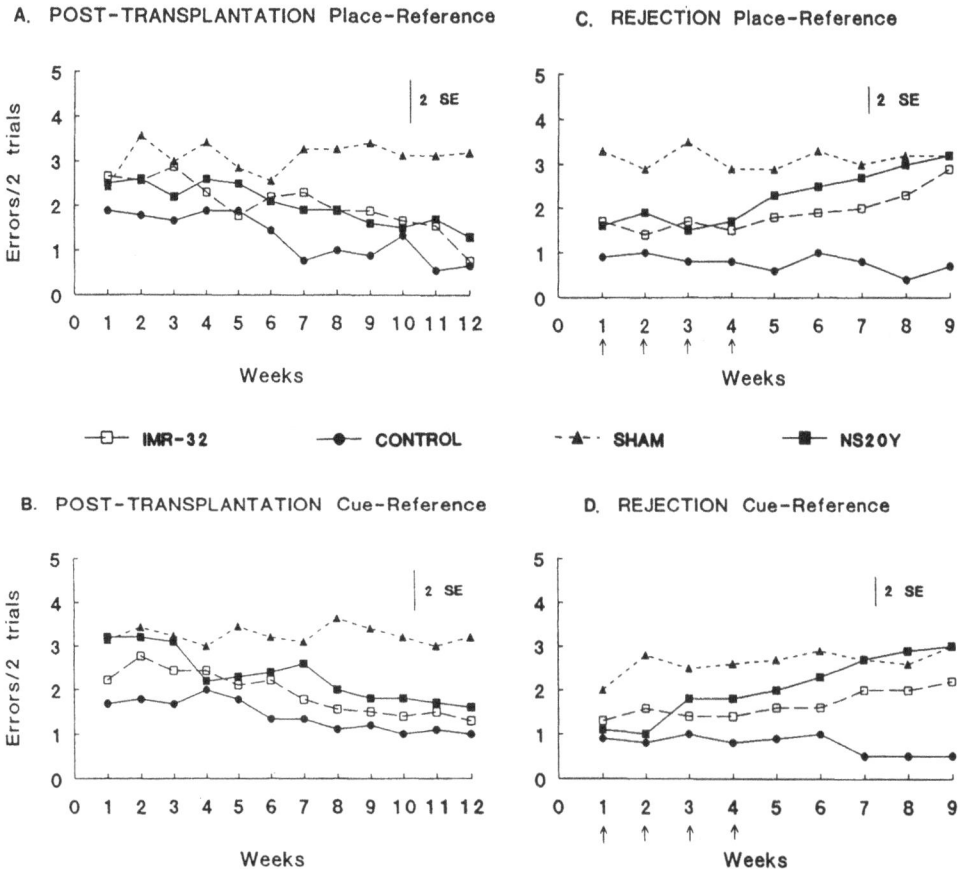

Figure 2. Effects of grafts of amitotic IMR-32 and NS20Y neuroblastoma cell lines into terminal regions following excitotoxic lesions of the FCPS. Mean numbers of place (A,C) and cue (B,D) errors on the radial arm maze are presented for 12 weeks of post-graft testing (A,B). Both cell lines produced significant recovery of function. The rats were then injected systemically with the appropriate cell lines during maze testing every week for 4 weeks (arrows in C and D), and the rats were tested for a further 5 weeks. Rejection of the grafts removed their behavioral effectiveness. Adapted from Marsden[89]

The original xenogeneic (human or mouse) source of these cell line grafts provided an opportunity to establish whether or not the grafts were operating through trophic effects on host brain. Although tissue transplanted to the brain may be able to enjoy a relatively high degree of immunological privilege compared to tissue grafted to the periphery[97,147], recent research suggests that cross-species and even cross-strain established neural transplants are immunologically unstable. If the host animal is sensitized to antigens from the donor species or strain, e.g. by peripheral skin grafts, then rapid rejection of the neural graft can ensue[118,119]. Therefore, a specific and non-invasive form of graft removal may be possible by sensitization of the grafted rats to the appropriate peripherally applied cell lines.

At the end of 12 weeks of post-graft testing, when asymptotic improvements in radial maze performance were seen in the IMR-32 and NS20Y groups, the appropriate neuroblastoma cells were irradiated and subcutaneously injected to the grafted and control groups. Rats were tested weekly on the radial maze during this time and for a further five weeks. The grafted rats' performance declined progressively over the nine weeks to the level of the lesioned controls, although performance in the other groups was unchanged (Fig 2, c and d)[89]. *Post-mortem* investigation showed substantial signs of graft rejection including an elevated peripheral lymphocyte response and, in the grafted cortical and hippocampal areas, mononuclear cell infiltration and high levels of MHC class I and II antibody staining, particularly in the NS20Y graft group[89]. Thus, dysfunction in or destruction of the grafted cells by the immune rejection removed the grafts' behavioural efficacy, indicating that the grafted cells themselves and not changes to host brain were responsible for the efficacy. Since neither grafted cell line affected ChAT activity *in vivo*[89], further studies on the *in vivo* neurochemical properties of these cells are required to determine how these grafts produce their effects on cognitive function.

The evidence that neural transplants can produce recovery of function in animals with denervating lesions by release of the appropriate lost neurotransmitter or its precursors is very well established. Whether the grafted neurons need to operate in the same way as the host neurons would operate or whether the transmitter release needs to be synaptically regulated (graft-host and/or host-graft) depends partly on the degree of circuit integration required for the control of the given behavior and partly on our understanding (or ignorance) of the neural mechanisms involved in that behavior. It is noteworthy that in the most commonly studied lesion models, the neurochemical system implicated (dopaminergic or cholinergic) appears to act in a diffuse, distributed and tonic manner rather than by point-to-point transmission of specific information. Intuitively, one would expect unregulated paracrine mechanisms to substitute more readily for the former than the latter. While synaptic connectivity and neuronal regulation are often features of fetal transplants rich in dopaminergic and cholinergic neurons, it is unproven that these features are important in behavioural recovery experiments.

It is important to note that in many experiments employing transplants in damaged neurochemical systems, fetal grafts can grow substantially as a dense, cellular mass with distinct glial boundaries. Transplant masses can often distort the normal structure of the brain, block ventricular spaces and alter the blood-brain barrier. One functional consequence of graft overgrowth that has been occasionally reported is the so-called 'overshoot' effect, where the graft produces the transmitter at levels well above the physiological range[148]. This may result in behavioural impairments over and above the lesion alone deficits in grafted animals, particularly at long post-graft intervals and where the denervating lesions are only partial, such that host and graft innervation of the target structure may interact in an abnormal fashion[26]. We have recently found that in rats subjected to long-term chronic alcohol consumption (which results in changes to a number of neurochemical systems[5,61], see above), frontal cortex grafts of either fetal basal forebrain, ventral mesencephalon (VM) or hippocampus all produced about 10-fold elevations in the levels of dopamine in frontal cortex, although the DA utilisation ratios suggested that the excess DA was not functional[61]. Since only the VM grafts contained TH-positive cells and processes, it appears that all grafts may have triggered sprouting of host frontal cortex dopaminergic afferents. A vital area of research for the eventual clinical application of neural grafting will be to ensure that any aberrant neurochemical effects of the procedure do not produce unwanted side effects, e.g. cytotoxicity from neurochemical hyperactivity[148] and also to determine the minimum number of grafted cells that can produce behavioural recovery, and not result in adverse transplant overgrowth.

Neural Circuit Reconstruction and Recovery of Function

There are a number of advantages to be gained from targeting neural transplants to instances of brain damage which involve destruction of neural circuitry. First, unlike cases where damage is made to, or occurs, in ascending projection systems, such as the nigro-striatal dopamine system or the FCPS, resulting in a consequent widespread denervated area, focal damage to neural circuits can involve quite a limited area. The data reviewed above indicate that although many transplanted fetal neurons can operate in a 'normal' physiological manner, their potential for axonal outgrowth is always limited. Transplants applied to a restricted neural circuit would obviate the need for long axonal growth (which is difficult to obtain) and large graft volumes (which can produce a range of adverse side effects). A second advantage is that one can more directly examine tissue-type specificity, by comparing the effects of grafts of homotypic versus heterotypic tissue, often where the same neurochemical profile applies. Third, if the graft is reconstructing a neural circuit, it must be located at the damaged site where it can receive undamaged host afferent inputs; thus, small changes in a graft position can provide important controls for efficacy. A final advantage is that because many specific neural circuits are anatomically well described, there is greater scope for assessing point-to-point connectivity[124] and determining whether such connectivity is required for behavioural recovery.

Neural circuit damage that has well-described behavioural effects can range from the relatively complex and poorly understood, e.g. neocortex, to the more straightforward, e.g. cerebellum. As the data reviewed in the Overview above would suggest, the transplant-induced recovery that occurs for a limited post-grafting period in rats with neocortical lesions is difficult to ascribe to circuit reconstruction, whereas transplants into mutant *pcd* cerebellum have provided the clearest evidence for point-to-point circuit reconstruction. This distinction suggests the hypothesis that in many complex circuits there is a high level of parallel processing, such that alternative circuits may often supervene to restore function following brain damage; hence grafts may operate to support this process trophically, or, if they make connections, actually interfere with recovery. However, in circuits that are anatomically simpler, where processing is dependent on a particular limited set of neuronal connections, there is a greater likelihood that grafted neurons will organize themselves for effective circuit reconstruction.

A number of anatomical studies of homotypic cortical grafts after cortical lesions have shown that the grafts receive highly organized afferent innervation from contralateral cortex, thalamus, brainstem (e.g. refs. 81 and 122) and even from basal forebrain neurons that were deafferented by the prior lesion[123]. Grafts of homotypic somatosensory cortex have been shown to contain neurons that respond to peripheral nerve or vibrissae stimulation[20]. However, evidence for outgrowth from cortical grafts is very limited. One exception is entorhinal cortex grafts placed in damaged entorhinal cortex where some perforant path input to the hippocampus has been identified[54,154]. Further, the intrinsic laminar organisation of cortical grafts is abnormal[95]. Hence, the absence of normal circuit reconstruction following neocortical grafts provides the most likely explanation for the failures of recovery in sensorimotor function[122] and the exacerbation of lesion deficits in some cognitive tasks[37,77].

Much recent interest in graft-induced restoration of neural circuits has focused again on the nigro-striatal system, in an attempt to develop a potential transplant therapy for Huntington's disease. This disease is an autosomal genetic disorder characterized by a progressive neuronal loss occurring principally in the striatum. Excitotoxic lesions of the striatum in the rat result in a similar profile of neuronal degeneration, sparing striatal axons and terminals[12]. The behavioral sequelae of these lesions are wide-ranging, including: nocturnal hyperactivity, seen as an analogue of the choreoathetoid hyperactivity of Huntington's disease; sensorimotor dysfunctions similar to those seen following DA denervation of the striatum; and cognitive deficits, due to the striatum's close functional relationship with frontal cortex[114].

The lesion-induced motor abnormalities following both DA denervation and intrinsic striatal damage have permitted elegant experimental comparisons between, respectively, the effects of transplants that operate ectopically to restore the DA input to the undamaged striatum and those that may restore intrinsic circuitry when the target structure is lesioned. In contrast to the failure of ectopic DA-rich grafts to restore a skilled paw-reaching task[39] (see above), rats with striatal grafts to lesioned striatum showed substantial improvement in their accuracy of paw reaching, as well as recovery of the lesion-induced motor asymmetries[35,92]. Together with a large body of anatomical evidence showing that striatal graft neurons receive extensive innervation from host substantia nigra[145] and cortex[144], and that the grafts establish efferent connections with host globus pallidus[146], these results suggest that the graft-induced restoration of a functional circuit is required for global recovery in motor function. It also indicates that striatal grafts into Huntington's patients may be a more rational therapy, at least for the motor consequences of the disease, than substantia nigra grafts for Parkinson's patients.

Evidence for recovery of cognitive function following striatal transplants in striatal lesioned animals is more limited. Deckel et al.[27] have shown some improvement in T-maze alternation performance three months after grafting, but without a control graft group it is not clear whether circuit reconstruction or trophic protection provided by the graft was responsible for the improvement. The effects of striatal lesions in spatial maze tasks may reflect damage to relays and/or motor initiation processes in this structure with its afferent connections from frontal cortex and hippocampal systems[56,114] and efferent connections to globus pallidus and motor cortex. Striatal lesions may, therefore, interrupt systems secondary to those directly responsible for the cognitive functions themselves. In our laboratory we have directly addressed the role of circuit reconstruction and recovery in spatial cognitive function, using lesions that selectively damage parts of the hippocampal circuit and transplants of fetal dissections of hippocampal subfields.

The normal hippocampus has well-defined routes of transmission along the 'trisynaptic circuit' organized in a laminar fashion. Entorhinal cortex afferents terminate at the distal parts of the granule and pyramidal cell dendrites. Mossy fibre afferents from dentate granule cells innervate the juxtacellular layer of field CA3. Afferents from CA3 to CA1, the Schaffer collaterals, innervate the proximal parts of CA1 dendrites. Using allelic differences between congenic mouse strains (Thy-1.1/Thy-1.2), Zhou et al.[154,155] were able to show immunohistochemically that fetal hippocampal and entorhinal cortex transplants reconstructed exactly these specific laminar projections after appropriate lesions, although the presence of synaptic connections has yet to be determined.

A number of studies have addressed the possibility that whole fetal hippocampal transplants can restore cognitive function following either extensive mechanical[73,149,150] or kainic acid[71,126] lesions to the hippocampal formation or colchicine injections that destroy dentate gyrus (DG) cells[10]. The evidence reviewed above has implied that improvements in performance depend on non-specific connectivity or trophic mechanisms rather than any selective circuit reconstruction. The combination of more selective lesions to hippocampal cell fields and subdissections of fetal hippocampus[41], however, is more likely to provide a means to study the neural organisation of cognitive function within the trisynaptic circuit and to determine the degree to which the anatomical specificity of intra-hippocampal graft-host connectivity is reflected in that function.

It is known that transitory occlusion of the major blood vessels to the brain of the rat produces ischemic damage to which the hippocampus is especially vulnerable[115]. We have found that 15 min of four vessel occlusion (4VO) in rats produces extensive damage to the CA1 cells in dorsal hippocampus and minimal damage in other intra- and extra-hippocampal forebrain regions (Netto et al., submitted). The selectivity of the 4VO ischemic lesion appears to mirror the well defined CA1 lesions in some patients suffering from anterograde memory loss after incidents of cardiac arrest or coronary artery occlusion[156].

Recently, we (Netto et al., submitted) have set out to determine whether the deficits in allocentric spatial learning in the water maze that are a consequence of 4VO ischemic CA1 damage can be improved by grafts of E19-20 fetal hippocampal cell suspensions derived from either the homotypic CA1 field or from heterotypic fetal DG. The DG cells, like those of CA1, are glutaminergic, so if the transplants promote functional recovery by neurotransmitter release, then both should be effective. It is also unlikely that CA1 and DG cells should differ in terms of any trophic influence they may exert on the host. A further control transplant tissue was used, that of E15 basal forebrain (BF). The grafts were placed in the alveus, just above the dorsal CA1 area of maximal cell loss.

The pattern of deficits in spatial learning in the water maze produced by the ischemic lesion was quite complex. There was an initial deficit in learning the hidden platform position. In further testing over the several training phases, which included reversal learning, working memory and transfer to a novel pool, the ischemic rats consistently showed much less flexibility in adapting to the changing requirements for successful orientation in the maze. After a post-grafting interval when the transplants would have fully developed and possibly formed new connections, the CA1 transplant group was almost always as efficient at learning as the sham controls and differed significantly from the ischemia-only and, in most of the testing phases, the DG and BF transplant groups. Figure 3 shows the different groups' retention of the previously trained platform position 9 weeks post-grafting.

These results are consistent with the view that cognitive recovery is highly specific to the subfield from which transplanted neurons are derived. The finding that only CA1 grafted cells were effective implies point-to-point circuit restoration, rather than release of glutamate, which would also have been supplied by the DG grafts. However, at the time of writing we must be cautious in drawing this conclusion because the CA1-containing grafts in this experiment were larger and more flourishing than the DG grafts, and some of the latter showed large patches of microglial invasion. This might arise because the CA1 lesioned host environment was more favourable to homotypic CA1 than DG cell growth. Alternatively, the timing of the dissection (E19-20, the time of CA1 - but too early for DG - neurogenesis) was more favourable to survival of CA1 cells. Further experiments will test these alternatives.

The evidence for field-specific behavioural recovery is reinforced by our parallel study in rats with selective colchicine lesions of the dorsal dentate gyrus[151], which also exhibited spatial learning deficits in the water maze. However in these animals solid grafts of E19-20 fetal DG but not CA1 tissue produce a selective improvement in performance, so that we have the suggestion of a double dissociation of functional recovery. Subsequent Timm staining in this experiment[151] demonstrated that the DG but not CA1 grafts increased the density of mossy fibre innervation of host CA3. We were also able to demonstrate in the DG-grafted animals host lateral and medial perforant path innervation and AChE lamination when the grafts were in contact with the lesioned DG, similar to observations by Tonder et al.[135] of neonatal dentate grafts following ibotenate lesions of hippocampus and dentate gyrus. Thus careful homotypic placement of the grafts is necessary before full connectivity can be assured.

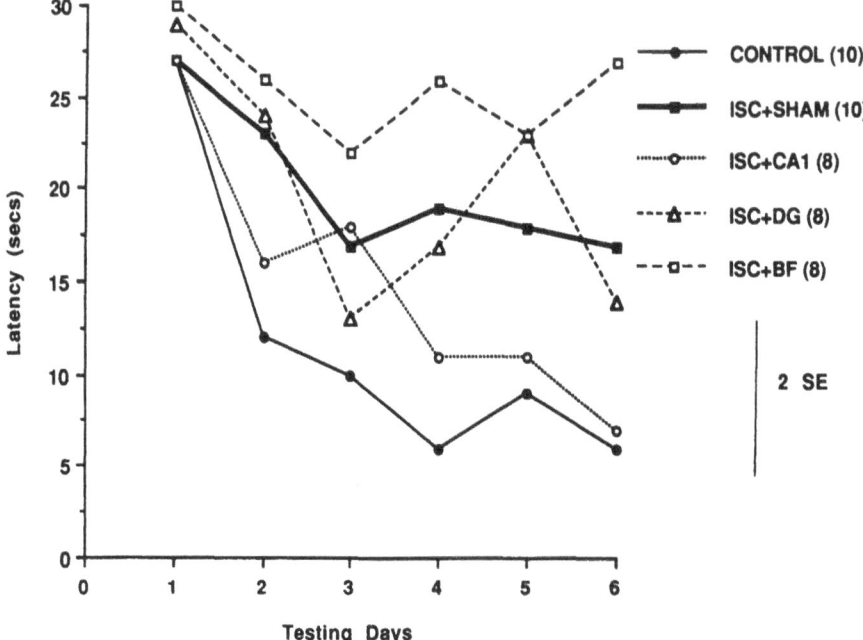

Figure 3. Effects of grafts of fetal cell suspensions of CA1, dentate gyrus (DG) and basal forebrain (BF) on retention of a hidden platform position in the water maze following ischemic lesions to CA1. Latency to find the platform for the ischemic rats with CA1 grafts (ISC+CA1) was not significantly different from unlesioned controls, whereas the other ischemic groups with or without grafts were significantly impaired in a number of measures of spatial learning compared to the controls. Adapted from Netto et al. (submitted).

Overall, the comparatively small amount of data on behavioural recovery following circuit reconstruction reviewed here suggests that where transplants are capable of reestablishing near-normal patterns of afferent and efferent innervation with the host brain, then behavioral recovery can be shown to depend on this reinnervation. It is possible that unlike the case for grafts that deliver neurotransmitters, successful recovery of neuronal circuits may depend on grafted neurons operating in a highly auto- and host-regulated fashion. In the hippocampal lesion and graft experiments reviewed here, we can hypothesize that grafted neurons may show relatively normal patterns of physiological potentiation and inhibition. For example, grafted dentate neurons may show long-term potentiation following host perforant path tetanic stimulation. We would thus predict that non-neuronal cell lines would be ineffective in this model. However, there is excellent scope for testing the efficacy of neuronal cell lines, such as the oncogenetically transformed hippocampal and cerebellar stem cell lines[108,121] and hippocampal neuron - neuroblastoma cell fusions[80] currently under development. One or more of these may provide an immortal source of non-fetal cells that demonstrate normal physiological properties and may thereby be behaviourally effective in lesioned circuits following implantation.

CONCLUSION

Neural transplants are capable of producing recovery of function after a variety of forms of brain damage. The effects obtained in many of the experimental models are tissue- and type-specific and involve some combination of trophic support to damaged systems, replacement of tonic neurotransmitter levels and/or circuit reconstruction. The extent to which fetal transplants operate through each of these mechanisms to produce recovery is becoming increasingly understood, and providing a developing scientific base for the application of genetically engineered cells suitable for transplantation. The long-term goal of establishing the required properties of a cell-line capable of restoring function is one of the most exciting scientific prospects in this field, allowing us both to see how normal cell development produces functional change and permitting the development of an effective therapy both for neurodegeneration and for acute brain damage.

ACKNOWLEDGEMENTS

We are grateful to Jeffrey Gray for many helpful discussions and to John Stephenson for his comments on an earlier draft. We would also like to thank the U.K. Medical Research Council for supporting this review, and, with the Wellcome Trust and the British Heart Foundation, for supporting our own research reviewed here.

REFERENCES

1. Aigner, T. G., Mitchell, S. J., Aggleton, J. P., DeLong, M. R., Struble, R. G., Price, D. L., Wenk, G. L., Pettigrew, K. L., and Mishkin, M., 1991, Transient impairment of recognition memory following ibotenic-acid lesions of the basal forebrain in macaques, *Exp. Brain Res.*, **86**, 18-26.

2. Alheid, G. F., and Heimer, L., 1988, New perspectives in basal forebrain organization of special relevance for neuropsychiatric disorders: The striatopallidal, amygdaloid, and corticopetal components of substantia innominata, *Neurosci.*, **27**, 1-39.

3. Annett, L. E., Dunnett, S. B., Torres, E. M., Ridley, R. M., Baker, H. F., and Marsden, C. D., 1991, Behavioural assessment of embryonic nigral grafts placed in the caudate nucleus and/or putamen of 6-OHDA lesioned marmosets, *Eur. J. Neurosci.*, Suppl **4**, 248-248.

4. Arendash, G. W., Millard, W. J., Dunn, A. J., and Meyer, E. M., 1987, Long-term neuropathological and neurochemical effects of nucleus basalis lesions in the rat, *Science,* **23**, 952-956.

5. Arendt, T., Allen, Y., Marchbanks, R., Schugens, M. M., Sinden, J., Lantos, P. L., and Gray, J. A., 1989, Cholinergic system and memory in the rat: effects of chronic ethanol, embryonic basal forebrain transplants and excitotoxic lesions of cholinergic basal forebrain projection systems, *Neurosci.*, **33**, 435-462.

6. Arendt, T., Allen, Y., Sinden, J., Schugens, M. M., Marchbanks, R. M., Lantos, P. L., and Gray, J. A., 1988, Cholinergic-rich brain transplants reverse alcohol-induced memory deficits, *Nature*, **332**, 448-450.

7. Arendt, T., Bigl, V., Arendt, A., and Tennstedt, A., 1983, Loss of neurons in the nucleus basalis of Meynert in Alzheimer's disease, paralysis agitans and Korsakoff's disease, *Acta Neuropathol.*, **61**, 101-108.

8. Augusti-Tocco, G., and Sato, G., 1969, Establishment of functional clonal lines of neurons from mouse neuroblastoma, *Proc. Nat. Acad. Sci. USA*, **64**, 311-315.

9. Backlund, E. O., Granberg, P. O., Hamberger, B., Knutsson, E., Martensson, A., Sedvall, G., Seiger, A., and Olson, L., 1985, Transplantation of adrenal medullary tissue to striatum in parkinsonism. First clinical trials, *J. Neurosurg.*, **62**, 169-173.

10. Barone Jr., S., Tandon, P., McGinty, J. F., and Tilson, H. A., 1991, The effects of NGF and fetal cell transplants on spatial learning after intradentate administration of colchicine, *Exper. Neurol.*, **114**, 351-363.

11. Bartus, R. T., Dean, R. L., Beer, B., and Lippa, A. S., 1982, The cholinergic hypothesis of geriatric memory dysfunction, *Science*, **217**, 408-417.

12. Beal, M. F., Kowall, N. W., Ellison, D. W., Mazurek, M. F., Swartz, K. J., and Martin, J. B., 1986, Replication of the neurochemical characteristics of Huntington's disease by quinolinic acid, *Nature*, **321**, 168-171.

13. Björklund, A., Gage, F. H., Stenevi, U., and Dunnett, S. B., 1983, Intracerebral grafting of neuronal cell suspensions. IV. Survival and growth of intrahippocampal implants of septal cell suspensions, *Acta Physiol. Scand.*, Suppl. **522**, 49-58.

14. Björklund, A., Schmidt, R. H., and Stenevi, U., 1980, Functional reinnervation of the neostriatum in the adult rat by use of intraparenchymal grafting of dissociated cell suspensions from the substantia nigra, *Cell Tiss. Res.*, **212**, 39-45.

15. Björklund, A., and Stenevi, U., 1984, Intracerebral neural transplants: neuronal replacement and reconstruction of damaged circuitries, *Ann. Rev. Neurosci.*, **7**, 279-308.

16. Björklund, A., Stenevi, U., Schmidt, R. H., Dunnett, S. B., and Gage, F. H., 1983, Intracerebral grafting of neuronal cell suspensions. 1. Introduction and general methods of preparation, *Acta Physiol. Scand.*, Suppl. **522**, 1-7.

17. Bohn, M. C., Cupit, L., Marciano, F., and Gash, D. M., 1987, Adrenal medulla grafts enhance recovery of striatal dopaminergic fibers, *Science*, **237**, 913-916.

18. Bolam, J. P., Freund, T. F., Björklund, A., Dunnett, S. B., and Smith, A. D., 1987, Synaptic input and local output of dopaminergic neurons in grafts that functionally reinnervate the host neostriatum, *Exp. Brain Res.*, **68**, 131-146.

19. Bowen, D. M., Smith, C. B., White, P., and Davison, A. N., 1976, Neurotransmitter-related enzymes and indices of hypoxia in senile dementia and other abiotrophies, *Brain*, **99**, 459-496.

20. Bragin, A. G., Bohne, A., Kitchigina, V. F., and Vinogradova, O. S., 1990, Functional integration of neurons in homotopic and heterotopic intracortical grafts with the host brain, *Prog. Brain Res.*, **82**, 287-300.

21. Brion, J. P. 1990, Molecular pathology of Alzheimer amyloid and neurofibrillary tangles, *Sem. Neurosci.*, **2**, 89-100.

22. Carder, R. K., Snyder-Keller, A. M., and Lund, R. D., 1988, Behavioral and anatomical correlates of immunologically induced rejection of nigral xenografts, *J. Comp. Neurol.*, **277**, 391-402.

23. Clarke, D. J., Gage, F. H., and Björklund, A., 1986, Formation of cholinergic synapses by intrahippocampal septal grafts as revealed by cholineacetyltransferase immunocytochemistry, *Brain Res.*, **369**, 151-162.

24. Clarke, D. J., Nilsson, O. G., Brundin, P., and Björklund, A., 1990, Synaptic connections formed by grafts of different types of cholinergic neurons in the host hippocampus, *Exp. Neurol.*, **107**, 11-22.

25. Collerton, D., 1986, Cholinergic function and intellectual decline in Alzheimer's disease, *Neurosci.*, **9**, 1-28.

26. Dalrymple-Alford, J. C., Kelche, C., Cassel, J. C., Toniolo, G., Pallage, V., and Will, B. E., 1988, Behavioral deficits after intrahippocampal fetal septal grafts in rats with selective fimbria-fornix lesions, *Exp. Brain Res.*, **69**, 545-558.

27. Deckel, A. W., Moran, T. H., Coyle, J. T., Sanberg, P. R., and Robinson, R. G., 1986, Anatomical predictors of behavioral recovery following fetal striatal transplants, *Brain Res.*, **365**, 249-258.

28. Dekker, A. J. A. M., Connor, D. J., and Thal, L. J., 1991, The role of cholinergic projections from the nucleus basalis in memory, *Neurosci. Biobehav. Rev.*, **15**, 299-317.

29. Drachman, D. A., and Leavitt, J., 1974, Human memory and the cholinergic system, *Arch. Neurol.*, **30**, 113-121.

30. Dunn, E. H. 1917, Primary and secondary findings in a series of attempts to transplant cerebral cortex in the albino rat, *J. Comp. Neurol.*, **27**, 565-582.

31. Dunnett, S. B., 1990, Neural transplantation in animal models of dementia, *Eur. J. Neurosci.*, **2**, 567-587.

32. Dunnett, S. B., 1991, Transplantation of embryonic dopamine neurons - what we know from rats, *J. Neurol.*, **238**, 65-74.

33. Dunnett, S. B., Björklund, A., Stenevi, U., and Iversen, S.D., 1981, Behavioral recovery following transplantation of substantia nigra in rats subjected to 6-OHDA lesions of the nigrostriatal pathway. 1. Unilateral lesions, *Brain Res.*, **215**, 147-161.

34. Dunnett, S. B., Everitt, B. J., and Robbins, T. W., 1991, The basal forebrain-cortical cholinergic system: interpreting the functional consequences of excitotoxic lesions, *Trends Neurosci.*, **14**, 494-501.

35. Dunnett, S. B., Isacson, O., Sirinathsinghji, D. J. S., Clarke, D. J., and Björklund, A., 1988, Striatal grafts in rats with unilateral neostriatal lesions - III. Recovery from dopamine-dependent motor asymmetry and deficits in skilled paw reaching, *Neurosci.*, **24**, 813-820.

36. Dunnett, S. B., Low, W. C., Iversen, S. D., Stenevi, U., and Björklund, A., 1982, Septal transplants restore maze learning in rats with fornix-fimbria lesions, *Brain Res.*, **251**, 335-348.

37. Dunnett, S. B., Ryan, C. N., Levin, P. D., Reynolds, M., and Bunch, S. T., 1987, Functional consequences of embryonic neocortex transplanted to rats with prefrontal cortex lesions, *Behav. Neurosci.*, **101**, 489-503.

38. Dunnett, S. B., Toniolo, G., Fine, A., Ryan, C. N., Björklund, A., and Iversen, S. D., 1985, Transplantation of embryonic ventral forebrain neurons to the neocortex of rats with lesions of nucleus basalis magnocellularis - II. Sensorimotor and learning impairments, *Neurosci.*, **16**, 787-797.

39. Dunnett, S. B., Whishaw, I. Q., Rogers, D. C., and Jones, G. H., 1987,

Dopamine-rich grafts ameliorate whole body motor asymmetry and sensory neglect but not independent limb use in rats with 6-hydroxydopamine lesions, *Brain Res.*, **415**, 63-78.

40. Ernfors, P., Ebendal, T., Olson, L., Mouton, P., Stromberg, I., and Persson, H., 1989, A cell line producing recombinant nerve growth factor evokes growth responses in intrinsic and grafted central cholinergic neurons, *Proc. Nat. Acad. Sci. USA*, **86**, 4756-4760.

41. Field, P. M., Seeley, P. J., Frotscher, M., and Raisman, G., 1991, Selective innervation of embryonic hippocampal transplants by adult host dentate granule cell axons, *Neurosci.*, **41**, 713-727.

42. Fischer, W., Wictorin, K., Björklund, A., Williams, L. R., Varon, S., and Gage, F. H., 1987, Amelioration of cholinergic neuron atrophy and spatial memory impairment in aged rats by nerve growth factor, *Nature*, **329**, 65-68.

43. Fisher, L. J., Jinnah, H. A., Kale, L. C., Higgins, G. A., and Gage, F. H., 1991, Survival and function of intrastriatally grafted primary fibroblasts genetically modified to produce L-dopa, *Neuron*, **6**, 371-380.

44. Freed, W. J., 1983, Functional brain tissue transplantation: reversal of lesion-induced rotation by intraventricular substantia nigra and adrenal medulla grafts, with a note on intracranial retinal grafts, *Biol. Psychiat.*, **18**, 1205-1261.

45. Freed, W. J., Perlow, M. J., Karoum, F., Seiger, A., Olson, L., Hoffer, B. J., and Wyatt, R. J. 1980, Restoration of dopaminergic function by grafting of fetal rat substantia nigra to the caudate nucleus: Long-term behavioral, biochemical and histochemical studies, *Ann. Neurol.*, **8**, 510-519.

46. Freed, W. J., Poltorak, M., and Becker, J. B., 1990, Intracerebral adrenal medulla grafts: a review, *Exp. Neurol.*, **110**, 139-166.

47. Freund, T. F., Bolam, J. P., Björklund, A., Dunnett, S. B., and Smith, A. D., 1985, Efferent synaptic connections of grafted dopaminergic neurons reinnervating the host neostriatum: a tyrosine hydroxylase immunohistochemical study, *J. Neurosci.*, **5**, 603-616.

48. Gage, F. H., 1990, Intracerebral grafting of genetically modified cells acting as biological pumps, *Trends Pharmacol. Sci.*, **11**, 437-439.

49. Gage, F. H., and Björklund, A., 1986, Cholinergic septal grafts into the hippocampal formation improve spatial learning and memory in aged rats by an atropine-sensitive mechanism, *J. Neurosci.*, **6**, 2837-2847.

50. Gage, F. H., Björklund, A., Stenevi, U., Dunnett, S. B., and Kelly, P.A.T., 1984, Intrahippocampal septal grafts ameliorate learning impairments in aged rats, *Science*, **225**, 533-536.

51. Gage, F. H., Dunnett, S. B., Stenevi, U., and Björklund, A., 1983, Aged rats: recovery of motor impairments by intrastriatal nigral grafts, *Science*, **221**, 966-969.

52. Gage, F. H., and Fisher, L. J., 1991, Intracerebral grafting: a tool for the neurobiologist, *Neuron*, **6**, 1-12.

53. Gash, D. M., Notter, M. F. D., Okawara, S. H., Kraus, A. L., and Joynt, R. J., 1986, Amitotic neuroblastoma cells used for neural implants in monkeys, *Science*, **233**, 1420-1422.

54. Gibbs, R. B., Harris, E. W., and Cotman, C. W., 1985, Replacement of damaged cortical projections by homotypic transplants of entorhinal cortex, *J. Comp. Neurol.*, **237**, 47-65.

55. Goedert, M., Fine, A., Hunt, S. P., and Ullrich, A., 1986, Nerve growth factor mRNA in peripheral and central rat tissues and in the human central

nervous system. Lesion effects in the rat brain and levels in Alzheimer's disease, *Mol. Brain Res.*, **1**, 85-92.

56. Gray, J. A., Feldon, J., Rawlins, J. N. P., Hemsley, D. R., and Smith, A. D., 1991, The neuropsychology of schizophrenia, *Behav. Brain Sci.*, **14**, 1-84.

57. Gray, J. A., Sinden, J., and Hodges, H., 1990, Cognitive function: neural degeneration and transplantation, *Sem. Neurosci.*, **2**, 133-142.

58. Hansen, J. T., Notter, M. F. D., Okawara, S. H., and Gash, D. M., 1988, Organization, fine structure and viability of the human adrenal medulla: considerations for neural transplantation, *Ann. Neurol.*, **24**, 599-609.

59. Hodges, H., Allen, Y., Kershaw, T., Lantos, P. L., Gray, J. A., and Sinden, J., 1991, Effects of cholinergic-rich neural grafts on radial maze performance of rats after excitotoxic lesions of the forebrain cholinergic projection system. 1. Amelioration of cognitive deficits by transplants into cortex and hippocampus but not into basal forebrain, *Neurosci.*, **45**, 587-607.

60. Hodges, H., Allen, Y., Sinden, J., Lantos, P. L., and Gray, J. A., 1991, The effects of cholinergic-rich neural grafts on radial maze performance of rats after excitotoxic lesions of the forebrain cholinergic projection system. 2. Cholinergic drugs as probes to investigate lesion-induced deficits and transplant-induced functional recovery, *Neurosci.*, **45**, 609-623.

61. Hodges, H., Allen, Y., Sinden, J., Mitchell, S. N., Lantos, P. L., and Gray, J. A., 1991, The effects of cholinergic drugs and cholinergic-rich foetal neural transplants on alcohol-induced deficits in radial-maze performance in rats, *Behav. Brain Res.*, **43**, 7-28.

62. Hodges, H., Sinden, J., Turner, J. J., Netto, C. A., Sowinski, P., and Gray, J. A., 1992, Nicotine as a tool to characterise the role of forebrain cholinergic projection system in cognition, in *The Biology of Nicotine*, P. M. Lipiello, A. C. Collins, J. A. Gray, and J. H. Robinson, eds., pp. 157-180, Raven Press, New York.

63. Horellou, P., Brundin, P., Kalen, P., Mallet, J., and Björklund, A., 1990, In vivo release of DOPA and dopamine from genetically engineered cells grafted to the denervated rat striatum, *Neuron*, **5**, 393-402.

64. Horneykiewicz, O., 1966, Dopamine (3-hydroxytyramine) and brain function, *Pharmacol. Rev.*, **18**, 925-964.

65. Hyman, C., Hofer, M., Barde, Y. A., Juhasz, M., Yancopoulos, G. D., Squinto, S. P., and Lindsay, R. M., 1991, BDNF is a neurotrophic factor for dopaminergic neurons of the substantia nigra, *Nature*, **350**, 230-232.

66. Kawabata, S., Higgins, G. A., and Gordon, J. W., 1991, Amyloid plaques, neurofibrillary tangles and neuronal loss in brains of transgenic mice overexpressing a C-terminal fragment of human amyloid precursor protein, *Nature*, **354**, 476-478.

67. Kawaja, M. D., Fagan, A. M., Firestein, B. L., and Gage, F. H., 1991, Intracerebral grafting of cultured autologous skin fibroblasts into the rat striatum: assessment of graft size and ultrastructure, *J. Comp. Neurol.*, **307**:695-706.

68. Kawaja, M. D., and Gage, F. H., 1991, Reactive astrocytes are substrates for the growth of adult CNS axons in the presence of elevated levels of nerve growth factor, *Neuron*, **7**, 1019-1030.

69. Kershaw, T. R., Sinden, J. D., Allen, Y. S., Gray, J. A., and Lantos, P. L., 1990, Behavioural recovery following transplantation of the neuroblastoma cell line IMR-32, *Prog. Brain Res.*, **82**, 47-53.

70. Kesslak, J. P., Nieto-Sampedro, M., Globus, J., and Cotman, C. W., 1986, Transplants of purified astrocytes promote behavioral recovery after frontal cortex ablation, *Exper. Neurol.*, **92**, 377-390.

71. Kesslak, J. P., Walencewicz, A., Calin, L., Nieto-Sampedro, M., and Cotman, C. W., 1988, Hippocampal but not astrocyte transplants enhance recovery on a forced choice alternation task after kainate lesions, *Brain Res.*, **454**, 347-354.

72. Kimble, D. P., 1990, Functional effects of neural grafting in the mammalian central nervous system, *Psychol. Bull.*, **108**, 462-479.

73. Kimble, D. P., Bremiller, R., and Stickrod, G., 1986, Fetal brain implants improve maze performance in hippocampal lesioned rats, *Brain Res.*, **363**, 356-363.

74. Kirschner, N., 1975, Functional organisation of the adrenal chromaffin vesicles, *Adv. Biochem. Psychopharmacol.*, **13**, 95-107.

75. Knusel, B., Winslow, J. W., Rosenthal, A., Barton, L. E., Seid, D. P., Nikolics, K., and Hefti, F., 1991, Promotion of central cholinergic and dopaminergic neuron differentiation by brain-derived neurotrophic factor but not neurotrophin-3, *Proc. Nat. Acad. Sci. USA*, **88**, 961-965.

76. Kolb, B., 1984, Functions of the frontal cortex of the rat: a comparative review, *Brain Res. Rev.*, **8**, 65-98.

77. Kolb, B., Reynolds, B., and Fantie, B., 1988, Frontal cortex grafts have opposite effects at different postoperative recovery times, *Behav. Neural Biol.*, **50**, 193-206.

78. Kordower, J. H., Notter, M. F. D., and Gash, D. M., 1987, Neuroblastoma cells in neural transplants: a neuroanatomical and behavioral analysis, *Brain Res.*, **417**, 85-98.

79. Labbe, R., Firl Jr., A., Mufson, E. J., and Stein, D. G., 1983, Fetal rat brain transplants: Reduction of cognitive deficits in rats with frontal cortex lesions, *Science*, **221**, 470-472.

80. Lee, H. J., Hammond, D. N., Large, T. H., Roback, J. D., Sim, J. A., Brown, D. A., Otten, U. H., and Wainer, B. H., 1990, Neuronal properties and trophic activities of immortalized hippocampal cells from embryonic and young adult mice, *J. Neurosci.*, **10**, 1779-1787.

81. Lee, S. M., and Ebner, F. F., 1990, Response characteristics of neocortical graft neurons to host somatosensory input, *Prog. Brain Res.*, **82**, 301-308.

82. Le Gros Clark, W. E., 1940, Neuronal differentiation in implanted foetal cortical tissue, *J. Neurol. Psychiat.*, **3**, 263-272.

83. Le Roch, K., Riche, D., and Sara, S. J., 1987, Persistence of habituation deficits after neurological recovery from severe thiamine deprivation, *Behav. Brain Res.*, **26**, 37-46.

84. LeVere, T. E., and LeVere, N. D., 1985, Transplants to the central nervous system as a therapy for brain pathology, *Neurobiol. Aging*, **6**, 151-152.

85. Lishman, W. A., 1986, Alcoholic dementia: a hypothesis, *Lancet*, **1**, 1184-1186.

86. Low, W. C., Lewis, P. R., Bunch, S. T., Dunnett, S. B., Thomas, S. R., Iversen, S. D., Björklund, A., and Stenevi, U., 1982, Functional recovery following neural transplantation of embryonic septal nuclei in adult rats with septohippocampal lesions, *Nature*, **300**, 260-262.

87. Lund, R. D., and Hauschka, S. D., 1976, Transplanted neural tissue develops connections with host rat brain, *Science*, **193**, 582-584.

88. Madrazo, I., Drucker-Colin, R., Diaz, V., Martinez-Mata, J., Torres, C., and Becerril, J. J., 1987, Open microsurgical autograft of adrenal medulla to the right caudate nucleus in two patients with intractable Parkinson's

disease, *New Eng. J. Med.*, **316**, 831-836.

89. Marsden, K. M., 1992, "Transplantation of neuroblastoma cell lines: a behavioural and histological analysis", PhD Thesis, University of London.

90. Marsden, K. M., Kershaw, T. R., Sinden, J. D., and Lantos, P. L., 1991, Survival and distribution of transplanted human IMR-32 neuroblastoma cells, *Brain Res.*, **568**, 76-84.

91. McKhann, G., Drachman, D., Folstein, M., Katzman, R., Price, D., and Stadlan, E. M., 1984, Clinical diagnosis of Alzheimer's disease: report on the NINCDS-ADRA work group under the auspices of Department of Health and Human Services task force on Alzheimer's disease, *Neurology*, **34**, 939-944.

92. Montoya, C. P., Astell, S., and Dunnett, S. B., 1990, Effects of nigral and striatal grafts on skilled forelimb use in the rat, *Prog. Brain Res.*, **82**, 459-466.

93. Morris, R. G., and Kopelman, M. D., 1986, The memory deficits in Alzheimer-type dementia: a review, *Q. J. Exper. Psychol.*, **38a**, 575-602.

94. Mudrick, L. A., and Baimbridge, K. G., 1991, Hippocampal neurons transplanted into ischemically lesioned hippocampus: anatomical assessment of survival, maturation and integration, *Exp. Brain Res.*, **86**, 233-247.

95. Mufson, E. J., Labbe, R., and Stein, D. G., 1987, Morphological features of embryonic neocortex grafts in adult rats following frontal cortical ablation, *Brain Res.*, **401**, 162-167.

96. Muller, H. W., and Seifert, W., 1982, A neurotrophic factor released from primal glial cultures supports survival and fiber outgrowth of cultured hippocampal neurons, *J. Neurosci. Res.*, **8**, 195-204.

97. Nicholas, M. K., and Arnason, B. G. W., 1989, Immunological considerations in transplantation to the central nervous system, in *Neural Regeneration and Transplantation*, Seil, F. J., ed., pp. 239-284, Alan R. Liss, New York.

98. Nieto-Sampedro, M., Manthorpe, M., Barbin, G., Varon, S., and Cotman, C. W., 1983, Injury-induced neuronotrophic activity in adult rat brain: correlation with survival of delayed implants in the wound cavity, *J. Neurosci.*, **3**, 2219-2229.

99. Nilsson, O. G., Kalen, P., Rosengren, E., and Björklund, A., 1990, Acetylcholine release from intrahippocampal septal grafts is under control of the host brain, *Proc. Nat. Acad. Sci. USA*, **87**, 2647-2651.

100. Olson, L. A., Seiger, A., Freedman, R., and Hoffer, B., 1980, Chromaffin cells can innervate brain tissue: Evidence from intraocular double grafts, *Exper. Neurol.*, **70**, 414-426.

101. Olton, D. S., Becker, J. T., and Handelman, G. E., 1979, Hippocampus, space and memory, *Behav. Brain Sci.*, **2**, 315-365.

102. Otto, D., and Unsicker, K., 1990, Basic FGF reverses chemical and morphological deficits in the nigrostriatal system of MPTP-treated mice, *J. Neurosci.*, **10**, 1912-1921.

103. Pearlman, S. H., Levivier, M., Collier, T. J., Sladeck Jr., J. R., and Gash, D. M., 1991, Striatal implants protect the host striatum against quinolinic acid toxicity, *Exp. Brain Res.*, **84**, 303-310.

104. Perlow, M. F., Freed, W. F., Hoffer, B. J., Seiger, A., Olson, L., and Wyatt, R. J., 1979, Brain grafts reduce motor abnormalities produced by destruction of nigrostriatal dopamine system, *Science*, **204**, 643-647.

105. Perry, E. K., Perry, R. H., Blessed, G., and Tomlinson, B. E., 1977, Necropsy evidence of central cholinergic deficits in senile dementia, *Lancet*, **I**, 189-189.

106. Plunkett, R. J., Bankiewicz, K. S., Cummins, A. C., Miletich, R. S., Schwartz, J. P., and Oldfield, E. H., 1990, Long-term evaluation of hemiparkinsonian monkeys after adrenal autografting or cavitation alone, *J. Neurosurg.*, **73**, 918-926.

107. Price, D. L., 1986, New perspectives on Alzheimer's disease, *Ann. Rev. Neurosci.*, **9**, 489-512.

108. Renfranz, P. J., Cunningham, M. G., and McKay, R. D. G., 1991, Region-specific differentiation of the hippocampal stem cell line HiB5 upon implantation into the developing mammalian brain, *Cell*, **66**, 713-729.

109. Ridley, R. M., and Baker, H. F., 1991, Can fetal transplants restore function in monkeys with lesion-induced behavioural deficits?, *Trends Neurosci.*, **14**, 366-370.

110. Ridley, R. M., Murray, T. K., Johnson, J. A., and Baker, H. F., 1986, Learning impairment following lesion of the basal nucleus of Meynert in the marmoset: modification by cholinergic drugs, *Brain Res.*, **376**, 108-116.

111. Robbins, T. W., Everitt, B. J., Marston, H. M., Wilkinson, J., Jones, G. H., and Page, K. J., 1989, Comparative effects of ibotenic acid- and quisqualic acid-induced lesions of the substantia innominata on attentional function in the rat: further implications for the role of the cholinergic neurons of the nucleus basalis in cognitive processes, *Behav. Brain Res.*, **35**, 221-241.

112. Robbins, T. W., Everitt, B. J., Ryan, C. N., Marston, H. M., Jones, G. H., and Page, K. J., 1989, Comparative effects of quisqualic and ibotenic acid-induced lesions of the substantia innominata and globus pallidus on the acquisition of a conditional visual discrimination: Differential effects on cholinergic mechanisms, *Neuroscience*, **28**, 337-352.

113. Rosenberg, M. B., Friedmann, T., Robinson, R. C., Tuszynski, M., Wolff, J. A., Breakefield, X. O., and Gage, F. H., 1988, Grafting of genetically modified cells to the damaged brain: restorative effects of NGF expression, *Science*, **242**, 1575-1578.

114. Rosvold, H. E., 1968, The prefrontal cortex and caudate nucleus. A system for effecting correction in response mechanisms, in *Mind as a Tissue*, C. Rupp, ed., pp. 21-38, Harper & Row, New York.

115. Schmidt-Kastner, R., and Freund, T. F., 1991, Selective vulnerability of the hippocampus in brain ischemia, *Neuroscience*, **40**, 599-636.

116. Siman, R., Card, J. P., Nelson, R. B., and Davis, L. G., 1989, Expression of ß-amyloid precursor protein in reactive astrocytes following neuronal damage, *Neuron*, **3**, 275-285.

117. Sinden, J. D., Allen, Y. S., Rawlins, J. N. P., and Gray, J. A., 1989, The effects of ibotenic acid lesions of the nucleus basalis and cholinergic-rich neural transplants on Win-stay/Lose-shift and Win-shift/Lose-stay performance in the rat, *Behav. Brain Res.*, **36**, 229-249.

118. Sloan, D. J., Baker, B. J., Puklavec, M., and Charlton, H. M., 1990, The effect of site of transplantation and histocompatability differences on the survival of neural tissue transplanted to the CNS of defined inbred rat strains, *Prog. Brain Res.*, **82**, 141-152.

119. Sloan, D. J., Wood, M. J., and Charlton, H. M., 1991, The immune response to intracerebral neural grafts, *Trends Neurosci.*, **14**, 341-346.

120. Smith, G., 1988, Animal models of Alzheimer's disease: experimental cholinergic denervation, *Brain Res. Rev.*, **13**, 103-118.

121. Snyder, E. Y., Deitcher, D. L., Walsh, C., Arnold-Aldea, S., Hartwieg, E. A., and Cepko, C. L., 1992, Multipotent neural cell lines can engraft and

participate in development of mouse cerebellum, *Cell*, **68**, 33-51.

122. Sofreniew, M. V., Dunnett, S. B., and Isacson, O., 1990, Remodelling of intrinsic and afferent systems in neocortex with cortical transplants, *Prog. Brain Res.*, **82**, 313-320.

123. Sorenson, J. C., Wanner-Olsen, H., Tonder, N., Danielsen, E., Castro, A. J., and Zimmer, J., 1990, Axotomized, adult basal forebrain neurons can innervate fetal frontal cortex grafts: a double fluorescent tracer study in the rat, *Exp. Brain Res.*, **81**, 545-551.

124. Sotelo, C., and Alvarado-Mallart, R. M., 1987, Reconstruction of the defective cerebellar circuitry in adult purkinje cell degeneration mutant mice by purkinje cell replacement through transplantation of solid embryonic implants, *Neurosci.*, **20**, 1-22.

125. Sotelo, C., and Alvarado-Mallart, R. M., 1991, The reconstruction of cerebellar circuits, *Trends Neurosci.*, **14**, 350-355.

126. Sprick, U., 1991, Transient and long-lasting beneficial behavioral effects of grafts in the damaged hippocampus of rat, *Behav. Brain Res.*, **42**, 187-199.

127. Stein, D. G., Labbe, R., Attella, M. J., and Rakowsky, H. A., 1985, Fetal brain tissue transplants reduce visual deficits in adult rats with bilateral lesions of the occipital cortex, *Behav. Neural Biol.*, **44**, 266-277.

128. Stenevi, U., Björklund, A., and Svengaard, N. A., 1976, Transplantation of central and peripheral monoamine neurons to the adult rat brain: techniques and conditions for survival, *Brain Res.*, **114**, 1-20.

129. Stromberg, I., Hultgardh-Nilsson, A., Hedin, U., and Ebendal, T., 1988, Fate of intraocular chromaffin cell suspensions: Role of initial nerve growth factor support, *Cell Tiss. Res.*, **254**, 487-497.

130. Stromberg, I., Van Horne, C., Bygdeman, M., Weiner, N., and Gerhardt, G. A., 1991, Function of intraventricular human mesencephalic xenografts in immunosuppressed rats: an electrophysiological and neurochemical analysis, *Exper. Neurol.*, **112**, 140-152.

131. Thal, L. J., Mandel, R. J., Terry, R. D., Buzsaki, G., and Gage, F. H., 1990, Nucleus basalis lesions fail to induce senile plaques in the rat, *Exper. Neurol.*, **108**, 88-90.

132. Thoenen, H., 1991, The changing scene of neurotrophic factors, *Trends Neurosci.*, **14**, 165-170.

133. Thompson, W. G., 1980, Successful brain grafting, *N.Y. Med. J.*, **51**, 701-702.

134. Tomlinson, B. E., Blessed, G., and Roth, M., 1970, Observations on the brains of demented old people, *J. Neurol. Sci.*, **11**, 205-242.

135. Tonder, N., Sorensen, T., and Zimmer, J., 1989, Enhanced host perforant path innervation of neonatal dentate tissue after grafting to axon sparing, ibotenic acid lesions in adult rats, *Exp. Brain Res.*, **75**, 483-496.

136. Ungerstedt, U., 1971, Adipsia and aphagia after 6-hydroxydopamine induced degeneration of the nigro-striatal dopamine system, *Acta Physiol. Scand.*, Suppl **367**, 95-122.

137. Ungerstedt, U., 1971, Postsynaptic supersensitivity after 6-hydroxydopamine induced degeneration of the nigro-striatal dopamine system, *Acta Physiol. Scand.*, Suppl **367**, 69-93.

138. Ungerstedt, U., 1971, Striatal dopamine release after amphetamine or nerve degeneration revealed by rotational behaviour, *Acta Physiol. Scand.*, Suppl **367**, 49-68.

139. Varon, S., Hagg, T., and Manthorpe, M., 1989, Neuronal growth factors, in: *Neural Regeneration and Transplantation*, F.J. Seil, ed., pp. 101-121, Alan R. Liss, New York.

140. Victor, M., Adams, R. D., and Collins, G. H., 1971, *The Wernicke-Korsakoff Syndrome*, F.A. Davis, Philadelphia.

141. Wets, K. M., Sinden, J., Hodges, H., Allen, Y., and Marchbanks, R. M., 1991, Specific brain protein changes correlated with behaviourally effective brain transplants, *J. Neurochem.*, **57**, 1661-1670.

142. Whitehouse, P. J., Price, D. L., Struble, R. G., Clark, A. W., Coyle, J. T., and DeLong, M. R., 1982, Alzheimer's disease and senile dementia: loss of neurons in the basal forebrain, *Science*, **215**, 1237-1239.

143. Wictorin, K., Brundin, P., Gustavii, B., Lindvall, O., and Björklund, A., 1990, Reformation of long axon pathways in adult rat central nervous system by human forebrain neuroblasts, *Nature*, **347**, 556-558.

144. Wictorin, K., Clarke, D. J., Bolam, J. P., and Björklund, A., 1989, Host corticostriatal fibres establish synaptic connections with grafted striatal neurons in the ibotenic acid lesioned striatum, *Eur. J. Neurosci.*, **1**, 189-195.

145. Wictorin, K., Isacson, O., Fischer, W., Nothias, F., Peschanski, M., and Björklund, A., 1988, Connectivity of striatal grafts implanted into the ibotenic acid-lesioned striatum. I. Subcortical afferents, *Neurosci.*, **27**, 547-562.

146. Wictorin, K., Simerly, R. B., Isacson, O., Swanson, L. W., and Björklund, A., 1989, Connectivity of striatal grafts implanted into the ibotenic acid lesioned striatum. III. Efferent projecting graft neurons and their relation to host afferents within the grafts, *Neurosci.*, **30**, 313-330.

147. Widner, H., and Brundin, P., 1988, Immunological aspects of grafting in the mammalian central nervous system. A review and speculative synthesis, *Brain Res. Rev.*, **13**, 287-324.

148. Will, B., Cassel, J. C., and Kelche, C., 1989, Deleterious and "overshoot" effects of intracerebral transplants, in: *Neuronal Grafting and Alzheimer's Disease*, F. Gage, A. Privat, and Y. Christen, eds., pp. 189-198, Springer-Verlag, Berlin.

149. Woodruff, M. L., Baisden, R. H., and Nonneman, A. J., 1990, Transplantation of fetal hippocampus may prevent or produce behavioral recovery from hippocampal ablation and recovery persists after removal of the transplant, *Prog. Brain Res.*, **82**, 367-376.

150. Woodruff, M. L., Baisden, R. H., Whittington, D. L., and Benson, A. E., 1987, Embryonic hippocampal grafts ameliorate the deficit in DRL acquisition produced by hippocampectomy, *Brain Res.*, **408**, 7-117.

151. Xavier, G. F., Kershaw, T. R., Gray, J. A., and Sinden, J. D., 1991, Foetal dentate and CA1 subfield transplants and spatial orientation following colchicine lesions of the dentate gyrus, *Eur. J. Neurosci.*, **4**, 103-103.

152. Yamaguchi, F., Richards, S. J., Beyreuther, K., Salbaum, M., Carlson, G. A., and Dunnett, S. B., 1991, Transgenic mice for the amyloid precursor protein 695 isoform have impaired spatial memory, *Neuroreport*, **2**, 781-784.

153. Yoshida, K., and Gage, F. H., 1991, Fibroblast growth factors stimulate nerve growth factor synthesis and secretion by astrocytes, *Brain Res.*, **538**, 118-126.

154. Zhou, C. F., Li, Y., and Raisman, G., 1989, Embryonic entorhinal transplants project selectively to the deafferented entorhinal zone of adult mouse hippocampi, as demonstrated by the use of Thy-1 allelic immunohistochemistry. Effect of timing of transplantation in relation to deafferentation, *Neurosci.*, **32**, 349-362.

155. Zhou, F. C., Raisman, G., and Morris, R. J., 1985, Specific patterns of fibre

outgrowth from transplants to host mice hippocampi, shown immunohistochemically by the use of allelic forms of THY-1, *Neurosci.*, **16**, 819-833.

156. Zola-Morgan, S., Squire, L. R., and Amaral, D. G., 1986, Human amnesia and the medial temporal region: enduring memory impairment following a bilateral lesion limited to field CA1 of the hippocampus, *J. Neurosci.*, **6**, 2950-2967.

NEURAL IMPLANTS AND RECOVERY OF FUNCTION: HUMAN WORK

Edward Hitchcock

Department of Neurosurgery
University of Birmingham
MCNN, Smethwick
West Midlands, England

INTRODUCTION

Organ transplantation is an accepted treatment for renal, hepatic and cardio-respiratory diseases and the principles of harvesting and transplantation technique, together with the maintenance of organ function are well established. The ethical aspects of harvesting have been widely debated[52,61] and, in most countries, appropriate regulations have been formulated which support and, indeed, may encourage organ donation. As regards neural transplantation, however, these principles are yet to be agreed and the clinical value established. Consequently, the management of patients with neural degenerative disease, who potentially have much to gain, is uncertain and, the ethical issues are still hotly debated.[23,43,47,52,55,61]

The first, and unsuccessful, brain transplantation was performed by Thomson[59] in 1890 when he transplanted cerebral cortex between adult dogs and from adult rats to dogs. In the following years it became clear that effective neural transplantation was more likely to be successful using foetal donors and even more so using young rather than adult recipients[14,17,20,33]. Synaptic connection between the embryonic graft and neonatal host brain was demonstrated by Lund and Hauska in 1976[37]. Two years later Das and Hallas (1978)[15] demonstrated successful transplantation of embryonic neural tissue into adult rat brain. That was an important experiment as it implied that neural degenerative diseases which largely occur in adults could possibly be treated by embryonic neural transplants. In their attempts to establish a model of Parkinson's disease (PD) laboratory experiments gradually focused on the effects of dopaminergic neurone grafts into the striatum of rats lesioned by 6-OHDA (6-hydroxydopamine) injections into the substantia nigra[2,46]. In 1979 Perlow et al[45] transplanted foetal mesencephalon into the striatum of such PD rats and observed a reduction in apomorphine and induced improvement in the abnormal, contraversive, rotation. In the same year, Björklund and Stenevi[9] reported that rotation could not only be stopped, but that it could actually be reversed after foetal mesencephalic grafting. This effect could also be produced by transplantation of other dopaminergic (DA) cells such as those within the adrenal medulla[25]. It was known that Parkinson's disease was accompanied by death of dopaminergic cells within the substantia nigra and those experiments suggested that the human condition may be improved by transplantation of a suspension of embryonic adrenal medullary grafts.

HUMAN NEURAL TRANSPLANTATION

The first clinical attempt was made by Backlund[3] in 1981, when he transplanted autologous adrenal tissue into the head of the caudate nucleus, using a stereotactic technique. This procedure produced a definite but, unfortunately, transient improvement in the condition of four patients with Parkinson's disease. Work on human transplantation was then suspended until Madrazo[38] in 1987 described striking improvement in Parkinson's disease patients using autologous adrenal medullary transplantation via an open craniotomy technique. His reported successes encouraged others to repeat this procedure but the mortality and morbidity rates were high when the procedure was used in elderly patients, which many were, and it fell into disrepute. Whilst recent reports suggest that it is not without value and work continues in this area[1, 44], animal studies have shown that foetal dopaminergic transplants produce more consistent improvement in spontaneous behaviour than do adrenal grafts.[10,11,25,45]. In 1985 the first clinical attempt at foetal neural transplantation was made in China by Jiang[30] but not reported until 1987. After creating a cavity in the caudate nucleus the transplantation was performed 20 days later with tissue obtained from the ventral mesencephalon of a 20 week foetus; this was a stereotactic procedure and brief improvement was noted. Madrazo[38] used a ventral mesencephalon and the adrenal medulla from a 13 week spontaneous abortion and, in September 1988[39], implanted the mesencephalon in one and the adrenal medulla into another two young patients with Parkinson's disease. An open craniotomy method was used with implantation of the foetal fragments into a cavity in the head of the caudate nucleus. In subsequent months, Swedish workers[35] used a stereotactic technique to perform foetal transplantation into two 55 year old women with Parkinson's disease. Multiple injection implantation sites were chosen, two putaminal and two caudate contralateral to the extremities with the most severe symptoms, and each procedure required four foetuses aged 8 to 10 weeks. Although definite physiological improvements were recorded, no major clinical improvement was observed unfortunately, and it was not possible to reduce the anti-Parkinsonism medication. At 12 months PET Scans suggested increased 18f-dopa intake at the caudate transplant site in one patient and at the putaminal site in the other but this was not subsequently confirmed. The United Kingdom Neural Transplantation group's interest began in 1982 with an application to the hospital ethical committee for approval of a transplantation protocol. It was not obtained until 1987, however, and the first foetal transplantation was performed in 1988[27]. A series of experiments was planned to explore the various uncertain factors in the treatment.

FACTORS INFLUENCING TRANSPLANTATION SUCCESS

Age of Foetus

In this first foetal transplantation in the UK[27] the material was obtained from therapeutically aborted foetuses but, with "separation" between the transplanters and clinicians performing the abortion. In all matters the Peel Code[58] was followed and the protocol met all of the recommendations of the subsequent Polkinghorne Committee[48].

Material was obtained from first and second trimester donors; first trimester donor material was obtained by vacuum suction and, since it was not ethical to influence the manner in which the abortion was performed, examination showed that the donor material was fragmented and brain tissue was usually lost. This problem has been circumvented in the countries which do not follow the codes already mentioned by modifying the abortion technique using a larger cannula and trap with ultrasound to direct the cannula to the exact site of the embryo. Using this method it is possible to obtain excellent specimens in about 40% of cases but, unfortunately, in this country unless this is the usual method of termination it is contrary to the Polkinghorne Recommendations. (A number of U.K. clinics are beginning to use the ultrasound trap technique routinely and it is likely that intact first trimester tissue will become more readily available). Whilst other groups without these difficulties were able to use this younger material, we concentrated our research on second trimester foetuses.

There was some concern and criticism of that approach since it was suggested that the substantia nigra neurones are no longer proliferating in the second trimester and also that they are more vulnerable to dissociation. Björklund and his fellow workers[10] performed a series of important experiments on the factors influencing transplantation of human foetal substantia nigra grafts into rats; they reported that human foetal substantia nigra grafts between 9 and 11 gestational weeks transplanted as xenografts into immunosuppressed rats survived and reinervated denervated striatum. Thus there appeared to be a transplantation "window" in that later gestational tissue did not survive[11,27,35]. On the other hand, primate studies[49,56,57] showed that successful transplantation could be achieved using very mature foetuses comparable with third trimester foetuses in human and the primate "window" thus appeared to be larger than the rodent "window". These non-human primate studies are particularly relevant to clinical experiments since the primate MPTP model has a close resemblance to Parkinson's disease in humans and the species difference is less than between rat and man. On that basis we felt justified in continuing our experiments with older foetuses.

Tissue Preparation

Björklund et al 1979[8] had shown that solid fragments survived successfully in neonatal, but rather less successfully in adult, host brains which were cavitated at the donor sites. The graft was rapidly revascularised 4 to 6 weeks later and more than 95% survival was achieved. Unfortunately this method was less successful at deep implantation sites but, if the cells were dissociated, there was a possibility of their dissemination throughout the target areas. A technique of cell dissociation was developed which involved incubating the tissue with trypsin and subsequently mechanically producing complete cellular dissociation which appeared to give the same results as the cavitation solid graft method[21]. In animal experiments this proved successful for first trimester cells but second trimester cells appeared more vulnerable possibly because developing neural processes could be damaged by the technique[7]. Our method of tissue preparation for clinical implantation has been non-enzymatic using a gentle mechanical dissaggregation technique which produces clumps of viable cells. Work in our laboratory has shown that second trimester human neurones are vulnerable to the enzymatic technique but that mechanical dissaggregation produces cell clumps which retain their viability for long periods[19].

Immune Reaction

Xenografts of human foetal substantia nigra cells to rodent striatum were expected to produce an immune response and, necessarily, immunosuppression was used[11]. The brain has a comparatively privileged immunological status[40] but antigenicity has been demonstrated[32] and, therefore, some workers have used immunosuppression in their clinical cases[6,24,36,38,41,62]. The work of Sladek and co-workers[49,50,51] and Fine et al[22] however, showed that successful homologous transplantation could be achieved without immunosuppression and we have not used this with our patients. The dangers of immunosuppression are well known and its use is to be avoided if possible.

Number of Foetuses

The small amount of tissue obtained from first trimester specimens has forced clinicians using this age group to transplant a number of different foetal substantiae nigrae into a single patient. Bankiewicz[4] pointed out the potential danger of inter-donor antigenic reactions and although there have been no reported antigenic responses from the clinical use of multiple donors we have continued to use a single donor.

Target Site

Although it was evident that the transplantation had to be into the striatum there has been considerable discussion as to whether the caudate nucleus or the putamen is the best site. The putamen is more severely affected by dopaminergic neurone loss in Parkinson's disease than is the caudate nucleus and the major disorders in Parkinsonism have been attributed to the predominantly putaminal loss.

It could be expected, therefore, that putaminal implantation would have a more beneficial effect than caudate implantation although, conversely, the less severely affected caudate neurones might be more capable of responding to dopaminergic neurone transplants than the more depleted putamen. Another factor which has received very small consideration is the surgical risks of implanting material into the deep putamen traversed by perforating blood vessels compared to implantation into the comparatively superficial and less vascular caudate nucleus.[28]

The difficulty of distinguishing any clinical or physiological effect as being due to a caudate or putaminal implantation in multiple implantations is obvious and, in our patients, we have chosen to transplant to a single and consistent side, irrespective of the side of maximal symptomatology which, in fact, was bilateral in all cases, rather than do multiple implantations. Furthermore, we have chosen to implant at a single site i.e. either the caudate or putamen. The plan of stereotactic neural transplantation for the UK trial is summarised in Table 1.

Surgical Technique - Open Versus Stereotactic

Although the open technique of craniotomy gives unequivocal identification of the transplant site in the case of caudate implantation it is clearly impractical and dangerous for deep implantations into the putamen. Additionally, it has the disadvantage of adding a more major procedure in patients who are often in poor general health apart from their Parkinson's disease. Nevertheless, a number of workers have used this technique largely for adrenal transplantation,[39] but sometimes for foetal transplantation[41]. The advantage of the stereotactic technique is that intracranial structures can be targeted with accuracy and it is the only feasible approach for multiple implantations in deep structures such as the putamen. The whole procedure is performed under local anaesthesia and thus the additional hazard of general anaesthesia is avoided and it is possible to determine what if any effect is produced by simple placement of the cannula in the target and the subsequent implantation of tissue[36].

Table 1. Stereotactic Neural Implantation. Plan for U.K. trial.

	1988	1989			1990	1991
	Pilot	**Matched Pairs**				
Series	I	II	III	->	III	IV
Site	R. caudate	R. putamen	Control		R. caudate	Bilateral p /c
Age	> 3 / 12	> 3 / 12	-		> 3 / 12	> 3 / 12
Tissue Genotype	Single	Single	-		Single	Single
Immuno-suppression	0	0	-		0	0

U.K. EXPERIENCE

To date we have operated on 36 patients. The criteria for acceptance in the trial are as follows:

1. Parkinson's Disease confirmed by 2 Neurologists
2. Continued deterioration despite optimal drug treatment
3. All stage 4/5 Hoehn and Yahr
4. Positive response to levadopa

A number of clinical assessments were made, using internationally recognised scales[12,13] and physiological tests of motor function.

Table 2. Summary of clinical assessments of patients used in the U.K. trial.

Webster rating scale - **W.R.S.**

North Western University Scale (modified) - **N.U.D.S.**

Birmingham Parkinsonian Rating Scale; (extremity rating for tremor, rigidity, and bradykinesia).

Dyskinesia scale; limbs, trunk, neck and face.

Timed motor responses.

On and Off records.

Video recordings (standard timing and conditions - Pre. and Post. Levodopa).*

Speech Assessments.*

Physiotherapy Assessments.*

* These assessments performed after overnight omission of levodopa, and again 2 hours later after levodopa, i.e. "OFF" and "ON" phases.

Series I

This comprised a pilot series of 12 patients (see Table 3) who were all grafts into the right caudate nucleus. Three patients were lost to follow-up, but the remaining 9 patients were followed up for more than 1 year[26,28]. Of those, three showed marked improvement with lengthening "on" periods and decreased "off" periods and a great reduction in l-dopa dosage. Those improvements have been well maintained for more than 3 years. Three patients had only transient improvement returning to their pre-operative gradual decline. Two of those patients have since died and their brains are presently being studied.

Table 3. Details of patients in Series I. - Right Caudate Implantation 1988

Patient No.	Sex	Age Years	Duration Disease Years	Duration L-Dopa Therapy Years	Daily L-Dopa Dose (Mgs)	Disability Hoehn & Yahr "OFF"
1	F	60	26	21	700	5
2	M	41	7	6	1000	5
3	F	58	12	10	2000	4
4	M	58	12	10	1050	4
5	M	60	15	14	1500	5
6	M	53	25	6	1600	4
7	M	67	25	20	2000	5
8	M	54	18	16	700	5
9	M	54	18	12	800	4
10	F	54	18	16	500	4
11	M	60	11	10	1000	4
12	M	53	20	17	2400	5
Range		41-67	7-26	6-21	700-24000	
Mean (SD)		56(6.2)	17 (6.1)	13(4.9)		

Series II and III

In 1989, aided by a grant from the Parkinson's Disease Society, a group of Parkinson's disease patients were matched and, on a random basis assigned to either Series II or III. Series II patients had putaminal implantations while Series III acted as control[5]. Whilst this work is still being analysed it is our impression that, although there were some improvements in skilled motor function in the patients receiving the putaminal implants, there was not the same generalised improvement in bradykinesia as we had seen after caudate implantation.

Series III

After serving as controls for Series II, these patients were then treated by right caudate implantation. Their results will be compared with the matched putaminal series. We have now completed our series of unilateral transplantation which, interestingly, often showed a bilateral beneficial effect. We intend to continue our experimental therapy with bilateral caudate implantations. We have thus engaged in a progressive series of experimental treatments designed to determine the relative effects of caudate or putaminal injections and the effect of unilateral placement. All these procedures have been done without immunosuppression so that this factor too has been explored.

The reported experience of clinical foetal transplantations internationally to date is divided between those who perform stereotactic implantation and those who perform the implantation using the open craniotomy and Madrazo technique. In general the results can be regarded as encouraging; in the Swedish series two out of six patients have had modest but definite improvement as judged by physiological motor testing. In our own series (I and II), a much larger number of patients using mature foetuses, we have obtained significant clinical and physiological improvement in the same proportion. The remaining series only recently completed their follow-up and fully documented results are not yet available. Molina et al[41], who also have operated upon a large number of cases, have reported a higher success rate using the open method with the first trimester foetal implantations. Undoubtedly, there is a great deal more work to be done in determining the optimal age for donor tissue and the need for immunosuppression. An important series of primate experiments by Bankiewicz et al[5] has provided strong evidence that at least a part of the transplantation effect could be due to induced sprouting of striatal neurones. Some degree of functional recovery in the primate PD model has also been seen following transplantation of such non-dopaminergic tissue as spinal cord, placenta, amnion and cerebellum.

NEURAL TRANSPLANTATION FOR OTHER NEURODEGENERATIVE DISEASES

Laboratory experiments and the encouraging results of neural transplantation for Parkinson's disease have encouraged consideration of neural transplantation for other neuro-degenerative diseases. The following are examples of such applications.

Huntington's Disease

An animal model of Huntington's disease has been attempted, utilising the injection of kainic acid into the rodent striatum. This causes striatal neuronal loss and motor hyperactivity which resembles some of the symptoms of Huntington's disease[16]. The transplantation of foetal striatum into the striatum of this animal model reversed the disorder but, in contrast to the effects of substantia nigra grafts in animal models in Parkinson's disease, the graft appeared to replace damaged pathways[16,29]. There is also some evidence that an initial striatal graft may offer some a protection against subsequent administration of quinolinic acid[34]. Transplantations in patients with Huntington's disease have not been reported to date but a number of groups are planning this in the near future.

Alzheimer's Disease

In an increasingly ageing population Alzheimer's disease is becoming more common. The disease affects cortex, hippocampus and limbic regions, and so the use of neural transplantation in this condition must be very speculative. However, some of these defects in an animal model can be corrected by neuronal transplantations of dopaminergic neurones into the striatum and septal cholinergic neurones into the hippocampus.

Cerebellar Degenerations

Of more than fifty forms of spino-cerebellar degeneration none have effective treatment. Cell suspensions of embryonic cerebellum injected into the degenerate cerebellum of an adult mouse are selectively attracted to the molecular layer, inducing sprouting of host fibres, and actually show synaptic integration in the cerebellar cortex and the deep nuclei[53,54]. Although there has been no clinical work in this area undoubtedly it is well worthy of consideration.

Cortical Injuries

Foetal neurones can also be successfully transplanted into cortex damaged by ischaemia[31,42] and there are isolated accounts of the use of foetal transplantation in treating certain mental disorders, cerebral palsy and spinal cord damage. However, some of these attempts have not been based on good experimental evidence. There is little scientific description and so the procedure must still be regarded as premature.

CONCLUSION

The plasticity of the adult neurone has only recently been appreciated[18] but it holds the promise that neural implantation may be a material advance in clinical neuroscience. The ethical debates, whilst a prerequisite, should not detract from the considerable potential that this field may offer millions of people with neurological disorders. There is clearly a great deal of work remaining, for example in delineating the contributions of neurotransmitter and structural regeneration, and the effects of concurrent drug regimes upon successful implants. Neural implantation is a fitting example of the problems encountered in the clinical application of experimental theory and practice which, nonetheless, offers tremendous challenge from a substantial base.

ACKNOWLEDGEMENTS

I am grateful to my colleagues in the U.K. Neural Transplantation Group for their support and encouragement and to the Robert Nursing Home, the staff of the Midland Centre for Neurosurgery and Neurology and Department of Cancer Studies, University of Birmingham for their continued help and to Marilyn Parkes for typing the manuscript. The clinical assessment of patients with Parkinson's Disease were made by B. Henderson as Parkinson's Disease Research Fellow on a grant from the Parkinson's Disease Society.

REFERENCES

1. Allen, G.S., Burns, R.C., Tulipan, N.B., and Parker, R.A., 1988, Adrenal medullary transplantation to the caudate nucleus in Parkinson's Disease, *Arch. Neurol.*, **46**, 487-491.

2. Anden, N.E., Dahlstrom, A., Fuxe, K., and Larsson, K., 1966, Functional role of the nigroneostriatal dopamine neurones, *Acta. Pharmacol. Toxicol.*, **24**, 263-274.

3. Backlund, E.O., Granberg, P.O., Hamberger, B., Gedvall, G. Seigar, A., and Olsen, L., 1985, Transplantation of adrenal mdedullary tissue to striatum in Parkinsonism. First clinical trials, *J. Neurosurg.*, **62**, 169-173.

4. Bankiewicz, K.S., Jacobowitz, D.M., Plunkett, R.J. Oldfield, E.H., and Kopen, I.J., 1987, Injury induced sprouting into the caudate nucleus, after solid tissue implantation in MPTP-induced Parkinsonism monkeys, *Soc. of Neurosc. Abs.*, **46**, 16.

5. Bankiewicz, K.S., Plunkett, R.J., Mefford, I. Kopin, I.J., and Oldfield, E.G., 1990, Behavioural recovery from MPTP-induced Parkinsonism in monkeys after intracerebral tissue implants is not related to CSF concentrations of dopamine metabolites, *Prog. in Brain Research*, **82**, 561-671, Elsevier, Amsterdam.

6. Barker, R.A., Cahn, A.P., 1988, Parkinson's Disease: an autoimmune process, *Int. J. Neurol.*, **43**, 1-7.

7. Björklund, A., Dunnett, S.B., Stenevi, U., Lewis, M.E., and Iverson, S.D., 1980, Reinnervation of the denervated striatum by substantia nigra transplants: functional consequences as revealed by pharmacological and sensorimotor testing, *Brain Res.*, **199**, 307-333.

8. Björklund, A., Kromer, L.F., and Stenevi, U., 1979, Cholinergic reinnervation of the rat hippocampus by septal implants is stimulated by perforant path lesion, *Brain Res.*, **173**, 57-64.

9. Björklund, A., and Stenevi, U., 1979, Regeneration of monoaminergic and cholinergic neurones in the mammalian central nervous system, *Physiol. Rev.*, **59**, 62-100.

10. Björklund, A., Stenevi, U., Dunnett, S.B., and Gage, F.H., 1982, Cross species neural grafting in a rat model of Parkinson's Disease, *Nature*, **298**, 652-654.

11. Brundin, P. Nilsson, O.G., Strecker, R.E., Lindvall, O. Astedt, B., and Björklund, A., 1986, Behavioural effects of human foetal dopamine neurons grafted in a rat model of Parkinson's Disease, *Exp. Brain Res.*, **65**, 235-240.

12. Canter, C.J., De La Torrer, D., Mier, M., 1961, A method for evaluating disability in patients with Parkinson's Disease, *J. Nerv. Ment. Dis.*, **122**, 143-147.

13. Collier, T.J., Gash, D.M., and Sladek, J.R., 1988, Transplantation of norepinephrine neurons into aged rats improves performance of a learned task, *Brain Res.*, **448**, 77-87.

14. Das, G.D. 1974, Transplantation of embryonic neural tissue in the mammalian brain. Growth and differentiation of neuroblasts from various regions of the embryonic brain in the cerebellum of neonate rats, *J. of Life Sci.*, 93-124.

15. Das, G.D., and Hallas, H.B., 1978, Transplantation of brain tissue in the brain of adult rat, *Experimentia*, **34**, 1304-1306.

16. Deckel, A.W., Robinson, R.G., Coyle, J.T., and Sanberg, P. R., 1983, Reversal of long term locomotor abnormalities in the Kainic Acid model of Huntington's Disease by day 18 foetal striatal implants, *European J. Pharmacol.*, **93**, 287-288.

17. Del Conte, G., 1907, Empflanzungen von embryonalem Gewebe ins Gehurn, *Beatr Path Anat. Allg. Pathol.*, **42**, 193-203.

18. Detta, A. Grabham, P., and Hitchcock, E.R., 1992, Phenotypic plasticity of mature human foetal mesencephalic dopaminergic neurones, *Restorative Neurol. and Neurosci.*, (in press).

19. Detta, A., Hitchcock, E.R., 1990, The selective viability of human foetal brain cells, *Brain Res.*, **520**, 277-283.

20. Dunn, E.H., 1917, Primary and secondary findings in a series of attempts to transplant cerebral cortex in albino rat, *J. Comp. Neurol.*, **271**, 565-582.

21. Dunnett, S., Björklund, A., and Stenevi, U., 1983, Transplant-induced recovery from brain lesions. A review of the nigro-striatal model, in *Neural Tissue Transplantation Research*, R. B. Wallace, and G. D. Das, eds., pp. 191-216, Springer-Verlag, New York.

22. Fine, A., Hunt, S.P., Oertal, W.H., Nomoto, M. Chong, P.N., Bond, A. Waters, C., Temlett, J.A., Annett, L., Dunnett, S.B., Jenner, P., and Marsden, C.D., 1987, Transplantation of embryonic marmoset dopaminergic neurons to the corpus striatum of marmosets rendered Parkinsonian by 1-methyl-4-phenyl-1,2,3,6-tetrahydropyridine, *Prog. in Brain Res.*, **78**, 479-489, Elsevier, Amsterdam.

23. Foetuses and Foetal Material, March 1988, *Hansard*, p. 243.

24. Freed, C.R., Breeze, R.E., Rosenberg, N.L., Barrett, J.N., and Rottenberg, D.A., 1989, Therapeutic effects of human foetal dopamine cells transplanted in a patient with Parkinson's Disease, in Neural transplantation: from molecular bases to clinical application, *Restorative Neurol. and Neurosci. Suppl.*, p. 231.

25. Freed, W.J., Morihisa, J.M. Spoor, E., Hoffer, B.J. Olson, L., Seiger, A., and Wyatt, R.J., 1981, Transplanted adrenal chromaffin cells in rat brain reduces lesion induced rotational behaviour, *Nature*, **292**, 351-352.

26. Henderson, B.T.H., Clough, C.G., Hughes, R.C., Hitchcock, E.R., and Kenny, B.G., 1991, Implantation of human foetal ventral mesencephalon to the right caudate nucleus in advanced Parkinson's Disease, *Arch. Neurol.*, **48**, 822-827.

27. Hitchcock, E.R., 1989, Recent experiences with dopamine transplantation for Parkinson's Disease, in Proceedings of Society of British Neurological Surgeons, Oxford, *J. Neurosurg. Psychiat.*, **52**, 141.

28. Hitchcock, E.R., Kenny B.G., Clough C.G., Hughes, R.C., Henderson, B.T.H., and Detta, A., 1990, Stereotactic implantation of foetal mesencephalon (STIM): the U.K. experience, *Prog. in Brain Res.*, **82**, 723-728, Elsevier, Amsterdam.

29. Isacson, O., Dunnett, S.B., and Björklund, A., 1986, Graft-induced behavioural recovery in an animal model of Huntington's Disease, *Proc. Nat. Acad. Sci.*, U.S.A., **83**, 27-32.

30. Jiang, N, Jiang, C., Tang, Z., Zhung, F., and Jiang Li, S.D., 1987, Human foetal brain transplant trials in the treatment of Parkinsonism, *Acta Academial Medicinae Shanghai*, **14**, No.1.

31. Justice, A., Deckel, W., and Robinson, R.G., 1986, Foetal neocortical tissue survives transplantation into an ischaemic cortical site, *Neurosci. Abs.*, **12**, 1471.

32. Lampson, L.A., 1987, Molecular bases of the immune response to neural antigens, *Trends in Neurosci.*, **10**, 211-216.

33. Le Gros Clarke, W.E., 1940, Neuronal differentiation in implanted foetal cortical tissue, *Journal of Neurol. Psychiat.*, **3**, 262-272.

34. Levivier, M., Sladek, Jr., J.R., Collier, T., Hagenmeyer-Houser, S.H., and Gash, D.M., 1989, The protective effect of various striatal implants on intrastriatal quinolinic application, *Restorative Neurol. Neurosci.* Suppl. 1.

35. Lindvall, O., Rehncrona, S., Brundin, P., Gustavi, B., Astedt, B. Widner, H., Lindholm, T., Björklund, A., Leenders, K., Rothwell, J.C., Frackowiak, R., Marsden, C.D., Johnels, B., Steg, G., Freedman, R., Hoffer, B.J., Seiger, A., Bygdeman, M., Stromberg, I., and Olson, L., 1989, Human foetal dopamine neurones grafted into the striatum in two patients with severe Parkinson's Disease, *Arch. Neurol.*, **46**, 615-631.

36. Lindvall, O., Rehncrona, S., Gustavi, B., Brundin, P., Astedt, B., Widner, H., Linkholm, T., Björklund, A., Leenders, K.L., Rothwell, J.C., Frackowiak, R., Marsden, C.D., Johnels, B., Steg, G., Freedman, R., Hoffer, B.J., Seiger, A.,Stromberg, I., Bygdeman, M., and Olson, L., 1988, Foetal dopamine-rich mesencephalic grafts in Parkinson's Disease, *Lancet*, **1**, 1483-1483.

37. Lund, R.D., and Hauschka, S.D., 1976, Transplanted neural tissue develops connections with host rat brain, *Science*, **193**, 582-584.

38. Madrazo, I., Drucker-Colin, R., Diaz, V., Martinez-Mata, J., Torres, C., and Becurri, J.J., 1987, Open microsurgical autograft of adrenal medulla to the right caudate nucleus in two patients with intractable Parkinson's Disease, *New Eng. J. Med.*, **316**, 831-834.

39. Madrazo, I., Leon, V., Torres, C. Aguilera, M.J.C., Valera, G., Alvarez, F., Fraga, A., Colin-Drucker, R., Ostrosky, F., Skurorich, M., and Franco, R. 1988, Transplantation of foetal substantia nigra and adrenal medulla to the caudate nucleus in two patients with Parkinson's Disease, *New Eng. J. Med.*, **318**, 51.

40. Medawer, P.B., 1948, Immunity to homologous grafted skin: III The fate of skin homografts transplanted to the brain to subcutaneous tissue, and to the anterior chamber of the eye, *Brit. J. Exp. Path.*, **29**, 58-59.

41. Molina, H., 1989, Neurotransplantation in Parkinson's Disease: The Cuban Experience, in Neuro transplantation: from molecular bases to clinical application, *Restor. Neurol. and Neurosci.*, Suppl. **1**, 230.

42. Mundrick, L.A., Leung, P.P.H., Baimbridge, K.G., and Miller, J.J., 1988, Neuronal transplants used in the repair of acute ischaemic injury in the central nervous system, *Prog. in Brain Res.*, **78**, 87-95, Elsevier, Amsterdam.

43. Parkinson's Disease Society Newsletter, 1988,Issue No. 65.

44. Penn, R.D., Goetz, C. G.,, Tanner, C. M. Klawans, H. L., Shannon, K.M., Comella, C.L., and Witt, T.R., 1988, The adrenal medullary transplant operation for Parkinson's Disease: clinical observations if five patients, *Neurosurg.*, **22**, 999-1004.

45. Perlow, M.J., Freed, W. J., Hoffer, B.J., Seiger, A., Olson, L. and Wyatt, R.J., 1979, Brain grafts reduce motor abnormalities produced by destruction of nigro-striatal dopamine systems, *Science*, **204**, 643-646.

46. Pycock, C.J., 1980, Turning behaviour in animals, *Neuroscience*, **5**, 461-514.

47. Report of Board of Social Responsibility, 1990, Human Transplants, *Church of Scotland and Social Work*.

48. Review of the guidance on the research use of foetuses and foetal material, 1989, *Report of the Polkinghorne Commission*, HMSO CM, 762.

49. Sladek, J.R., Collier, J.J., Haber, S. N., Roth, R.H., and Redmond, E., 1986, Survival and growth of foetal catecholamines neurones transplanted into primate brain, *Brain Res. Bull.*, **17**, 809-818.

50. Sladek, J.R., and Gash, D.M., 1988, Nerve cell-grafting in Parkinson's Disease, *J.of Neurosurg.*, **68**, 337-351.

51. Sladek, J.R., Redmond, D.E., Collier, T.J., Haaber, S.N., Elsworth, J.D., Deutsche, A.Y., and Roth, R.H., 1987, Transplantation of foetal dopamine neurons in primate brain reserves MPTP-induced Parkinsonism, *Prog. in Brain Res.*, **71**, 309-323, Elsevier, Amsterdam.

52. Sladek, J.R. and Shoulson, I., 1988, Neural transplantation: a call for patience rather than patients, *Science*, **240**, 1386-1388.

53. Sotelo, C., and Alvarado-Mallart, R.M., 1988, Integration of grafted Purkinje cell into the host cerebellar circuitry in Purkinje cell degeneration mutant mouse. *Prog. in Brain Res.*, **78**, 141-154, Elsevier, Amsterdam.

54. Sotelo, S., and Alvarado-Mallart, R.M., 1987, Cerebellar transplantation in adult mice with heredo-degenerative ataxia. In cell and tissue transplantation into the adult brain, eds., E.C. Azmita, and A. Björklund, *Annals. N. Y. Acad. of Sci.*, **495**, 242-167.

55. Statement of the Administrative Council of the World, 1989, *Federation of Neurosurgical Societies.*

56. Stromberg, I., Almquist, P., Bygdeman, M., Finger, T.E., Gerhardt, G., Granholme, A-Ch., Mahalik, T.J., Seiger, A., Hoffer, B., and Olson, L., 1988, Intracerebral zenografts of human mesencephalic tissue into athymic rats: immunocytochemical and in vivo electrochemical studies, *Proc. Nat. Acad. Sci.*, USA, **85**, 8331-8334.

57. Stromberg, I., Bygdeman, M., Goldstein, M., Seiger, A., and Olson, L., 1986, Human substantia nigra grafted to the dopamine denervated striatum of immunosuppressed rats: evidence for functional reinnervation, *Neurosci. Letters*, **71**, 271-276.

58. The use of foetuses and foetal material for research, 1972, *The Peel Report*, HMSO.

59. Thompson, W.G., 1890, Successful brain grafting, *New York Med. J.*, **51**, 701-702.

60. Webster, D.D., 1968, Critical analysis of the disability in Parkinson's Disease, *Mod. Treat.*, **5**, 257-282.

61. Weiss, R., 1988, Forbidding fruits of foetal cell research, *Science News*, **134**, 289-304.

62. Woodruff, M. F. A., Hitchcock, E.R., and Whitehead, V.L., 1977, Effect of C parvum and active specific immunotherapy on intracerebral transplantation of a murine fibrosarcoma, *Br. J. Cancer*, **35**, 687-692.

ENVIRONMENTAL APPROACHES TO RECOVERY OF FUNCTION FROM

BRAIN DAMAGE: A REVIEW OF ANIMAL STUDIES (1981 to 1991)

Bruno Will and Christian Kelche

Laboratoire de Neurophysiologie et Biologie des Comportements
UPR 419 du CNRS - Centre de Neurochimie
Strasbourg, France

INTRODUCTION

During the sixties and seventies there has been a major shift in our beliefs about brain plasticity and, more specifically, about the effects of environment on both brain and behavior. This shift in beliefs concerns not only intact subjects in the course of development and adaptation but also, more recently, subjects having sustained brain or spinal cord injury. During the late seventies it became clear that the environment may play an important role in brain-damaged subjects, and this has led to an effort to "treat" disturbances induced by central nervous system (CNS) injury by means of environmental "therapy" (e.g. references 25, 33, 44, 87). In 1981, at the first E.B.B.S. workshop on "recovery of function from brain damage", we came to the conclusion that "there exists.... strong evidence that a postoperative or post-traumatic enriched experience significantly aids functional recovery after various kinds of brain injuries", but we also acknowledged and even stressed "that a few studies have also obtained negative findings"[88]. In this latter case, we were referring to studies which failed to demonstrate any beneficial effects of postoperative enrichment or sensory stimulation.

Although several studies have been conducted during the last decade on the effects of preoperative experience on recovery from brain damage and of childhood or adult experience on aging-related impairments, we will consider only, as in the 1981 review, the effects of postoperative experience on recovery. We adopt this approach because modifying the environment of brain-injured animals or patients may be considered as a "therapeutic" procedure, which may have a greater relevance for clinical purposes than preoperative environmental manipulations. This chapter will thus review literature since 1981 on the effects of postoperative environmental factors on recovery of function in animals and will address the following questions. What is new in this area of research? What are the trends? What are the questions to address and to answer? What are the lines of research to develop?

From a statistical point of view, the overall picture has not been dramatically modified by 10 years of research; indeed, the initial trends have actually been confirmed (for some recent reviews, see 16, 26, 70, 71, 75, 83, 90, 92). As shown in figure

1, there is still a large majority of publications reporting either "positive" effects or, depending on the task used, both "positive" effects and "no" effects of enriched housing on recovery of function[a] following various kinds of brain damage. There are also a few additional reports of neither beneficial nor detrimental effects of a socially and/or physically enriched postoperative experience. Finally, what does not appear in figure 1 and should be underlined is that, over the entire 30-year period considered, there are only three reports indicating truly although slightly negative (deleterious) effects of such an experience; actually, these three publications reported mixed results, both "negative" and either neutral or "positive", depending on the behavioral task used. Furthermore, three truly "negative" findings out of more than fifty other outcomes can be considered as a matter of chance. Thus, from a rather superficial point of view, one may now consider postoperative environmental enrichment as a potential "therapeutic" tool of low risk; but is it an efficacious tool? Is it as efficacious as it could be?

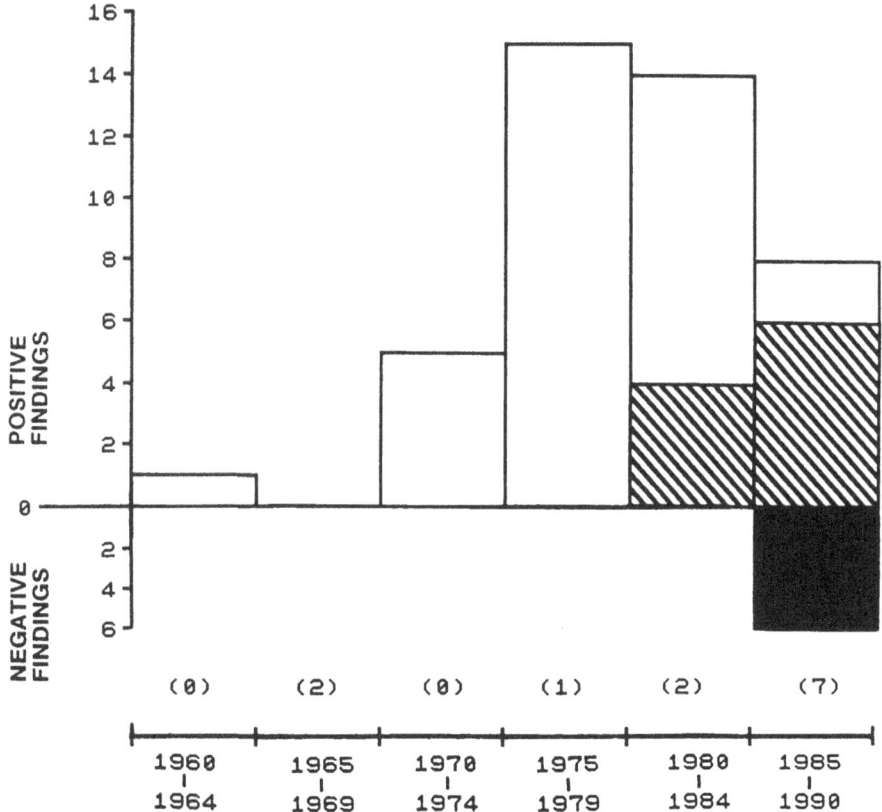

Figure 1. Number of publications reporting significant effects of enriched housing or training on behavioral recovery after brain damage. Open histograms: positive findings; hatched histograms: mixed "positive" findings (positive effects and no significant effects, according to task); black histograms: mixed "negative" findings (negative findings with either no significant effect and/or positive effects, according to task); between brackets: no significant effects.

---

[a] Note that, unless otherwise stated, by the expression "recovery of function" we refer in this chapter to sparing/or substitution and/or genuine restitution of function

In order to analyze the situation in a more subtle way and more carefully, we will consider first the generality and specificity of the effects of postoperative environmental factors. Second, we will analyze these effects to know what are the critical components involved. Third, we will concentrate on two lines of research which were developed during the last 10 years: one considered the interaction between differential housing and brain noradrenaline, the other considered the interaction between differential housing and intracerebral transplants. Finally, we will consider the underlying processes in the light of these two and of some other lines of research.

GENERALITY AND SPECIFICITY OF ENVIRONMENTAL EFFECTS

The earliest experimentation presenting an exclusive analysis of postoperative environmental effects on recovery of function was probably that conducted by Schwartz in the sixties. In order to take advantage of the greater plasticity of the neonatal brain, Schwartz made bilateral posterior cortical lesions in rats on their first postnatal day[79]. Rats given lesions and sham-operated controls were then reared from day 5 until day 95 in either enriched or standard conditions (EC and SC, respectively). When the rats were subsequently tested in the Hebb-Williams maze, both brain status (lesion or sham) and environment yielded significant effects; there was also a significant interaction between these factors due to the fact that enriched experience caused a greater absolute reduction of errors among the rats with lesions than among the sham-operated control rats. Early enriched experience offset the lesion effects so effficiently that rats with cortical lesions from the enriched condition made even fewer errors than intact rats reared in the standard condition.

The study by Schwartz had the merit of indicating that functional recovery was possible after brain damage, although with the limitation of given environmental and age conditions. The vast majority of the subsequent reports indicated at least some degree of improvement after brain damage in animals subjected to environmental enrichment. In most studies, as in the study by Schwartz, the differences between impoverished (or standard) and enriched groups were even larger in brain-damaged than in intact animals. Thus, during the seventies, similar effects to those reported by Schwartz were found (1) after various kinds of brain damage, (2) after various periods of differential housing, (3) with delayed onset of differential housing, (4) in various behavioral testing situations, (5) at different ages, (6) in various strains of rats and (7) in both genders. In 1981, there were, however, a few reports mentioning no effects of stimulating environmental conditions: (1) after certain kinds of lesions, (2) in certain specific behavioral tasks and (3) in certain species. Before analyzing such data, let us see what kind of information has been added to this picture over the last decade.

Generality

The generality of the picture showing "beneficial" effects of postoperative enriched housing on recovery of function has definitely been broadened, since similar effects have been reported during the eighties in other species and following other kinds of brain damage.

Whereas all the early studies were carried out in rats, mice and, exceptionally, in rabbits, some more recent studies, especially those concerned with the effects of exercise or training, have used cats and even monkeys (e.g. 13, 24, 42, 55, 56) showed that postoperative enriched housing (pen-rearing) facilitated Hebb-Williams maze learning in both normal kittens and kittens with neonatal lesions of the marginal and posterolateral gyri, although such experience did not facilitate form or grating discrimination either in normal or operated cats. In both cats and monkeys, Lacour[55] found that functional recovery following unilateral vestibular neurectomy developed only in unrestrained animals, i.e., when they had the possibility of using information elicited by active sensorimotor exploration; in contrast, recovery was blocked and delayed when the animals had no opportunity to interact behaviorally with their environment.

Similar effects of enviromnental conditions and experience on functional recovery were also reported in animals which sustained other kinds of brain damage, such as X-irradiation-induced microcephaly[80], monosodium-glutamate-induced brain lesions[78] or those induced by genetic deficiencies[5, 6, 7, 36, 37].

The data recently reported by Saari and coworkers[78] support the idea that the efficacy of "environmental therapy" may not be restricted to the kinds of surgical lesions which were initially studied. Saari and collaborators treated rat pups with monosodium -L-glutamate (MSG) for ten days starting on the second day after birth and housed them in either an enriched or an impoverished condition for 35 days after weaning. Such MSG treatment was shown to produce lesions of the inner layer of the retina, cingulate gyrus, arcuate nucleus of the hypothalamus, and other structures of the circumventricular organ system (e.g. 27). Associated with the lesions are both behavioral deficits and neurochemical disturbances (e.g. 27, 82). After differential housing, the rats were tested in an open field and in the Morris water maze, which consists of a water tank with a submerged platform generally located 1 cm below the surface of milky water; in the water maze task, the animals are tested for their ability to reach the platform after being released from various starting positions around the perimeter of the tank (generally, north, south, east, west, in a random order; e.g. 62). There was a housing by drug interaction in the place navigation task, but not in the open field test. In the water maze, MSG-treated impoverished rats were significantly slower to solve the task than the other three groups on all test days, whereas MSG-treated enriched rats mastered the task almost as effficiently as saline-injected control rats as can be seen in figure 2.

The effects of environmental conditions on recovery have also been studied in animals characterized by various hereditary cerebral syndromes, such as those observed in some mutant strains of mice. Bouchon and Will[5, 6, 7,] studied "dwarf" mice which are characterized by a primary deficiency of the anterior hypophysis and which exhibit, as adults, learning and memory deficits in various tasks. They showed that one month post-weaning differential housing of these mice was suffficient to alter their behavioral performances: in comparison to impoverished dwarf mice, the enriched group made fewer errors in the Hebb-Williams maze, and showed more spontaneous alternation in a T-maze and better performance in a passive avoidance task. In "staggerer" mice characterized by anatomical and physiological abnormalities of the cerebellum and aberrant gait,[36, 37] reported that tilted rotational stimulation, given two times per day from day 1 to day 21, increased the ability of these neurological mutant mice to ambulate on a holed floor. The mutants appeared to be even more sensitive to the enrichment factor than normal mice when considering their ability to avoid holes.

There are now many reports indicating at least some degree of improvement after brain damage in animals subjected to environmental enrichment. In many studies, the differences between impoverished and enriched groups are even larger among the brain-damaged than among intact control subjects. It may be that handicapped populations profit more from an enriched experience than do intact animals, because they may be hypersensitive to the effects of environmental conditions. However, the interaction between brain condition and environment may also be related to the characteristics of the behavioral tasks used: in most of these tasks, the performance improvement of brain-damaged animals is clearly less affected by a possible ceiling or floor effect than it is in intact controls.

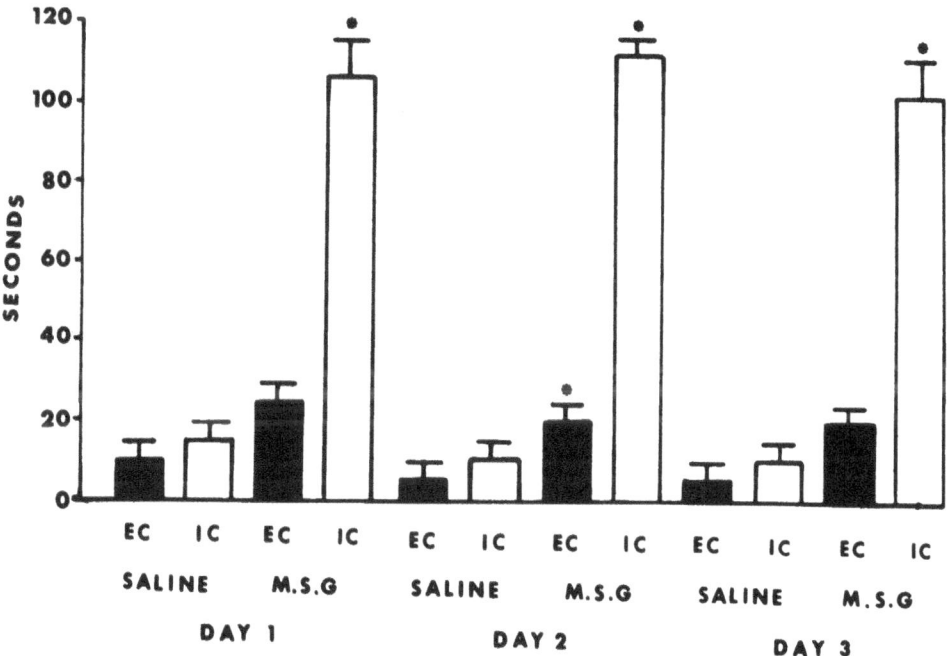

Figure 2. Latency to solve the place navigation task by isolation-reared monosodium-L-glutamate (MSG) injected, isolation-reared saline-injected, enrichment-reared MSG-injected and saline-injected enrichment-reared rats. *Differs significantly from all other groups. EC: Enriched Condition; IC: Impoverished Condition (from Saari et al.[78], with permission).

Specificity

If the generality of environmental effects on recovery has been extended to a few additional species and kinds of brain damage, somewhat paradoxically, over the last 10 years, their specificity has expanded too: it is becoming increasingly apparent that these effects may, indeed, be task-specific, lesion-specific, and age-specific, and this list is probably incomplete.

Several task specificities have already been mentioned incidentally (see 13, 78) and there are now more than ten reports of mixed results of enrichment, either "beneficial" or not, depending on the behavioral task used. Kolb (this volume) stresses the need for a broad functional evaluation and for using a large behavioral and neurologic test battery in order to determine more accurately the effects of any one factor on the general outcome of brain damage. For instance, in a recent study[53], the authors used a large battery of tests (see table 1) and found task specific environmental effects in rats which sustained unilateral or bilateral frontal cortex ablation. As shown in table 1, the lesions induced several deficits which were not all attenuated or compensated for by 90 days of postoperative environmental enrichment. One should note, however, that, in this study as in most others, the functional demands of the tasks were obviously quite different.

In our group, Dalrymple-Alford and co-workers[18] found that 10 days postoperative differential housing was suffficient to induce significant effects in rats which sustained dorsal hippocampal lesions at the age of 30 days. However, these effects were opposite in two behavioral tasks with quite similar functional demands, namely the Morris water maze task and a dry version of the same task. In the latter task a small food cup (same diameter as the platform in water maze) filled with dry food pellets was hidden underneath sawdust in a open circular arena of same diameter as the water maze; the water maze and the sawdust arena were located in the same

Table 1. Summary of the behavioral effects of bilateral frontal lesions, enrichment, and the interaction of lesion and enrichment (from Kolb and Gibb[53], with permission).

Measure	Lesion	Enrichment	Lesion X Enrichment
Body weight	*	*	
Claw cutting	*	*	
Water task	*		*
Tongue extension	*		*
Food hoarding	*		
Beam traversing		*	
Running activity		*	
Grooming			

Note: * indicates a significant difference either between bilateral frontals and controls (for lesion), between isolated and enriched groups (for enrichment), or a unique interaction of lesion and enrichment (interaction).

experimental room and, in both tasks, the rats had to reach the target - the platform or the food cup - as efficiently as possible. As shown in figure 3, enriched housing had no beneficial effect on performance in the water maze, but did exert beneficial effects in the same animals tested in the dry version of these two place navigation tasks. One may thus assume that the functional demands of these two tasks were not equivalent in all respects: while the spatial memory requirements to solve the tasks were virtually identical, other attributes (see 52) sensory, motor, response, time, motivational - may have differed importantly in these tasks. The "dry" and "wet" versions of this place navigation task may have differed, in particular, by their motivational features, since it is likely that the "dry" version was much less stressing than the "wet" version.

Lesion specificities were already documented during the seventies and have been analyzed in our previous reviews[16, 88]. We will not reconsider this topic here, since data accumulated during the eighties only confirm earlier findings showing that postoperative enrichment may be an efficient therapeutic tool after certain kinds of brain damage, such as hippocampal lesions, but not after certain others such as lesions of the afferent-efferent systems of the hippocampus[17, 49, 91]. A careful analysis of such specificities is fundamentally important and will necessitate comparison, within one single experiment, of animals with different lesions, but submitted to the same differential housing conditions and to the same functional (behavioral, neurological, etc...) assessments.

A few studies have considered the effects of postoperative experience in animals sustaining brain injury at different ages; some of these studies demonstrate age-specific effects. Whishaw and coworkers[86], for instance, reported that "beneficial" enrichment effects were observed in the water maze task only in the rats which underwent hemidecortication when adult, and not in those receiving virtually the same brain surgery when one day old. As shown in figure 4, the absence of environmental effects in those rats sustaining hemidecortication when 1 day old seems not to be due to a "floor" effect, since their performances were lower than those of control animals. However, in this particular example of neonatal lesions and lesions sustained in adulthood, one may question, whether the lesions can be considered as really identical.

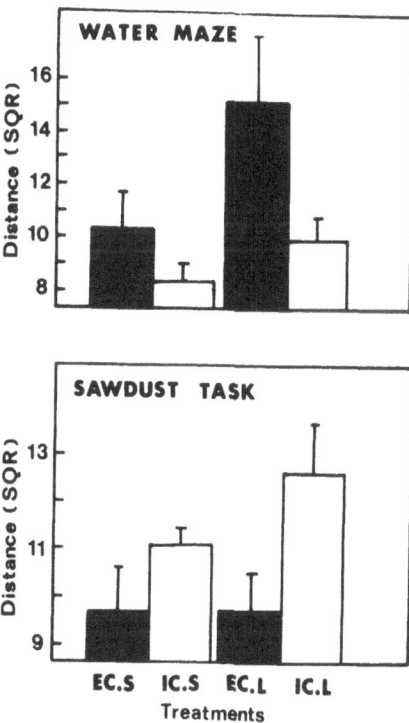

Figure 3. Effects of 10 day postoperative differential housing in rats with dorsal hippocampal lesions. Distance (Square root of means and S.E.M.) to hidden platform in the water maze and to hidden food cup in the sawdust task. EC: Enriched Condition; IC: Impoverished Condition; S: Sham Operated; L: Lesion (Dalrymple-Alford et al.[18]).

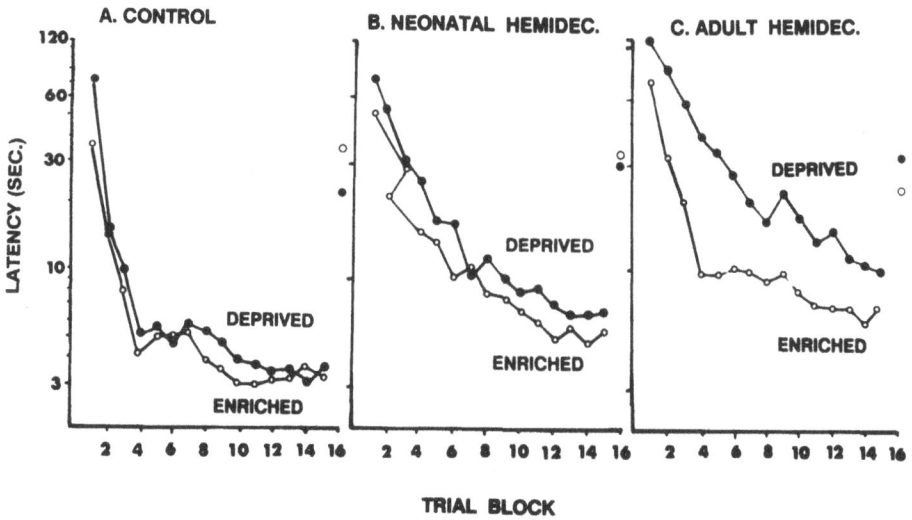

Figure 4. Mean latency per trial block (semilog graph) for (A) control enriched and control deprived groups, (B) neonatal hemidecorticate-enriched, neonatal hemidecorticate-deprived groups, and (C) adult hemidecorticate-enriched and adult hemidecorticate-deprived groups. The platform was moved 180° on Trial Block 16. (from Whishaw et al[86], with permission).

Perhaps should one relate the observations by Whishaw and collaborators[86] to others showing age-specific effects of differential housing on brain measures. Kolb and Elliott[54], for instance, reported that the effects of experience on brain anatomy following frontal lesions are age-dependent (fig. 5). Rats raised in an enriched condition developed thicker cortices following lesions at 5 days of age but not at 1 day of age (as was also the case in the study by Whishaw and coworkers). Moreover, in the Kolb and Elliott study, enriched housing also markedly attenuated the behavioral consequences of early lesions in the 5-day operates, even on tests such as tongue extension that would not be expected to benefit from specific practice in the complex environment. Parallel to the anatomical data, in the 1-day operates, the behavioral effects of enriched housing were much less pronounced than in the 5-day operates.

Thus, if "environmental therapy" can be considered as safe, its efficacy has some limitations. However, better analysis and understanding of its effects may well help to increase its efficacy.

ENRICHMENT VERSUS IMPOVERISHMENT: SOCIAL AND PHYSICAL COMPONENTS

Enriched and impoverished conditions may be distinguished by several factors or components, such as the amount of sensory stimulation, locomotor activity, handling and training. Each of these factors may be responsible for some of the reported effects of differential housing in impoverished and enriched conditions (e.g. 19, 24, 29, 31, 36, 37, 38, 39, 42, 55, 56). Impoverished and enriched conditions may also be distinguished by their social and physical components, as they generally differ both in the number of animals and the number of objects per cage. It makes sense, therefore, to look for an optimal combination of enrichment components in order to increase the efficacy of environmental therapy. However, before breaking down the enriched condition into its components, let us see whether the reported environmental effects on recovery are actually due to enrichment effects or to impoverishment effects.

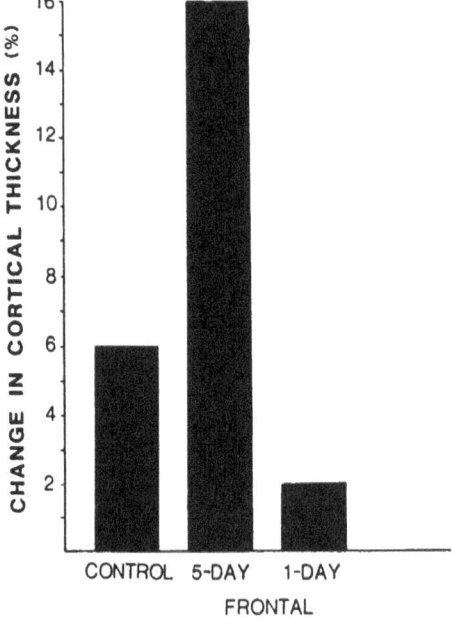

Figure 5. Summary of overall changes in cortical thickness represented as a percentage of lab-reared cortical thickness. (from Kolb and Elliott[54], with permission).

Attenuation or Increase of Symptoms

Since enriched brain-damaged animals generally exhibit attenuated symptoms, it is usually assumed that enriched housing fosters recovery. However, this interpretation may be questioned because, in most experiments, the behavioral performance was measured after only one single postoperative delay. Therefore, as shown on figure 6, there are two different possible interpretations for one behavioral outcome.

In order to verify whether environmentally-induced modifications correspond to an attenuation of symptoms or to an increase of symptoms we used a brief behavioral task which does not require any deprivation or training and which constitutes a good "barometer" of hippocampal dysfunction, namely spontaneous alternation[89]. Rats with dorsal hippocampal lesions and sham-operated control rats were tested pre- and postoperatively on a spontaneous alternation task. Four days after surgery, the group of rats with lesions alternated significantly less than the control group. Starting on the fifth postoperative day, the rats were assigned to three different environmental conditions - enriched, social or impoverished - in which they were placed for 7, 15 or 23 days. Environmental enrichment significantly increased

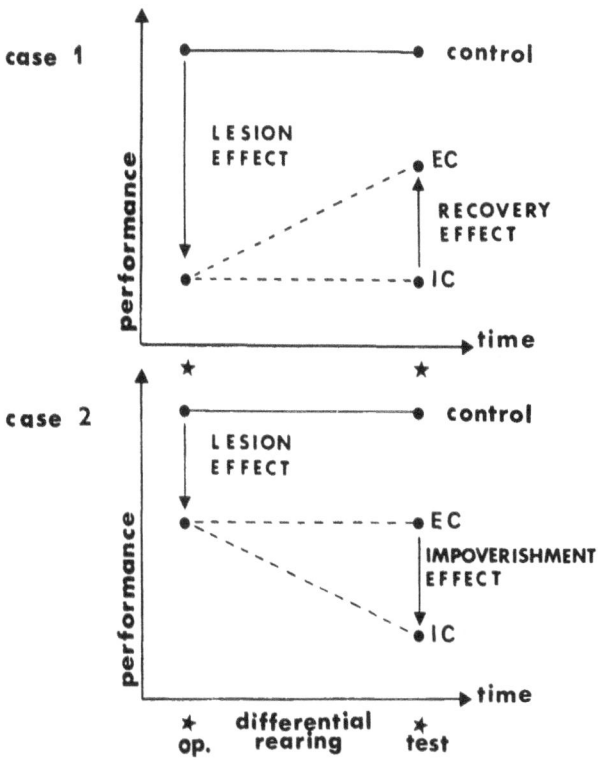

Figure 6. Two possible interpretations of differential housing (enrichment, EC, versus impoverishment, IC) effects in animals with lesions, when behavioral assessment is carried out after only one single postoperative delay.

spontaneous alternation in rats with lesions, even for the shortest enrichment period (7 days); impoverished housing did not exacerbate the lesion-induced symptoms. Although this result might be task and lesion-specific, it clearly indicates that postoperative enrichment can help to reduce postoperative symptoms in brain-damaged animals.

The Social Component

In the study by Will and co-workers[89], enriched housing differed from social housing only by its physical aspects; indeed, in both enriched and social conditions, the rats were housed in groups of 10 in virtually identical cages which differed only in the presence or absence of various junk objects, in enriched and social conditions, respectively. The results therefore suggest that the critical component for enrichment effects might be the physical component.

However, there are several reports showing that social grouping in comparison to isolation may be sufficient *per se* to foster recovery, especially when considering reactivity and social behavior following septal lesions (e.g. 1, 43); several experiments have compared the effects of enriched, standard and impoverished housing on behavioral expression, although both standard and impoverished conditions differ from enriched housing in both their social and physical components. Engellener and coworkers, for instance, found that enriched housing reduced handling hyperactivity in septal mice, but their experimental design (enrichment versus impoverishment) does not clarify whether the observed beneficial effect is due to social grouping or physical complexity[23, 32]. Only a few experiments have used a social (instead of a standard) condition differing from enrichment only in its physical aspects and from impoverishment only in its social aspects (e.g. 22, 66). These few studies suggest that the social and physical components of enrichment may have additive effects on the expression of at least some behavioral capacities. Indeed, in the study by Einon and co-workers[22], both social housing and environmental enrichment improved the performance of rats with hippocampal lesions in a radial maze task, but the improvement was greater when social grouping and physical complexity were combined.

The Physical Component

Even in isolated animals (which may constitute a model of some clinical situations), the postoperative physical environment may play a critical and unspecific role in the process of recovery of function. We have shown[95] that "enriching" the physical environment by introducing various objects into the home cage is a sufficiently potent factor for altering the behavior of isolated rats in a rather general way. The rats sustained dorsal hippocampal lesions at 30 days. After surgery, they were isolated for one month, either with or without objects in their cage. All rats were moved to new cages daily. The housing conditions affected (1) reactions towards a novel object in both lesioned and intact rats, (2) reactions towards a novel environment in intact rats only and (3) learning of a radial maze task in lesioned rats, although not significantly.

Thus, the addition of a few objects to the postoperative environment may change the behavioral outcome of brain injury, at least in some respects and if a genuine possibility for active interaction with the postoperative environment is provided (see 20).

Overall, it now appears that the effectiveness of environmental therapy, probably based on interaction between the brain-damaged subject and a socially and physically enriched environment has been corroborated. Nevertheless, as mentioned earlier, this effectiveness also appears limited under certain task, lesion and age (and perhaps other) conditions. In order to understand these limitations and to improve the efficacy of environmental therapy, analysis of the underlying processes is required.

THE UNDERLYING PROCESSES

Two interesting lines of research have developed during the last decade, both of which may help us to understand the processes underlying environmental influences on recovery from brain damage: one approach analyzes the interaction between postoperative differential housing and brain noradrenaline, the other explores the interaction between postoperative differential housing and intracerebral transplants. Both these lines of research consider brain state as a critical factor for the expression of environmental effects and, thus, may reveal some of the necessary conditions for such effects to occur.

Brain Noradrenaline

Periods during which the brain is shaped by experience may require intact functioning of the noradrenergic system. This hypothesis derives from Kasamatsu and Pettigrew[45], who have shown that the neurophysiological consequences (i.e., ocular dominance shift) of monocular eye occlusion in the developing kitten are prevented by depletion of brain catecholamines with 6-hydroxydopamine (6-0HDA). They also showed that this effect is reversed by cortical perfusion with noradrenaline, which renders the adult cat brain more susceptible to the effects of monocular occlusion[68]. Such observations (e.g., see also 81) have led to the suggestion that noradrenaline has a permissive role in cortical plasticity.

There is now, indeed, a large number of reports showing that noradrenaline depletion (but not dopamine depletion) abolishes or attenuates the effects of differential housing or training on both cerebral and behavioral measures (e.g. 8, 14, 59, 60, 65, 67, 77). As illustrated in figure 7[59], neonatal noradrenaline depletion induced by 6-OHDA treatment virtually abolishes the effects of differential housing on Hebb-Williams maze performance in rats; in contrast, dopamine depletion induced by the combined treatment of the noradrenaline uptake inhibitor desipramine followed by 6-OHDA, does not produce such an effect.

Consistent with such a role for noradrenaline are the pharmacological data reported by the groups of Feeney and of Davis, who showed that amphetamine treatment may exert beneficial effects on recovery if the animals are given practice or exercise[24, 31, 42]. However, in their initial study, Feeney and collaborators[24] found that haloperidol blocked the facilitation of recovery produced by amphetamine and practice, suggesting that the acceleration of recovery by amphetamine is dependent on dopamine.

There are also two reports which are not completely consistent with the noradrenaline hypothesis, one by Whishaw et al[85] and another by Murtha et al[63]. Whishaw and coworkers examined the contributions of forebrain noradrenaline and environmental enrichment to recovery of place navigation ability after hemidecortication sustained in rats either at the age of 7-9 days or in adulthood. In otherwise normal rats noradrenaline depletion failed to attenuate the beneficial effects of enriched housing, but among hemidecorticated rats maintained in impoverished conditions, the depleted rats displayed none of the recovery observed in the saline-treated control animals. The recent report by Murtha and co-workers[63] does not support a role for forebrain noradrenaline in the effects of environmental enrichment on rat cortex and behavior. There is therefore a need to explain the observed discrepancies in this important line of research, and to reconcile the majority of results which suggest at least a permissive role (if not a critical role) of noradrenaline in cortical plasticity and the few contradictory results. Several possibilities may be considered, such as the route of 6-0HDA administration (s.c. versus i.c.v., thus causing

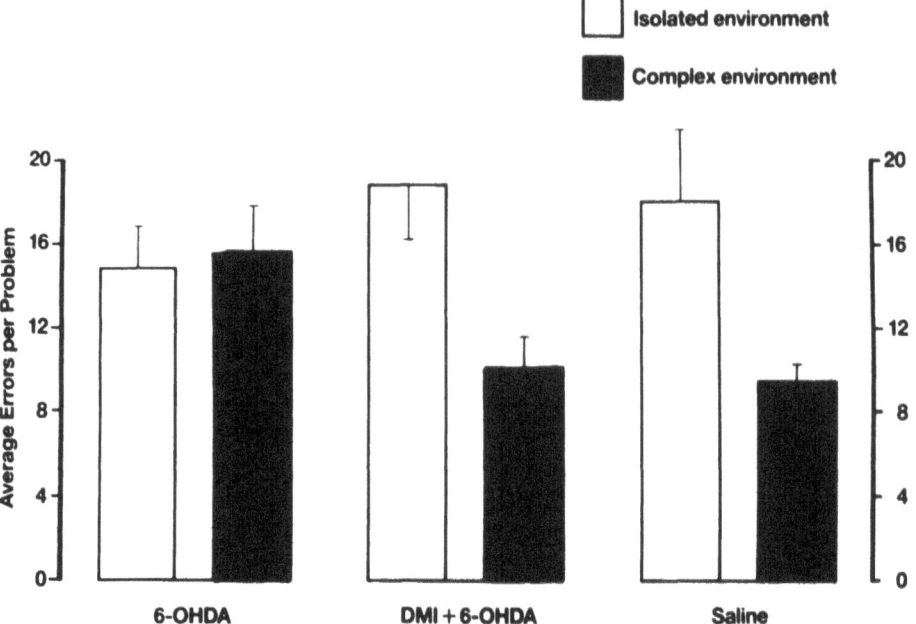

Figure 7. Median (quartiles) average errors per problem in the Hebb-William maze for 6 hydroxydopamine (6-OHDA), desipramine (DMI + 6-OHDA) and saline-treated rats housed in an Isolated (IC) or a Complex environment (EC) for 35 days following weaning. Saline- and DMI + 6-OHDA-treated rats raised in EC made significantly fewer errors than those raised in IC. Mann-Whitney U-tests, P < 0.01. Both 6-OHDA groups made more errors than the Complex environment groups in the saline and DMI + 6OHDA conditions. (from Mohammed et al[59], with permission).

damage or not to the peripheral sympathetic system) the age of the animals at the time of drug treatment, or the extent of noradrenaline depletion. The effects of noradrenaline depletion may depend on one or several of these factors.

Intracerebral Transplants

Another as yet embryonic line of research considers the interaction between the postoperative environment and intracerebral grafts. Some of the conditions under which fetal neural grafts survive, reinnervate denervated host tissue and affect the functional expression of the host have recently been identified (e.g. 3, 11, 28). Aspects of the graft microenvironment known to be important in this respect include trophic factors and possibly anti-trophic factors, and regional blood, hormonal, and cerebrospinal fluid supply (e.g. 28, 64, 69). One potentially important factor which has gone almost unstudied in this context is the macroenvironment of the graft recipient, namely its rearing or housing conditions. Other stimulatory factors such as electric stimulation of the lesion area (e.g. 40) pharmacological stimulation (e.g. 12, 57, 58, 84), mild stress produced by non-painful tail pinch[2, 96] or "active" sensory stimulation (e.g. 20) may also facilitate functional recovery after brain damage. An "enriched" macroenvironment, however, may be of easier clinical applicability and may provide a tool for modulating the functional outcome of intracerebral grafts which, indeed, may still not be optimal. Conversely, perhaps by forming bridges for host neurons, by setting the level of neurotransmitters above a given functional threshold, or by some other means, grafts may allow the effects of differential housing to be expressed in organisms which otherwise, because of the kind of brain lesions they have (e.g. 49), would not benefit from enriched housing.

There are only two published reports considering the possibility that housing conditions may modulate the effects of intracerebral transplants.

Kelche et al[50] conducted a study on the long-term behavioral expression of rats which sustained complete aspirative lesions of the fimbria-fornix pathways and received solid fetal septal transplants grafted into the lesion cavity. Control animals sustained either the lesion alone, or only sham surgery. Two days after transplantation surgery, half the rats were housed in an enriched condition, the other half remained in standard conditions (3 rats per cage). Two and ten months later, the rats were tested in a Hebb-Williams maze.

Two months after surgery, there was a highly significant detrimental lesion effect, no graft effect and no environmental effect except in sham-operated rats, "enriched" sham-operated rats making fewer initial errors than sham-operated rats housed in standard conditions.

Ten months after surgery, all rats with lesions showed some degree of recovery but still made more errors than sham-operated rats; furthermore, enriched sham-operated rats still made fewer initial errors than their counterparts housed in standard conditions. However, at this postsurgical delay, the lesion induced deficits were significantly attenuated in those animals which benefited from both intracerebral transplants and enriched housing (fig. 8). Thus, these data show that under similar lesion conditions in which both enriched housing[49] and the transplant[10] were unable alone to promote behavioral recovery, they reduced lesion-induced deficits when applied together. In this experiment, grafts partially reinnervated the hippocampus of rats with fimbria-fornix lesions (fig.8). It would thus be worthwile to verify whether this reinnervation (or perhaps the restoring by the grafts of a partial link between the septum and the hippocampus) is a condition for differential housing effects to be expressed.

Dunnett and colleagues[21] also ran an experiment aimed at analyzing the graft by environment interaction. In this case, embryonic ventral forebrain tissue was grafted into the neocortex of rats in which the intrinsic cortical cholinergic innervation had been removed by nucleus basalis lesions. Half the rats were housed in an enriched environment, and the other half in a "deprived" environment (standard housing with 4-6 rats per cage). The rats were killed either 4 or 10 weeks after transplantation surgery. Postoperative enriched housing produced a temporary enhancement of fibre outgrowth 4 weeks after transplantation, which was no longer apparent by 10 weeks survival (fig. 9). Unfortunately, there was no behavioral assessment of whether this transient enhancement of fibre outgrowth had any long term functional effects.

In a study not yet published, Kelche et al obtained preliminary evidence showing that training in a simple reinforced alternation task may also interact with grafts and facilitate recovery in animals which receive intracerebral transplants.

This line of research may help in the study of processes underlying the effects of both intracerebral grafts and differential housing in an original way. From both a fundamental and a clinical point of view, it deserves to be developed.

Environmentally-Induced Brain Modifications

Over the last 30 years, environmentally-induced cerebral modifications have been well documented in intact animals. For example, rats raised in enriched conditions develop heavier cerebral cortices, larger cell bodies, increased dendritic arborizations, greater numbers of dendritic spines and longer synaptic appositions (e.g. 70). Recently enriched housing was also shown to increase neurogenesis in the dentate gyrus[97] and to affect cerebral vasculature, with capillaries of "enriched" rats being closer together than those of "impoverished" rats[4].

In contrast, there are only a few reports on environmentally-induced brain modifications in brain damaged animals, and they provide a rather incomplete picture. As in some early experiments in which differential housing had been shown to

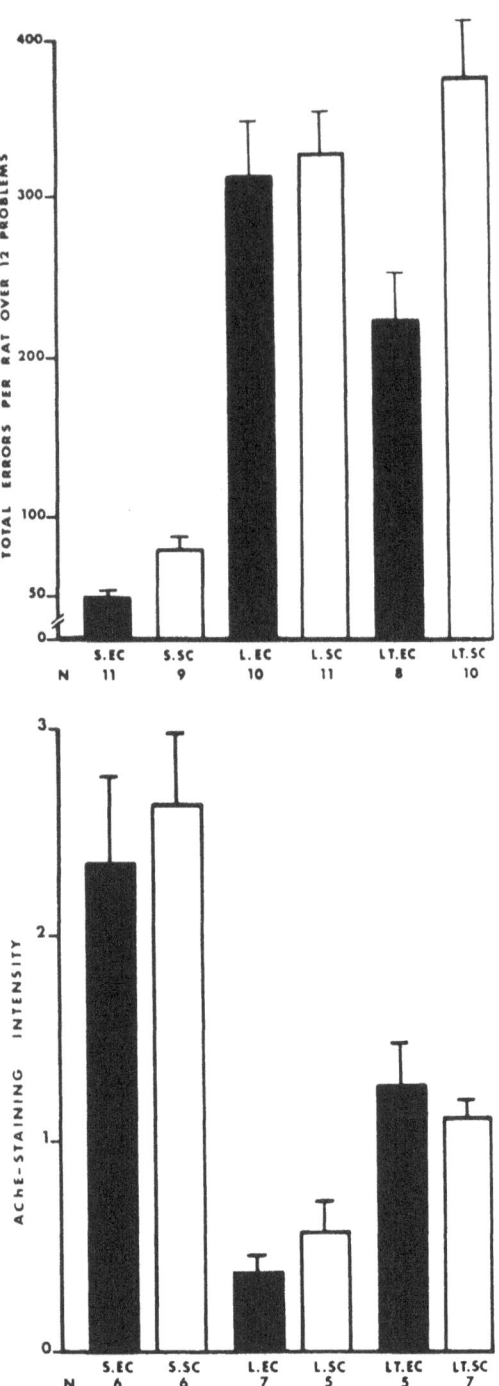

Figure 8. Total errors (means ± S.E.M.) over the 12 Hebb-Williams maze problems (6 trials a day) 10 months after transplantation surgery (upper part of the figure) and mean evaluation (performed by 3 evaluators) of AChE -staining intensity (rated on a 4 level scale) in the dorsal hippocampus of rats 11 months after surgery (lower part of the figure). S: Sham operation; L: Lesion; LT: Lesion + Transplant, EC: Enriched Condition; SC: Standard Condition; N: number of rats per treatment group (Kelche et al[50]).

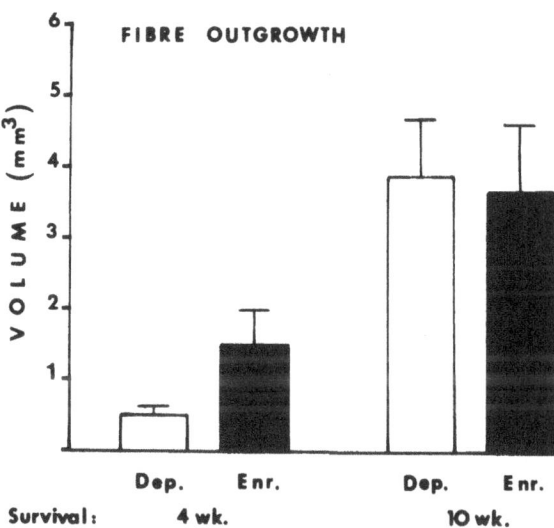

Figure 9. Fibre outgrowth (means and S.E.M.) of ventral forebrain grafts implanted in the deafferented dorsolateral, frontal cortex of rats subsequently housed in an enriched (Enr) or deprived (Dep) environment and killed after 4 or 10 weeks. (from Dunnett et al[21], with permission).

influence gross neuroanatomical measures following various cortical lesions and following malnutrition (e.g. 48, 76, 93, 94) several authors have reported such effects on brain weight and size or on cortical thickness. Rosenzweig[75] found that enriched experience increases the weight of residual cortex after various bilateral cortical lesions but, contrary to earlier speculation[94], he found no experiential effect on remote cell loss observed during the month or more following the lesions. Kolb and Elliott[54] showed that enriched postoperative experience can attenuate the thinning of cerebral cortex induced by neonatal frontal lesions, but they found this effect to be age-dependent: it was greatest in animals which sustained frontal decortication at 5 days of age and much less effective in animals with lesions sustained at 1 day of age (fig. 5). Enriched housing has also been shown to alter gross measures of brain morphology in noradrenaline-depleted rats[63], in malnourished rats (e.g. 9, 46, 47, 48) and vasopressin deficient rats of the mutant Brattleboro strain[34, 35]. However, other researchers using adult hemidecorticate rats[86], prenatally X-irradiated microcephalic rats[80], noradrenaline-depleted rats[8, 65], or malnourished rats[15] have failed to observe any influence of differential housing on gross neuroanatomy, although most of them found housing effects on behavior in brain-damaged animals or on neuroanatomical measures in intact control animals. The gross measures considered were possibly too gross to reveal subtle changes accompanying functional modifications.

In our study on environmental influences on dendritic branching and spines in the cortex of rats with hippocampal lesions, we found that dorsal hippocampal lesions decreased the branching and number of spines of basilar dendrites in layer V pyramidal cells of area 17, and that differential housing affected these measures only in sham-operated control rats[51]. However, as there was a significant main effect of housing conditions on spine density, we replicated this study with D. Cassel and found similar results (Kelche, Cassel and Will, unpublished). Taken together, the results of both experiments suggest that in rats with lesions differential housing tends to affect synaptic connectivity as indirectly measured by spine density, whereas in intact rats housing conditions affect both branching and spine density (fig. 10).

In their recent study Kolb and Gibb[53] found that enrichment increased brain weight and dendritic branching in layer II/III pyramidal cells of the occipital cortex similarly in normal rats and in rats with either unilateral or bilateral frontal lesions. In contrast, however, enriched experience affected parietal neurons in normal but not in

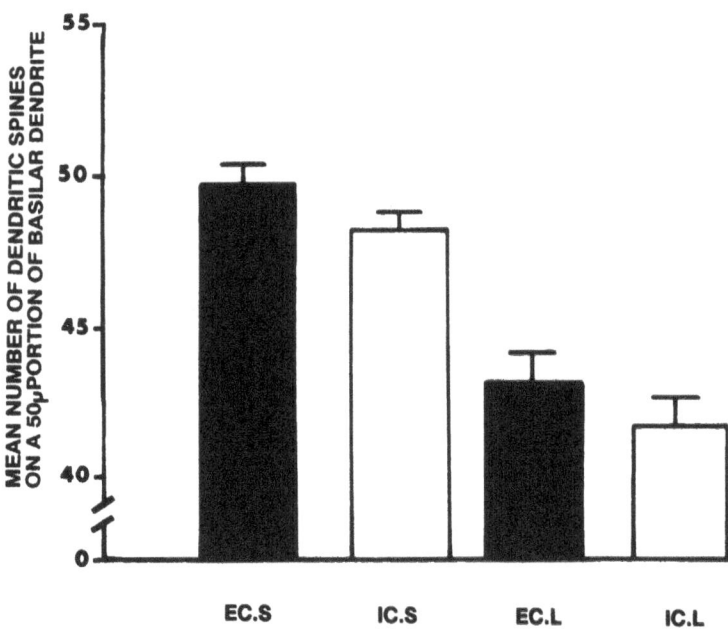

Figure 10. Number (means and S.D.) of dendritic spines on basilar dendrites of pyramidal neurons (layer V of area 17). Abbreviations as in Fig. 3 (Kelche and Will[51]; Kelche et al., unpublished).

brain-damaged animals. Instead, the frontal operates showed an increase in parietal branching irrespective of their rearing condition, which implies that the lesion itself may have led to some form of reactive synaptogenesis which was not affected by and which precluded environmental effects (fig. 11).

Environmentally induced morphological changes may be triggered by trophic factors. Ten years ago, Will[88] speculated that trophic factors such as NGF might be critically involved in the mediation of differential housing effects. This speculation has now received indirect support from research carried out by Mohammed and his colleagues[61] in Sweden. Indeed, they reported recently that NGF concentration may be changed in a subtle way in certain brain areas by differential housing, at least when some training experience was added to differential housing.

Obviously, research on underlying processes should be expanded. Such research might help us to better understand some of the reported data, particularly some of the specificities mentioned earlier. It might also help to increase the efficacy of postoperative environmental therapy, although it should not be forgotten, as mentioned by Rose[71], that "the major criterion of recovery of function must be behavioral".

DISCUSSION

The literature reviewed in this chapter demonstrates that: (1) both the generality and specificity of postoperative environmental effects have been extended over the last 10 years; (2) under many circumstances, postoperative enrichment constitutes a potentially powerful "therapeutic tool" which combines the additive effects of its various social and physical components; (3) modifying the brain state of brain-damaged animals by drugs or grafts modulates the effficacy of postoperative enrichment (or training) and, thus, may provide a better understanding of the underlying processes. Nevertheless, as stressed by Rose[71], differential housing research has failed so far to provide a very clear lead for those working in clinical situations, the diffficulty being essentially due to problems with definition and experimental design.

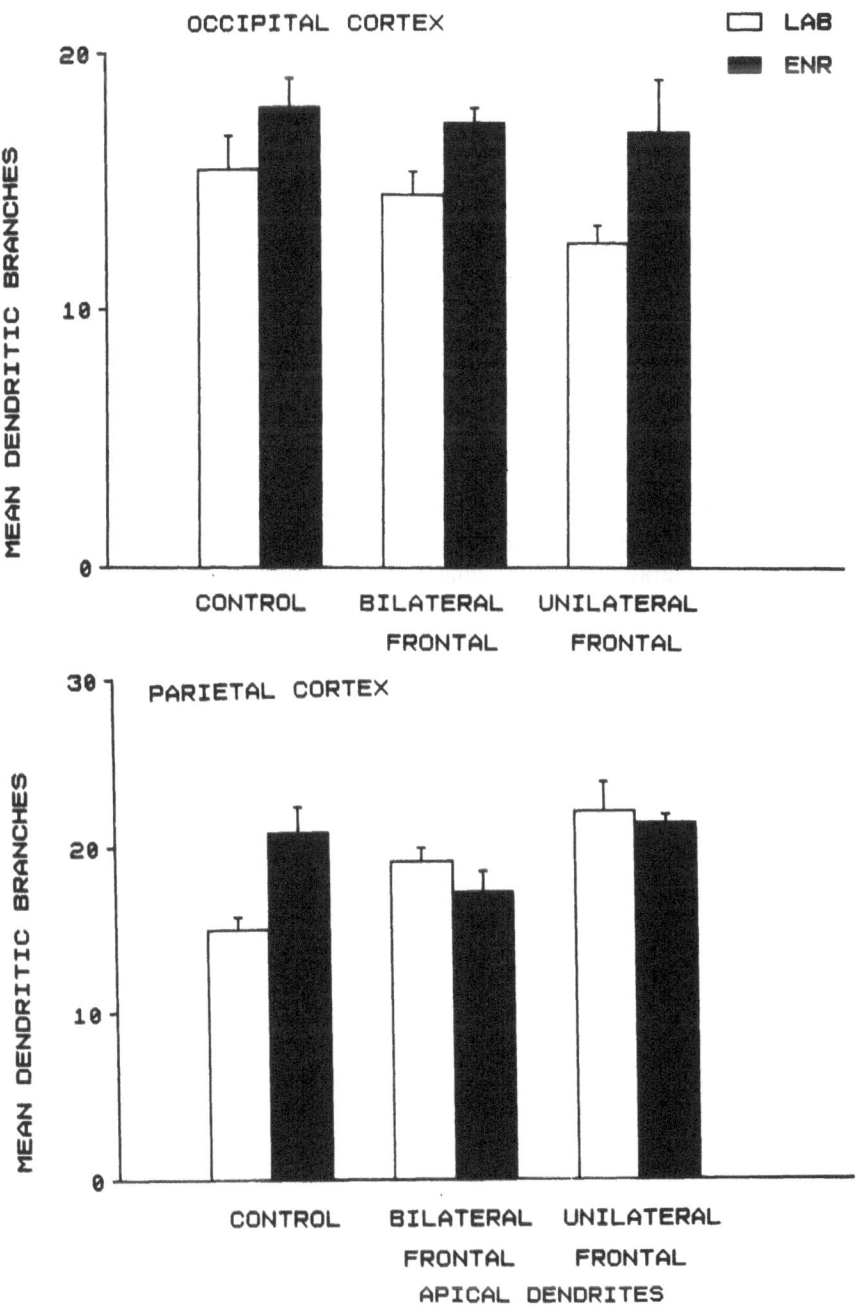

Figure 11. Dendritic branching (means and S.E.M.) in occipital and parietal cortices after either bilateral or unilateral frontal cortex lesions. LAB: lab cage housing; ENR: enriched housing. (adapted from Kolb and Gibb[53]; with permission).

Rose[71] has argued that one should agree on what, operationally, should be interpreted as recovery. He and his colleagues[72,73,74] have paid particular attention to distinguishing between the processes of recovery of lost function and compensation for lost function. In order to conclude that enrichment has aided recovery - and not only compensation - they emphasize the need for before-after designs, i.e., in which behavioral baselines are established pre-operatively and some measure of return to those baselines obtained postoperatively. Although this view makes sense, it would be difficult to avoid confrontation with certain problems of interference, especially when considering learned behaviours; in this case, enriched and impoverished experiences may differentially interfere with the processes underlying the behavior in question. Rose and his coworkers also rightly consider that enrichment has aided recovery when a significant interaction between pre-/postoperative performance and postoperative environment has been demonstrated among the lesioned animals. However, one should keep in mind that statistically significant interactions may result from "ceiling" or "floor" effects on the performances of only one of the treatment groups. In most of their experiments, Rose and his collaborators used unilateral lesions, thus avoiding total loss in any sensory modality, and examining behavioral deficits not thought to be primarily due to sensory loss. They concluded that their results were consistent with the view that any restorative value that postoperative environmental enrichment may have lies in facilitating compensatory mechanisms rather than in true recovery. This conclusion has been supported by the results of several other groups which compared the topology of motor responses (e.g 30, 41) used before and after brain surgery, or the cognitive strategies employed by lesioned and intact enriched animals. Held and coworkers[41], for instance, reported that both pre- and postoperative enriched housing attenuated beam-walking deficits in rats with bilateral sensorimotor cortex lesions, but normal response topology was observed only in pre-operatively enriched rats while aberrant topology characterized the behavior of postoperatively enriched rats, which without topological analysis might have been fallaciously considered as recovered. Compensation may also underly the neuromorphological data reported by Kolb and Gibb[53], who found that environmental enrichment produced similar effects in intact and brain-damaged animals without modifying the lesion-induced plastic processes.

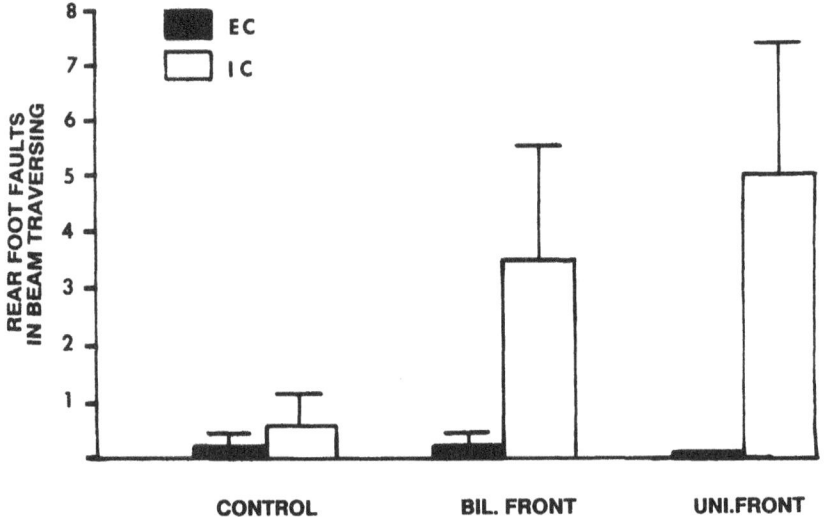

Figure 12. Total number (means and S.E.M.) of rear foot faults in beam traversing over 3 trials (adapted from Kolb and Gibb[53]).

However, these authors have found similar significant beneficial enrichment effects in a sensorimotor task in rats with either unilateral or bilateral frontal cortex lesions (fig. 12).

Apart from matters of concept definition, experimental factors, whether pre-surgical, surgical or postsurgical, may also be important for understanding some of the specificities and apparent inconsistencies mentioned earlier in this chapter. As indicated by Rose[71], it is beyond the scope of any laboratory to systematically assess the importance of all of these factors, and there is a need to promote more active collaborative efforts between laboratories involved in research on recovery of function. During the EBBS workshop on recovery of function (1991), a network organization was even considered as one possible solution. Such an organization would help researchers both to analyze existing data more synthetically and to standardize some of their experimental designs; finally, it would also facilitate communication between clinicians and researchers involved in basic research.

Overall, the situation has not changed dramatically over the last 10 years, although environmental enrichment increasingly appears to be a potential tool of high efficacy and certainly of low risk, the major risk being that of inefficacy. However, the therapeutic efficacy of environmental enrichment, whether compensatory or not, needs to be assessed finally by the clinicians themselves, and is likely to require adaptation of both concepts and methods to man (see Diller, this volume).

ACKNOWLEDGEMENTS

Our research was supported by grants from the Fondation Simone et Cino Dell Duca, the Fondation pour la Recherche Médicale and from the Centre National de la Recherche Scientifique (A.T.P. 4780). The authors are highly indebted to Dr. J. Anderson for reviewing the manuscript and to Bernadette Malycha for her technical assistance in preparing the manuscript.

REFERENCES

1.   Albert, D.J., Walsh, M.L., and Longley, W., 1985, Group rearing abolishes hyperdefensiveness induced in weanling rats by lateral septal or medial accumbens lesions but not by medial hypothalamic lesions, *Behav. Neural Biol.*, **1**, 101-109.

2.   Antelman, S.M., Rowland, N.E., and Fisher, A.E., 1976, Stress related recovery from lateral hypothalamic aphagia, *Brain Res.*, **102**, 346-350.

3.   Björklund, A., Gage, F.H., and Stenevi, U., 1983, Intracerebral grafting of neuronal cell suspensions. VI. Survival and growth of intrahippocampal implants of septal cell suspensions, *Acta Physiol. Scand. Suppl.*, 48-58.

4.   Black, J.E., Sirevaag, A.M., and Greenough, W.T., 1987, Complex experience promotes capillary formation in young rat visual cortex, *Neurosci. Lett.*, **83**, 351-355.

5.   Bouchon, R., and Will, B., 1982, Effects of early enriched and restricted environments on the exploratory and locomotor activity of dwarf mice, *Behav. Neural. Biol.*, **35**, 174-186.

6.   Bouchon, R., and Will, B., 1982, Effets des conditions d'élevage après le sevrage sur les performances d'apprentissage des souris "Dwarf", *Physiol. Behav.*, **28**, 971-978.

7.   Bouchon, R., and Will, B., 1983, Effects of post-weaning environment and

apparatus dimension on spontaneous alternation as a function of phenotype in "Dwarf" mice, *Physiol. Behav.*, **30**, 213-219.

8. Brenner, E., Mirmiran, M., Uylings, H.B.M., and Van Der Gugten, J., 1983, Impaired growth of the cerebral cortex of rats treated neonatally with 6-hydroxydopamine under different environmental conditions, *Neurosci. Lett.*, **42**, 13-17.

9. Carughi, A., Carpenter, K., and Diamond, M. C., 1989, Effect of environmental enrichment during nutritional rehabilitation on body growth, blood parameters and cerebral cortical development of rat, Amer. Inst. Nutr., *Growth, Development and Aging*, 2005-2016.

10. Cassel, J.C., Kelche, C., Hornsperger, J.M., Jakisch, R., Hertting, G., and Will B., 1990, Graft-induced learning impairment despite graft-enhanced cholinergic functions in the hippocampus of rats with septohippocampal lesions, *Brain Res.*, **534**, 295-298.

11. Cassel, J.C., Kelche, C., Majchrzak, M., and Will, B., 1992, Factors influencing structure and function of intracerebral grafts in the mammalian brain: a review, *Restor. Neurol. Neurosci.*, **4**, 65-96.

12. Cole, D.D., Sullins, W.R., and Isaac, W., 1967, Pharmacological modification of the effects of spaced occipital ablations, *Psychopharmacol.*, **11**, 311-316.

13. Cornwell, P., and Overman, W., 1981, Behavioral effects of early rearing conditions and neonatal lesions of the visual cortex in kittens, *J. Comp. Physiol. Psychol.*, **6**, 848-862.

14. Cornwell-Jones, C.A., Velasquez, P., Wright, E.L., and McGaugh, J.L., 1988, Early experience influences adult retention of aversively motivated tasks in normal, but not DSP4-treated rats, *Develop. Psychobiol.*, **2**, 177-187.

15. Crnic, L., 1982, Effects of nutrition and environment on brain biochemisty and behavior, *Develop. Psychobiol.*, **2**, 129-145.

16. Dalrymple-Alford, J.C., and Kelche, C., 1985, Behavioural effects of preoperative and postoperative differential housing in rats with brain lesions: A review, in *Brain Plasticity, Learning and Memory. Advances in Behavioral Biology,* B. Will, P. Schmitt, J.C. Dalrymple-Alford eds., pp. 441-458, Plenum Press, New York.

17. Dalrymple-Alford, J.C., and Kelche, C., 1987, Behavioral effects of differential postoperative housing after septal lesions made in weanling rats, *Psychobiol.*, **3**, 255-260.

18. Dalrymple-Alford, J.C., Kelche, C., and Will, B., 1985, Is place learning impaired after lesions of the dorsal hippocampus? *Behav. Brain Res.*, **20**, EBBS meeting, Oxford, UK.

19. Delay, E.R., 1988, Facilitative effects of cross-modality training on recovery of a conditioned avoidance response following striate cortex ablations in the rat, *Neurolpsychol.*, **5**, 661-671.

20. Dru, D., Walker, J.P., and Walker, J.B., 1975, Self-produced locomotion restores visual capacity after striate lesions, *Science,* **187**, 265-266.

21. Dunnett, S.B., Wishaw, I.Q., Bunch, S.T., and Fine, A., 1986, Acetylcholine-rich neuronal grafts in the forebrain of rats: effects of environmental enrichment, neonatal noradrenaline depletion, host transplantation site and acetylcholinesterase-positive fibre outgrowth, *Brain Res.*, **378**, 357-373.

22. Einon, D.F., Morgan, M.J., and Will, B.E., 1980, Effects of postoperative environment on recovery from dorsal hippocampal lesions in young rats: tests of spatial memory and motor transfer, *Quart. J. Exp. Psychol.*, **32**, 137-148.

23. Engellenner, W.J., Goodlett, C.R., Burright, R.G., and Donovick, P.J., 1982, Environmental enrichment and restriction: effects on reactivity, exploration and maze learning in mice with septal lesions, *Physiol. Behav.*, **29**, 885-893.

24. Feeney, D.M., Gonzalez, A., and Law, W.A., 1982, Amphetamine, haloperidol, and experience interact to affect rate of recovery after motor cortex injury, *Science*, **217**, 855-857.

25. Finger, S., 1978, Environmental attenuation of brain-lesion symptoms, in *Recovery from Brain Damage. Research and Theory*, S. Finger, ed., pp. 3, 297-329.

26. Finger, S., and Stein, D.G., 1982, Environmental and experiential determinants of recovery of function, in *Brain Damage and Recovery*, S. Finger, D.G. Stein, eds., pp. 175-202, Academic Press, New York.

27. Freed, L.A., Dow-Edwards, D.L., and Milhorat, T.H., 1986, A 2-deoxyglucose study of female and male rats neonatally treated with monosodium glutamate, *Soc. Neurosci. Abstr.*, **2**, 1409.

28. Gage, F.H., Buzsaki, G., and Nilsson, O., 1987, Grafts of fetal cholinergic neurons to the deafferented hippocampus, in *Progress in Brain Research*, Seil F.J., Herbert E. and Carlson B.M., eds., chapter 27, pp. 335-347. Elsevier, Amsterdam.

29. Gage, P.D., 1985, Performance of hippocampectomized rats in a reference/working-memory task: effects of preoperative versus postoperative training, *Physiol. Psychol.*, **4**, 235-242.

30. Gentile, A.M., Beheshti, Z., and Held, J., 1987, Enrichment versus exercise effects on motor impairments following cortical removals in rats, *Behav. Neural. Biol.*, **3**, 321-332.

31. Goldstein, L.B., and Davis, J.N., 1990, Post-lesion practice and amphetamine-facilitated recovery of beam-walking in the rat, *Rest. Neurol. Neurosci.*, **1**, 311-314.

32. Goodlett, C.R., Engellenner, W.J., Burright, R.G., and Donovick, P.J., 1982, Influence of environmental rearing history and postsurgical environmental change on the septal rage syndrome in mice, *Physiol. Behav.*, **28**, 1077-1081.

33. Greenough, W.T., Fass, B., and De Voogd, T.J., 1976, The influence of experience on recovery following brain damage in rodents: Hypotheses based on development research, in *Environments as Therapy for Brain Dysfunction*, R. Walsh, W.T. Greenough, eds., pp. 1-50, Plenum Press, New York.

34. Greer, E.R., Diamond, M.C., and Tang, J.M.W., 1981, Increase in thickness of cerebral cortex in response to environmental enrichment in brattleboro rats deficient in vasopressin, *Exp. Neurol.*, **72**, 366-378.

35. Greer, E.R., Diamond, M.C., and Murphy, M., 1982, Correlation between water intake and dendritic branching in homozygous brattleboro rats: a golgi study, *Exp. Neurol.*, **78**, 15-25.

36. Guastavino, J.M., 1983, A tilted rotational stimulation improves the gait of a cerebellar mutant mouse: the staggerer, *Behav. Process.*, **9**, 79-84.

37. Guastavino, J.M., and Larsson, K., 1983, Quand un mutant surmonte ses handicaps, *La Recherche*, 1440-1442.

38. Handelmann, G.E., and Olton, D.S., 1981, Spatial memory following damage to hippocampal CA3 pyramidal cells with kainic acid: Impairment and recovery with preoperative training, *Brain Res.*, **217**, 41-58.

39. Handelmann, G.E., and Olton, D.S., 1981, Recovery of function after neurotoxic

damage to the hippocampal CA3 region: Importance of postoperative recovery interval and task experience, *Behav. Neurol. Biol.*, **4**, 453-464.

40. Harrell, L.E., Raubeson, R., and Balagura, S., 1974, Acceleration of functional recovery following lateral hypothalamic damage by means of electrical stimulation in the lesioned areas, *Physiol. Behav.*, 897-899.

41. Held, J.M., Gordon, J., and Gentile, A.M., 1985, Environmental influences on locomotor recovery following cortical lesions in rats, *Behav. Neurosci.*, **4**, 678-690.

42. Hovda, D.A., and Feeney, D.M., 1984, Amphetamine with experience promotes of locomotor function after unilateral frontal cortex injury in the cat, *Brain Res.*, **298**, 358-361.

43. Johnson, D.A., Spiker, M., and Carlson, K., 1984, Open-field social behavior in rats as a function of septal lesions in infancy and group versus isolated rearing conditions, *Physiol. Psychol.*, **1**, 14-16.

44. Jones, D.G., and Smith, B.J., 1980, Morphological analysis of the hippocampus following differential rearing in environments of varying social and physical complexity, *Behav. Neural. Biol.*, **30**, 135-147.

45. Kasamatsu, T., and Pettigrew, J.D., 1976, Depletion of brain catecholamines: failure of ocular dominance shift after monocular occlusion in kittens, *Science*, **194**, 206.

46. Katz, H.B., and Davies, C.A., 1982, The effects of early-life undernutrition and subsequent environment on morphological parameters of the rat brain, *Behav. Brain Res.*, **5**, 53-64.

47. Katz, H.B., and Davies, C.A., 1983, The separate and combined effects of early undernutrition and environmental complexity at different ages on cerebral measures in rats, *Develop. Psychobiol.*, **1**, 47-58.

48. Katz, H.B., Davies, C.A., and Dobbing, J., 1980, The effects of environmental stimulation on brain weight in previously undernourished rats, *Behav. Brain Res.*, **1**, 445-449.

49. Kelche, C., Dalrymple-Alford, J., and Will, B., 1987, Effects of postoperative environment on recovery of function after fimbria- fornix transection in the rat, *Physiol. Behav.*, **40**, 731-736.

50. Kelche, C., Dalrymple-Alford, J.C., and Will, B., 1988, Housing conditions modulate the effects of intracerebral grafts in rats with brain lesions, *Behav. Brain Res.* **3**, 287-295.

51. Kelche, C., and Will, B., 1982, Effects of postoperative environments following dorsal hippocampal lesions on dentritic branching and spines in rat occipital cortex, *Brain Res.*, **245**, 107-115.

52. Kesner, R.P., 1986, Neurological views of memory, in *Learning and Memory. A Biological View*, J.L. Martinez and P.K. Kesner, eds., pp. 399-438, Academic Press, Inc.

53. Kolb, B., and Gibb, R., 1991, Environmental enrichment and cortical injury: behavioral and anatomical consequences of frontal cortex lesions, *Cereb. Cortex*, **1**, 189-198.

54. Kolb, B., and Elliott, W., 1987, Recovery from early cortical damage in rats. II. Effects of experience on anatomy and behavior following frontal lesions at 1 or 5 days of age, *Behav. Brain Res.*, **26**, 47-56.

55. Lacour, M., 1984, Réapprentissage et période postopératoire sensible dans la restauration des fonctions nerveuses. Exemple de la compensation vestibulaire et implications cliniques, *Ann. Oto-Laryng.*, 177-187.

56. Lovely, R.G., Gregor, R.J., Roy, R.R., and Edgerton, V.R., 1986, Effects of training on the recovery of full-weight bearing stepping in the adult spinal cat, *Exp. Neurol.*, **92**, 421-435.

57. Macht, M.B., 1950, Effects of d-amphetamine on hemidecorticate, decorticate and decerebrate cats, *Fed. Proc.*, 731-732.

58. Meyer, P.M., Horel, J.A., and Meyer, D.R., 1963, Effects of DL-amphetamine upon placing responses in neodecorticate cats, *J. Comp. Physiol. Psychol.*, **56**, 402-404.

59. Mohammed, A., Jonsson, G., and Archer, T., 1986, Selective lesioning of forebrain noradrenaline neurons at birth at birth abolishes the improved maze learning performance induced by rearing in complex environment, *Brain Res.*, **398**, 6-10.

60. Mohammed, A., Luthman, J., Archer, T., and Winblad, B., 1988, Behavioural deficits induced by neonatal dopamine lesion are modified by enriched environment, *Psychopharmacol.*, **1**, S38.

61. Mohammed, A.K., Winblad, B., Ebendal T., and Larkfors, L., 1990 Environmental influence on behaviour and nerve growth factor in the brain, *Brain Res.*, **528**, 69-72.

62. Morris, R.G.M., 1983, An attempt to dissociate "spatial mapping" and "working memory" theories of hippocampal function, in *Neurobiology of the Hippocampus*, W. Seifert, ed., pp. 405-432, Academic Press, London.

63. Murtha, S., Pappas, B.A., and Raman, S., 1990, Neonatal and adult forebrain norepinephrine depletion and the behavioral and cortical thickening effects of enriched impoverished environment, *Behav. Brain Res.*, **3**, 249-261.

64. Nieto-Sampedro, M., Manthorpe, M., Barbin, G., Varon, S., and Cotman C.W., 1983, Injury-induced neuronotrophic activity in adult rat brain: correlation with survival of delayed implants in the wound cavity, *J. Neurosci.*, **3**, 2219-2229, 1983.

65. O'Shea, L., Saari, M., Pappas, B.A., Ings, R., and Stange, K., 1983, Neonatal 6-Hydroxydopamine attenuates the neural and behavioral effects of enriched rearing in the rat, *Eur. J. Pharmacol.*, **92**, 43-47.

66. Pacteau, C., Einon, D., and Sinden, J., 1989, Early rearing environment and dorsal hippocampal ibotenic acid lesions: long-term influences on spatial learning and alternation in the rat, *Behav. Brain Res.*, **34**, 79-96.

67. Pappas B. A., Saari M., Smythe J., Murtha S., Stange K., and Ings R., 1987, Forebrain norepinephrine and neurobehavioral plasticity: neonatal 6-hydroxydopamine eliminates enriched-impoverished experience effects on maze performance, *Pharmacol. Biochem. Behav.*, **27**, 153-158.

68. Pettigrew, J. D, and Kasamatsu, T., 1978, Local perfusion of noradrenaline maintains visual cortical plasticity, *Nature*, **271**, 761.

69. Raisman, G., Lawrence, J. M., Zhou, C. F., and Lindsay R. M., 1985, Some neuronal, glial and vascular interactions which occur when hippocampal primordia are incorporated into adult host hippocampi, in *Neural Grafting in the Mammalian CNS*, A. Björklund and U. Stenevi, eds., pp. 125-150 Elsevier, Amsterdam.

70. Renner, M.J., and Rosenzweig, M.R., 1987, *Enriched and Impoverished Environments. Effects on Brain and Behaviour*, Springer-Verlag, New York.

71. Rose, F.D., 1988, Environmental enrichment and recovery of function following brain damage in the rat, *Med. Sci. Res.*, **16**, 257-263.

72. Rose, F.D., Davey M.J., Love S., and Dell, P.A., 1987, Environmental

enrichment and recovery from contralateral sensory neglect in rats with large unilateral neocortical lesions, *Behav. Brain Res.*, **24**, 195-202.

73. Rose, F.D., Dell, P.A., Love, S., and Davey, M.J., 1988, Environmental enrichment and recovery from a complex Go/No-Go reversal deficit in rats following large unilateral neocortical lesions, *Behav. Brain Res.*, **31**, 37-45.

74. Rose, F.D., Dell, P.A., Love, S., and Davey, M.J., 1989, Post-surgical environmental enrichment and functional recovery in the hemidecorticate rat: alternative interpretations, *Med. Sci. Res.*, **17**, 481-483.

75. Rosenzweig, M.R., 1984, Experience, memory, and the brain, *Amer. Psychol.*, **4**, 365-376.

76. Rosenzweig, M.R., and Bennett, E.L., 1976, Enriched environments: Facts, factors and fantasies, in *Knowing, Thinking, and Believing*, L. Petrinovich and J.L. McGaugh, eds., pp. 179-213, Plenum Press, New York.

77. Saari, M.J., Armstrong, J., Nobrega, J., Chambers J., and Coscina, D., 1987, Neonatal forebrain norepinephrine (NE) depletion reduces the influence of the rearing environmental on learning and social behaviour, *Soc. Neurosci. Abstr.*, **406.**

78. Saari, M.J., Fong, S., Shivji, A., and Armstrong, J.N., 1990, Enriched housing masks deficits in place navigation induced by neonatal monosodium glutamate, *Neurotoxicol. Teratol.*, **1**, 29-32.

79. Schwartz, S., 1964, Effect of neonatal cortical lesions and early environmental factors on adult rat behavior, *J. Comp. Physiol. Psychol.*, **57**, 72-77.

80. Shibagaki, M., Seo, M., Asano, T., and Kiyono S., 1981, Environmental enrichment to alleviate maze performance deficits in rats with microcephaly induced by X-irradiation, *Physiol. Behav.*, **27**, 797-802.

81. Sutherland, R.J., Kolb, B., Whishaw, I.Q., and Becker, J.B., 1982, Cortical noradrenaline depletion eliminates sparing of spatial learning after neonatal frontal cortex damage in the rat, *Neurosci. Lett.*, **32**, 125-130.

82. Vorhees, C., Butcher, R., Brunner, R., and Sobotka, T., 1979, A developmental test battery for neurobehavioural toxicity in rats: a preliminary analysis using monosodium glutamate, calcium carageenan, and hydroxyurea, *Toxicol. Appl. Pharmacol.*, **50**, 267-282.

83. Walsh, R., 1981, Sensory environments, brain damage, and drugs: a review of interactions and mediating mechanisms, *Int. J. Neurosci.*, **3-4** 129-138.

84. Ward, A.A., and Kennard, M.A., 1942, Effect of cholinergic drugs on recovery of function following lesions of the central nervous system in monkeys, *Yale J. Biol. Med.*, **15**, 189-228.

85. Whishaw, I.Q., Sutherland, R.J., and Kolb, B., 1986, Effects of neonatal forebrain noradrenaline depletion on recovery from brain damage: performance on a spatial navigation task as a function of age of surgery and postsurgical housing, *Behav. Neural. Biol.*, **46**, 285-307.

86. Whishaw, I.Q., Zaborowski, J.A., and Kolb, B., 1984, Postsurgical enrichment aids adult hemidecorticate rats on a spatial navigation task, *Behav. Neural Biol.*, **42**, 183-190.

87. Will, B., 1977, Methods for promoting functional recovery following brain damage, in *Brain Foetal and Infant. Current Research on Normal and Abnormal*, S.R. Berenberg, ed., pp. 330-344, Martinus Nijhoff, La Haye.

88. Will, B., 1981, The influence of environment on recovery after brain damage in rodents, in *Functional Recovery from Brain Damage*, M.W. van Hof and G. Mohn eds., pp. 167-188, Elsevier/North-Holland, Amsterdam.

89. Will, B., Deluzarche, F. and Kelche, C., 1983, Does postoperative environment attenuate or exacerbate symtoms which follow hippocampal lesions in rats? *Behav. Brain Res.*, **7**, 125-132.

90. Will, B., and Eclancher, F., 1984, Environmental effects on recovery, in *Early Brain Damage and Early Environment,* S. Finger and C.R. Almli, eds., pp. 349-367, Academic Press.

91. Will, B., Kelche, C., Deluzarche, F., 1981, Effects of postoperative environment in functional recovery after entorhinal cortex lesions in the rat, *Behav. Neural. Biol.*, **33**, 303-316.

92. Will, B. and Kelche, C., 1990, Environnement, développement normal et restauration fonctionnelle après atteinte cérébrale, *Neuropsy.*, **9**, 510-520.

93. Will, B., Rosenzweig, M.R., Bennett, E.L., 1976, Effects of differential environments on recovery from neonatal brain lesions, measured by problem-solving scores, *Physiol. Behav.*, **16**, 603-611.

94. Will, B., Rosenzweig, M.R., Bennett, E.L., Hebert M., and Morimoto, H., 1977, Relatively brief environmental enrichment aids recovery of learning capacity and alters brain measures after postweaning brain lesions in rats, *J. Comp. Physiol. Psychol.*, **91**, 33-50.

95. Will, B., Toniolo, G., Kelche, C., Pallage, V., Deluzarche, F., and Misslin, R., 1986, The effects of postoperative physical environment on novelty seeking behaviour and maze learning in rats with hippocampal lesions, *Behav. Brain Res.*, **19**, 233-240.

96. Wolgin, D.L., and Teitelbaum, P., 1978, Role of activation and sensory stimuli in recovery from lateral hypothalamic damage in the cat, *J. Comp. Physiol. Psychol.*, **3**, 474-500.

97. York, A.D., Breedlove, S.M., Diamond M.C., and Greer, E.R., 1989, Housing adult male rats in enriched conditions increases neurogenesis in the dentate gyrus, *Soc. Neurosci. Abstr.*, **383**, 11.

NEUROPSYCHOLOGICAL REHABILITATION

Leonard Diller

Rusk Institute Rehabilitation Medicine
New York University Medical Center
New York, U.S.A.

INTRODUCTION

Students of recovery of CNS damage are generally interested in organismic and environmental factors and their interactions which influence behaviors of individuals. Major considerations pertain to age of onset and age of examination, time since onset, gender, and etiology, locus, and extent of brain damage. The major indicators of recovery are generally carefully calibrated situations with precise stimuli and response dimensions. The aims are generally to document CNS factors in recovery. Such studies usually use experimental methods to elucidate mechanisms of function e.g. the induction of an alternate way of handling or training an animal to alter a response. Since these approaches are well covered in other papers in this volume there is no reason to dwell further on them in this paper.

REHABILITATION : A FRAMEWORK FOR RECOVERY

The context in which rehabilitation services operate provide a somewhat different perspective for looking at recovery. The major innovation in rehabilitation after the second world war which helps define the modern era, is not in its techniques or theories, but in its perspective and aims. The goal of rehabilitation is to assist a person with CNS damage to facilitate recovery and adaptation so that the individual with residual impairments can perform optimally and reduce the burdens on his/her environment. This is usually done by organizing a team of specialists to assist the individual to develop skills to overcome the disability imposed by impairments and to organize environmental resources to aid the process. The aims are utterly pragmatic and "functional".

The constraint offered by the presence of brain damage is only one element in the picture[43]. When one speaks of functions in this context, the term does not refer to issues in underlying substrates of behavior (impairments). The term refers to the ability to carry out practical activities such as those involved in self care (disabilities).

A function is not a property of an organism such as memory or perception. It is an activity such as walking or talking to permit the individual to carry out normal demands of living independently.

Traditional sociologists have approached this from a framework of disease, sickness and illness[48]. Students of rehabilitation have used a different but analogous vocabulary - impairment, disability and handicap[52]. An impairment is a defect in the structure of the organism through disease or trauma; A disability is a difficulty in performing an activity in the environment without support; A handicap is a difficulty in conducting role expected demands as a result of or in association with an impairment and or disability. This vocabulary permits a more fine grained description of phenomena associated with attempts to have individuals resume normalized roles following disease or trauma which may result in residual deficits. Thus recent studies attempting to reduce consequences of spinal cord injury by methylpresdinolone[10] used measures of impairment e.g. changes in muscle tone as outcome indicators but not measures of disability ie ability to function independently in self care. This exciting finding for students of recovery is therefore incomplete for students of rehabilitation.

CLASSICAL CLINICAL NEUROPSYCHOLOGY

Neurologists and neuropsychologists in the classical medical framework have placed major emphasis on diagnoses and syndromes, particularly on elucidating brain behavior relationships. Working in this tradition neuropsychologists have developed carefully normed tests which are measures of impairments i.e. indicators of cognitive deficit to match diagnoses or syndromes associated with pathology. Neuropsychologists in rehabilitation settings are confronted with issues of disability and handicap. They use measures which approximate naturalistic situations as indicators of disability. In medical rehabilitation, measures of disability are related to the level of assistance needed to complete a task. They are measures of burden. The aim of rehabilitation, in this sense, is to reduce burden resulting from damage to the CNS, from more assistance to less assistance.

Given the attractiveness and practicality of this perspective, it is easy to see why rehabilitation is basically a pragmatic loosely defined enterprise with a strong appeal on a personal as well as public policy level. Although there is little experimental evidence for therapeutic procedures used in rehabilitation settings[6], there is a serious attempt towards accountability, by the application of scales sensitive to levels of assistance or reductions in burden[17] for populations receiving rehabilitation interventions. These scales are used to document benefits associated with interventions in rehabilitation.

The current efforts in our cost conscious era are to build a body of data to document and eventually justify the use of procedures and services. There is an emerging body of normative data on rehabilitation outcomes in terms of disability indicators with more than a hundred studies in adult hemiplegics resulting from stroke[13]. Despite the fact that the handful of controlled studies do not lend strong support for the efficacy of specific interventions; eligibility and outcome are being judged in terms of how hemiplegics do in comparison with other hemiplegics. The Uniform Data System (UDS)[49], for example, has logged a vast amount of cases in its data base of different kinds of neurologic populations as of this writing. Rehabilitation centers decide admissions and discharges, and in the future, will market their programs by outcome data which show improvement. Like promotions in other industries they will attribute their products to the procedures which they employ. In effect these outcome measures will govern policy.

REHABILITATION AND COGNITIVE DISABILITY

An important gap at this point is the absence of measures of cognitive disability. While there are many scales to assess cognitive impairments, e.g. neuropsychological tests, there are few measures of cognitive disability. For example, what are real world indicators of a perceptual or a memory problem? A person with brain damage may score poorly on a neuropsychological test, but the test results offer only very gross indication of specific areas of disturbance in daily life activities. Two people with identical patterns of scores will behave very differently in situations outside of the test. Psychometric guidelines for therapeutic interventions are therefore too nonspecific to be useful in remedial situations.

What to do about this problem? Several approaches are beginning to emerge:

1. Developing tests which yield samples which more closely approximate real world behavior such as the Rivermead batteries for memory which sample real life tasks in controlled circumstances.

2. Designing test batteries which sample the complaints is a second approach. In a questionnaire study, it was found that the most bothersome aspect of memory in a head injured population was prospective memory, a feature of memory seldom assessed in conventional testing[31].

From a theoretical standpoint, rehabilitation in a sense maybe seen as an example of a field moving to articulate the interplay between laboratory derived measures (Binet's psychometric tests originated in laboratories to measure individual differences) and contextually derived measures. This movement resonates with the current dispute between laboratory and field approaches to cognition[3,5,37]. It suggests that issues in cognitive rehabilitation ultimately feed back onto basic issues of cognitive and educational psychology[18, 47].

PREDICTION STUDIES

Neuropsychologists in the classical diagnostic tradition have approached rehabilitation as a domain of activity to be predicted from a prior knowledge base developed for the elucidation of impairment due to pathology and disease. The results have produced a substantial body of literature regarding outcome predictions in the rehabilitation of individuals with brain damage due to stroke[27, 33] and traumatic brain injury[1]. The common elements in these prediction studies are attempts to designate criteria in terms of outcomes at later points in time and utilize measures of demographic, neurologic, and neuropsychologic status as independent variables obtained at earlier points in time. The major results of these studies are, at best modest positive correlations. In general more competent people will do better than less competent people[23, 29]. While this might be useful for identifying classes of people, it is not adequate for the management of the individual case.

From the standpoint of rehabilitation a major criticism of these studies is, that they do not take into account the content of therapy or remediation. It is almost as if the particularities of the treatment are substitutable. The criteria are so gross that, important and key outcome differences between patients are ignored. For example, the well known Glasgow Coma Scale developed by Jennet, has been used to predict outcome on the Glasgow Outcome Scale[26]. Yet the categories on this outcome measure are extremely broad, from bare survival to independent functioning. Because major quality of life issues are bypassed, such predictions are of limited help in overall management in rehabilitation. This has lead to the development of alternate or more sensitive measures e.g. the Diagnostic Rating Scale, (DRS)[40] with more refined indicators, such as employment, as an outcome. Yet even the refined measures maybe too broad to assess the efficacy of a specific cognitive intervention. For example, it may be possible to improve an individual's thinking following brain damage, but this improvement may not be related to employment. Outcomes should reflect goals of interventions. They must be sensitive to important individual and contextual features of clinical situations, as well as other determinants of policy goals.

In rehabilitation settings, one typically assesses the individual on a sampling of tasks which are to be taught in the program. In a physical medicine setting, a therapist wishing to assess the patient's ability to transfer from a bed to a wheel chair will typically provide the patient with a trial experience. A vocational counselor will introduce a worker with a disability to a job sample in addition to, or rather than, a standardized vocational test. A special education teacher will sample a child's response to a learning situation rather than rely only on a widely normed standardized test and finally a speech pathologist will attempt to sample an aphasic's response in a conversational context in addition to a response to a standard test.

Prediction studies, in brief, have failed to engage specific contents of therapies involved in rehabilitation. Because of this they become less sensitive to the decisions which take place in clinical management. While they may ultimately be useful with regard to program evaluation issues, they are less useful in regard to the needs of individual patients.

In the case of traumatic brain injury, one approach is to identify behaviors which are central to the problems of the patient sample and treat these behaviors and test whether the samples predict outcomes. For example, in our setting while we have emphasized a variation of remediation for two major domains, divided into the cognitive and the social, we have also focussed on acceptance of disability as a central content and goal for the rehabilitation of individuals with severe brain injury. For these individuals with traumatic brain damage, with a combination of cognitive and behavioral disturbances which interfered with return to work, we set up a program which emphasized the following; the individual acknowledging and accepting the trauma, the disabilities which followed from the trauma, the consequences of these disabilities and most importantly engaging in a program to address the life changes brought about by the trauma. We were able to demonstrate that if one layers the independent variables gathered on admission and during the program, then one finds that neurological (duration of coma), demographic (age), neuropsychological (test scores) data gathered at the beginning of the program combine to yield a significant prediction of outcome. However, a measure of acceptance of disability based on observed ratings during participation in the program, significantly enhances the power to predict return to employment after the program had been completed[15].

COGNITIVE REMEDIATION

A decade ago, a colleague and I reviewed the state of knowledge with regard to interventions for cognitive deficits in individuals with brain damage[14,41]. At that time we found that there were approximately three dozen papers, with two thirds concerned with behavior modification to deal with behavioral symptoms of dysfunction across a wide band of neurologic syndromes. Only a handful were concerned with the alleviation of cognitive deficit and the development of skills to permit normal functioning in stroke and brain trauma. For the most part, the studies aimed at improving cognition were applications of cuing systems in right and left brain damaged people and the use of mnemonic devices to improve memory. Most of the studies were of a laboratory type, with little direct evidence for actually helping patients in the real world. Since the studies were too few to focus on results, it was more important to focus on methodologies. A most critical element noted, was a need to translate sound approaches in experimental design to capture events which could be public, repeatable, and measurable. Thus in rehabilitation the need was not only for a theory of brain damage as a platform for deductions about a given path of intervention. It was at least as important to spell out a theory of treatment in steps which took into account what was being treated i.e. the deficit state and how it was being operationalised, how the treatment occurred i.e. the precise instructions, the stimuli to be used and the rationale for given procedures, how were the treatment effects measured, what were the consequences of the treatment for real world functioning and who was being treated, i.e. the parameters of neuropsychologic dysfunction[14, 41]. Indeed except for the work of a few neuropsychologists most of the remediation attempts are addressed to the presenting behavioral impairments or disabilities associated with brain damage rather the brain damage itself[11].

Since the time of that review, there has been a considerable number of publications including review articles[7, 21, 50] and books on interventions for cognitive deficit[28]. Although remediation of perceptual problems, particularly difficulties associated with syndromes of visual neglect in patients with damage to the right hemisphere have received some attention, by far the greatest attention has been on interventions for individuals who have suffered traumatic head injury.

A Taxonomy for Interventions

A taxonomy for interventions might include the following ways of organizing the many studies.

1. **Direct remediation of cognitive impairments**. This approach basically identifies a deficit area such as attention, memory, perception, or thinking and formulates regimens to identify the deficit, presents tasks to patients which break the deficit area into component parts, teaches patients strategies to achieve success and offers a good deal of practice and feedback to build up skill levels. This approach may utilize computers as the major method of presenting materials or, as a supplementary modality for more precise control of stimuli and feedback for responses.

The underlying premise is that cognitive deficits reflect impairments of skill substrates such as the kind identified on psychometric or neuropsychologic tests. At more severe levels of brain damage, these impairments must be addressed. Correction of these substrates may be useful but it must be accompanied by practice of the new found skills in an actual life situation.

In 1989 Benedict[7] reviewed studies in cognitive remediation which covered most of the literature in this area. Analysis of 12 studies reported for improving attention and 11 studies reported for improving memory, reveals that nearly 60 % of the studies are single case reports, less than one quarter used formal single case designs, and only 13% involved experimental vs. control groups. While most studies show improvement as a result of training, the most striking impressions are the lack of replication in either assessment or treatment procedures. In the one replication[39] it is unclear whether failure to duplicate previous results[8] was due to fewer hours of treatment than in the first study. More recent studies have shown more sophisticated designs. Thus Ryan and Ruff[42] in a well controlled study, found that in a sample of "moderate to severely" impaired individuals with traumatic brain damage, the milder patients within their sample benefitted from an intensive cognitive retraining program in attention and memory. Neiman, Ruff, and Baser[36] found that attention training was more effective than memory training, when two groups who received different types of training were compared with each other. The procedures have been carefully developed. By way of contrast a study using computerized means to train in attention vs. reasoning found equal gains in both methods. Specific computer training did not have a differential effect on criteria[34].

If we regard Benedict's review as a reflection of a second generation of interest following the earlier review[14], one is struck by the explosion of clinical activity which is slowly being hammered out in a more scientific direction. Increasingly investigators are coming to grips with issues such as the recognition that:-

(a) a single deficit such as attention may encompass a series of subdeficits in attention. The treatment of an attention deficit requires the analysis and treatment of substrates of attention. Ben Yishay et al[8] proposed a hierarchy of subtasks to be remediated. This hierarchy was based on clinical observation and phenomenological analysis. Moore-Sohlberg and Mateer[35] proposed a hierarchy based on clinical observation. Their approach, postulates treatment to certain levels of skill before the introduction of the next level or domain of skill. This is analogous to the platform approach adopted in developing a package of skills for the treatment of visual neglect in stroke patients. While there have been attempts to apply more generic theories of the structure of attention to account for deficits in attention in individuals with traumatic brain injury e.g. Sternberg's theory (see 46) there has been little application to remediation.

(b) cognitive deficits generally coexist. It is rare to find a problem in attention existing in isolation from other cognitive deficits. Clinically, the treatment of a single deficit may be hampered by the presence of another deficit. In addition treating an isolated deficit may not bring about change which is clinically meaningful[20]. One approach to this problem is to combine treatments of coexisting deficits resulting in simultaneous multimodality treatments. In a formal experiment one can deal with the issue of the confounding of treatments by varying the hours or intensity of the treatment modalities in different groups of people.[9]

2.   Intervention in naturalistic contexts

(a)   It can be argued that learning takes place best via direct experience in a situation in which the task to be performed becomes the content of the training. Work samples, educational samples, and competency based types of examinations follow this line of reasoning. The argument takes on additional claim when one recognizes that concrete thinking and difficulty in generalization are hall marks of traumatic brain injury.

Several paths of remediation have been pursued along this way. Conducting a job sample of a specific task to be learned and training directly for each step in the task. Thus Mayer et al[32] found that toothbrushing is a task which can fractionated into steps which can be trained. A further example, is a method for training an individual to perform cleaning tasks through the use of a computer providing cuing in a hospital situation. Chaining a series of steps to develop skills to master more complex activities has been used to train severely impaired patients to be operate computers[44]. These studies are of interest not only for their practical value, but they assume in advance that brain damaged people are concrete in their thinking, that individuals are motivated to perform activities which are meaningful and relevant, but cannot generalize beyond specific domains in procedures used to perform a task. They also utilize different perspectives towards instruction. Thus Mayer's group[32] emphasizes correction of errors, which is related to examining response style or process approaches, in clinical neuropsychology. Schachter and Gliskey[44] use a method of fading cues derived from experimental cognitive psychology. They also draw on Shachter's well known notions of implicit memory remaining more intact than explicit memory in amnesics so that individuals who cannot recall well, recognize stimuli[45].

Less systematic, are applications of cuing and prompts for specific tasks in the expanding field of supportive employment. Supportive employment wherein individuals are placed directly in carefully monitored work situations under a job coach, is a major innovative approach in returning individuals with disabilities to work[51].

(b)   Individuals with impairments due to traumatic brain injury have been taught different kinds of strategies to overcome cognitive disability. Thus in one earlier study, Glasgow et al[19] taught a brain injured person with a problem in reading comprehension and retention, a strategy for improving both. Cicerone and Wood[12] helped manage impulse control in a patient by first teaching a strategy for self regulation in completing the Tower of Hanoi problem, and then applying this strategy in a social situation.

(c)   Problem solving is an emerging area. Simulations derived from work with other populations were successfully used with three traumaticallly brain injured patients[16]. Adamovich et al[2] point out that successful problem solving skills generally include methods for verbal reasoning skills (categorization, convergent thinking, divergent thinking) and executive functions involving self monitoring and modifying the smooth execution of action plans.

(d)   In dealing with remediation of cognitive activities such as problem solving, a combination of remedial exercises and applications in naturalistic situations appears to be the dominant mode. There is a growing trend to the study of learning and memory in naturalistic situations in non brain damaged people. Studies in strategies used in everyday problem solving and memory have not as yet been systematically codified and incorporated in rehabilitation. Aside from the field of health care, there has been study by commercial interests e.g. advertising agencies and public media which are potentially useful[25].

3.   **Prosthetic devices**. During the past decade there has been increasing attention to using prosthetic devices as cognitive aids[22,30]. Such devices, including commercial memory aids[24] range from simple dairies or electric timers to more sophisticated electronic aids adapted to cognitively impaired.   Many can be purchased commercially[38]. One problem in severely impaired patients, is that the use of such devices may require extensive training. It may be difficult, for example to train a person who forgets, to use a dairy, to keep appointments. At the present time prosthetic memory aids maybe used, but not without instruction and practice.

SOME FUTURE DIRECTIONS IN COGNITIVE REMEDIATION

The application of cognitive remediation as a treatment for traumatically brain injured over the past decade has seen two major corollary areas of growth.

1.   The development of strategies for improving cognitive functioning in diverse groups of cognitively disabled individuals, including learning disabled, mentally retarded, and other subgroups of neurologically disabled. Many of the concepts e.g. the role of metacognition and generalization in retraining, developed in working with other groups of cognitively impaired, are beginning to appear in the literature on traumatic brain injury.

2.   To be effective in rehabilitation, cognitive remediation must be tied to self efficacy[4]. In cognitive remediation it is clear that issues of motivation and self concept play an increasingly critical role as one moves away from training motoric components of daily living to the interpersonal, the vocational, and the 'well being 'components. Issues of awareness of cognitive disabilities play an enormous role in patient cooperation and engagement in procedures which may be perceived as disconnected from pre traumatic life expectations. Future studies will see attempts to develop outcome measures and training programs for brain damaged people building on advances in cognitive psychology and motivational psychology. It will incorporate not only programs for problem solving, but also develop programs acceptance and self efficacy. The latter fit well into notions of empowerment currently promoted as policy for individuals with disability.

ACKNOWLEDGEMENTS

This work was supported by a grant from the National Institute on Disability and Rehabilitation Research, Department of Education, Grant # HI 33BOO2894, to New York University, School of Medicine, as a Research and Training Center for traumatic brain injury.

REFERENCES

1. Acker, M., 1986, Relationships between test scores and everyday life, in *Neuropsychological Intervention*, B. P. Uzzel and Y. Gross, eds., pp. 85-118, Martinus Nijhoff, Boston.
2. Adamovich, B.B., Henderson, J.A., and Auerbach, S., 1985, *Cognitive Rehabilitation of Closed Head Injured Patients*, College Hill Press, San Diego.
3. Banaji, M.R., and Crowder, R.G., 1989, The bankruptcy of everyday memory, *Amer. Psychol.*, **44**, 1185-1196.
4. Bandura, A., 1986, *Social Foundations of Thought and Action; A Social Cognitive Theory*, Prentice-Hall, Englewood Cliffs, New Jersey.
5. Barrett, G. V., and Depinet, R. L., 1991, A reconsideration of testing for competence rather than for intelligence, *Amer. Psychol.*, **46**, 1012-1024.
6. Basmajian, J.V., 1989, The winter of our discontent: Breaking intolerable time locks for stroke survivors, *Arch. Phys. Med. Rehab.*, **70**, 92-95.
7. Benedict, R.H., 1989, The effectiveness of cognitive remediation strategies for victims of traumatic head injury, *Clin. Psychol. Review*, **9**, 608-626.
8. Ben-Yishay, Y., Piasetsky, E.B., and Rattok, J., 1987, A systematic method for ameliorating disorders in basic attention, in *Neuropsychological Rehabilitation*, M.J. Meier, A.L. Benton, and L. Diller, eds., pp. 165-181, Guilford Press, New York.
9. Ben-Yishay, Y., and Diller, L., (in press), Cognitive remediation in traumatic brain injury: Update and issues, *Arch. Phys. Med. Rehab.*
10. Bracken, M.B., Shepard, M.J., Collins, W.F., Holford, T.R., Young, W., Baskin, D.S., Eisenberg, H.M., Flamm, E., Leo-Summers, L., Maroon, J., Marshall,L.F., Perot, Jr., P.L., Peipmeier, J., Sonntag, V.K.L., Wagner, F.C., Wilberger, J.E.,and Winn, H.R., 1990, A randomized, controlled trial of methylprednisolone or naloxone in the treatment of acute spinal-cord injury, *New Eng. J. Med.*, **322**, 1405-1411.
11. Butler, R.H., and Namerow, N.S., 1988, Cognitive retraining in brain injury rehabilitation. A critical review, *J. Neurol. Rehab.*, **2**, 97-102.
12. Cicerone, K.D., and Wood, J.C., 1987, Planning disorder after closed head injury. A case study, *Arch. Phys. Med. Rehab.*, **68**, 111-115.
13. Diller, L., 1990, Outcomes in stroke rehabilitation, in *Third Annual Stroke on ference*, Spaulding Rehabilitation Center, Boston.
14. Diller, L., and Gordon, W.A., 1981, Interventions for cognitive deficits in brain-injured adults, *J. Cons. Clin. Psychol.*, **49**, 822-834.
15. Ezrachi, O., Ben-Yishay, Y., Kay,T., Diller, L. and Rattock, J., 1991, Predicting employment outcome after neuropsychological rehabilitation, *J. Head Trauma Rehab.*, **6**, 71-84.
16. Foxx, R.M., Martella, R.C., and Marchand-Martella, N.E., 1989, The acquisition,

maintenance, and generalization of problem-solving skills by closed head-injured adults, *Behavior Therapy*, **20**, 61-76.

17. Fuhrer, M.S., 1987, *Functional Outcomes*, Paul H. Brookes Co., Baltimore.

18. Gardner, H., 1991, Tensions between education and development, *J.Moral Develop.*, **20**, 113-125.

19. Glasgow,R.S., Zeiss, R.A., Barrera,M.D., and Lewinsohn, P., 1977, Case studies in remeding memory deficits in brain damaged individuals, *J.Clin.Psychol.*, **33**, 1049-1054.

20. Gordon, W.A., 1987, Methodological considerations in cognitive remediation, in *Neuropsychological Rehabilitation*, M.J. Meier, A.L. Benton, and L. Diller, eds., pp. 111-131, Guilford Press, New York.

21. Gordon,W.A., and Hibbard, M.R., 1991, The theory and practice of cognitive rehabilitation, in *Cognitive Rehabilitation for Persons with Traumatic Brain Injury*, J.S. Kreutzer, and P.H. Wehman, eds., pp. 13-22, Paul H. Brookes Co., Baltimore.

22. Harris, J.E. and Morris, P.E., eds., 1984, *Everyday Memory Actions and Absentmindedness*, Academic Press, London.

23. Heaton, R., and Pendleton, M., 1981, Use of neuropsychological tests to predict adult patients everyday functioning, *J.Cons.Clin.Psychol.*, **49**, 807-821.

24. Herrmann, D.J., and Petro, S.J., 1991, Commercial memory aids, *App. Cog. Psychol.*, **3**.

25. Herrmann, D.J. and Searleman, A., 1990, The new multimodal approach to memory improvement, *Psychol. Learn. Motivat.*, **26**, 175-205.

26. Jennett, B., and Bond, M., 1975, Assessment of outcome after severe brain damage. A practical scale, *Lancet*, **I**, 480-487.

27. Jongbloed, L., 1987, Prediction of function after stroke. A critical review, *Stroke*, **17**, 765-787.

28. Kreutzer, J.H. and Wehman, P.H., eds., 1991, *Cognitive Rehabilitation for Persons with Traumatic Brain Injury A Functional Approach*, Paul H. Brookes Co., Baltimore.

29. Lam, C.S., Priddy, D.A., and Johnson, P., 1991, Neuropsychological indicators of employability following traumatic brain injury, *Rehab. Psychol. Bulletin*, **35**, 69-75.

30. Levin, W., 1991, Computer applications in cognitive rehabilitation, in *Cognitive Rehabilitation for Persons with Traumatic Brain Injury: A Functional Approach*, J.S. Kreutzer, and P.H. Wehman, eds., pp. 163-180, Paul H. Brookes Co., Baltimore.

31. Mateer, C.A., and Sohlberg, M.M., 1988, A paradigm shift in memory rehabilitation, in *Neuropsychological Studies of Non Focal Brain Damage: Dementia and Trauma*, H. Whitaker, ed, pp. 209-214, Springer Verlag, New York.

32. Mayer, N., Keating,D.J., and Rapp, D., 1986, Skills, routines and activity patterns: A functional nested approach, in *Clinical Neuropsychology of Intervention*, B. Uzzel, and Y. Gross, Y., eds., pp. 205-222, Martinus Nijhuss, Boston.

33. Meier, M.J., Strauman, S., Thompson, W.G., 1987, Individual differences in psychological recovery: an overview, in *Neuropsychological Rehabilitation*, M.J. Meier, A.L. Benton, and L. Diller, eds., pp. 71-110, Guilford Press, New York.

34. Middleton, D.K., Lambert, M.J., and Seggar, L.B., 1991, Neuropsychological

rehabilitation: Microcomputor-assisted treatment of brain injured adults, *Percep. Mot. Skills*, **72**, 527-530.

35. Moore-Sohlberg, M., and Mateer, C.A., 1987, Effectiveness of an attentional training program, *J. Clin. Exper. Neuropsychol.*, **9**, 117-130.

36. Neiman, H., Ruff, R.M., and Baser, C.A., 1990, Computer-assisted attention retraining in head-injured individuals: A controlled efficacy study of an outpatient program *J. Consult. Clin. Psychol.*, **58**, 811-817.

37. Neisser, U., 1991, A case of misplaced nostalgia, *Amer. Psychol.*, **46**, 34-36.

38. Parente', R., and DiCesare, A., 1991, Retraining memory: Theory, evaluation, and applications, in *Cognitive Rehabilitation for Persons with Traumatic Brain Injury; A Functional Approach*, J.S. Kreutzer, and P.H. Wehman, eds., pp. 147-162, Paul H. Brookes, Baltimore.

39. Ponsford, J.L., and Kinsella, G., 1988, Evaluation of a remedial programme for attentional training following closed head injury, *J. Clin. Exper. Neuropsychol.*, **10**, 693-708.

40. Rappaport, M., Hall, K.M., Hopkins, K. & Belleza, T., 1982, Disability Rating Scale for severe head trauma patients: Coma to community, *Arch. Phys. Med. Rehab.*, **63**, 118-127.

41. Ruff, R.M. and Camenzuli,L.F., 1991, Research challenges for behavioral rehabilitation. Searching for solutions, in *Cognitive Rehabilitation for Persons with Traumatic Brain Injury. A Functional Approach*, J.S. Kreutzer, and P.H. Wehman, eds., pp. 23-34, Paul H. Brookes Co., Baltimore.

42. Ryan, T.V. and Ruff, R.M., 1988, The efficacy of structured memory retraining in a group comparison of head injured patients, *Arch. Clin. Neuropsychol.*, **3**, 165-179.

43. Sbdorne, R.J. Management of psychosocial and behavioral problems in cognitive rehabilitation, in *Cognitive Rehabilitation for Persons with Traumatic Brain Injury. A Functional Approach*, J.S. Kreutzer, and P.H. Wehman, eds., pp. 105-116, Paul H. Brookes, Co., Baltimore.

44. Schachter, D., 1987, Implicit memory: History and current status, *J. Exp. Psychol: Learn, Memory and Cognit.*, **13**, 501-518.

45. Schachter, D., and Glisky, E.L., 1986, Memory remediation: restoration, alleviation, and the acquisition of domain specific knowledge, in *Clinical Neuropsychology of Intervention*, B. P. Uzzel, and Y. Gross, eds., pp. 257-282, Martinus Nijhoff Co., Boston.

46. Shum, D.H.K., McFarland, K., Bain, J.D., and Humphreys,,M.S, 1990, Effects of closed head injury on attentional processes :an information - processing stage analysis, *J. Clin. Exper. Neuropsychol.*, **12**, 247-264.

47. Sternberg, R.J., 1990, T & T is an explosive combination: Technology and Testing, *Educat. Psychol.*, **25**, 201-222.

48. Susser, M., 1990, Editorial: Disease, illness, sickness: impairment, disability and handicap, *Psychol. Med.*, **20**, 471-473.

49. UDS Update, 1991, *Uniform Data System for Medical Rehabilitation*, Buffalo, New York: Department of Rehabilitation Medicine.

50. Volpe, B.P., and McDowell, F.H., 1990, The efficacy of cognitive rehabilitation in persons with traumatic brain injury, *Arch. Neurol.*, **47**, 220-222.

51. Wehman, P.J., and Kreutzer, J.S., 1991, *Vocational Rehabilitation of Persons with Traumatic Brain Injury*, Aspen, Rockville, MD.

52. World Health Organization, 1980, *International Classification of Impairments, Disabilities, and Handicaps. A Manual of Classification Relating it to the Consequences of Disease.* Geneva World Health Organization.

HEMIDECORTICATION AND RECOVERY OF FUNCTION: ANIMAL STUDIES

F D Rose
Department of Psychology
Goldsmiths' College
University of London
London, England

Ian Q Whishaw
Department of Psychology
University of Lethbridge
Alberta, Canada

M W van Hof
Department of Physiology I
Erasmus University
Rotterdam, The Netherlands

INTRODUCTION

Hemidecortication may be defined as the surgical removal of the entire neocortex on one side of the brain. Its use in the elucidation of brain behaviour relationships dates back to the latter part of the last century, for example, to the work of Vulpian[107], Carville and Duret[12], Soltmann[98] and Goltz[27] and the early years of the present century also saw a steady stream of relevant studies (for example, 5,17,23,24,34,39,48,54,73,90,101). However, some of these early reports are not easily available and mention of them in papers such as those of Tsang[103], Bromiley[6] and White et al.[122] rarely detail the exact extent of surgical intervention. Detailed accounts of the behavioural consequences of hemidecortication are nevertheless contained in several reports dating from the first half of the century[6,26,35,36,37,49,103,113]. More recently, as well as some isolated reports (e.g. 100,112), there have been further series of hemidecorticate studies carried out in the laboratories of Russell[60,61,62,63,64,65,91,92,93], Rose [16,81,82,83,84,85,86,87,88], van Hof[31,104,105,106] and Whishaw[40,41,43,44,46,116,117,118,121]

In total the literature detailing the behavioural impairments of surgically hemidecorticated animals is quite extensive and encompasses studies of numerous categories of behaviours in a variety of species (cats, rats, rabbits and primates). It is only recently, however, that the potential value of the hemidecorticate in investigating mechanisms underlying recovery of function has been acknowledged. In this chapter we shall examine hemidecortication as a model preparation for recovery of function research and focus upon some of the studies in which hemidecortication has been used to investigate recovery and related phenomena such as sparing of function and age effects in lesion deficits.

HEMIDECORTICATION AS A MODEL FOR STUDYING RECOVERY OF FUNCTION FOLLOWING BRAIN DAMAGE

Several arguments have been advanced for using hemidecortication in recovery of function research[82,83,84].

1. Not least of these is the sizeable literature on the behavioural effects of hemidecortication referred to above. From this literature we already have quite detailed knowledge of the sensory capacities and motor characteristics of hemi-decorticate animals and of both their learned and unlearned behaviours. In addition, the secondary effects of hemidecortication on the rest of the brain are quite well documented (see below). Overall this provides a valuable baseline profile against which to view recovery of function.

2. A second and more fundamental argument for the use of the hemidecorticate is that it provides a way of studying the aftermath of a large lesion without allowing the processes of recovery of lost function and sensory compensation for lost function to become conflated. Among those studying cortical involvement in learning and memory the resurgence of interest in the hemidecorticate in the late 1960's was due, in part, to the work of Russell[91,92]. He argued that the hemidecorticate provides a means of separating out genuine learning impairments from the consequences of the sensory channel loss[32] which follows extensive bilateral cortical lesions. Complete hemi-decortication, he argued, still spares a significant proportion of the pathways of all sensory modalities, and certainly a sufficient proportion to accommodate the sensory requirements of most learning tasks. If the hemidecorticate deficit in learning tasks could not be explained in terms of sensory channel loss it seemed reasonable to suppose it was due to impaired learning or memory. In the context of recovery of function research Rose and coworkers[82,83,84] have presented a rather similar argument. After bilateral cortical lesions it is often difficult to distinguish the contributions to any reduction in impairment of recovery of cognitive function and compensation for sensory channel loss inadvertently caused by the lesion. However, since after hemi-decortication there is significant sparing in all sensory channels there is neither need for, nor value in, a compensatory switch to a different sensory channel. Any reduction in a hemidecorticate impairment is correspondingly more likely to reflect genuine recovery of function, therefore.

In the light of recent discussion of lesion size effects on functional impairment [33,51,52] this line of argument for the use of the hemidecorticate might be extended still further. Indeed hemidecortication, in sparing a proportion of not just sensory and motor systems but all bilaterally symmetrical neural systems, may provide a unique opportunity to study recovery from a large lesion which does not spare any significant part of the target structure and yet which avoids triggering the type of "shift in neural systems" hypothesised by LeVere[52].

A final point, and one that is related to bilateral symmetry of neural systems, is that in a hemidecorticate preparation the intact hemisphere can be used as a control for the damaged one. This argument also formed part of Russell's case for the use of hemidecortication in relating brain structure and function[91,92] but it has just as much relevance to studies of the neural basis of recovery from lesion impairments. In both contexts the adequacy of the spared hemisphere as a control for the lesioned one depends upon the degree of structural and functional symmetry between the hemispheres in the species in question, of course, and this point will be taken up later in the present discussion.

3. A third potential advantage of using surgical hemidecortication in recovery of function studies lies in the existence of a sizeable parallel literature on the behavioural effects of "functional" hemidecortication[92] produced by cortical spreading depression. According to Marshall[55] and Ochs[66] although cortical spreading depression was first observed by Dusser de Barrenne and McCulloch[19] it was first described in detail by Leao[50]. It involves a wave of depression of normal electrical activity spreading outwards from the point of elicitation to encompass the whole of the neocortical mantle of that hemisphere. It can be elicited by electrical, mechanical, thermal or chemical stimuli although most usually, in behavioural studies, by topical application of dilute potassium chloride (KCl) to the dura. This depression of activity typically occurs within twenty minutes of KCl application and can be maintained for up to three or four hours[10] although the exact duration of the depression of activity depends on a number of factors[11]. In most behavioural studies which have utilised the cortical spreading depression technique the primary interest has been in interhemispheric transfer and lateralisation of learning. However, within this literature there is a considerable amount of information about the performance of the functional hemidecorticate in a variety of behavioural test situations[11,81].

As a functional hemidecortication, unilateral cortical spreading depression is not without its complications[81,87]. For example, it does not result in complete suppression of electrical activity in the affected hemineocortex and there is evidence that it spreads to other parts of the brain[11]. Nevertheless, Rose et al[86] have argued that the comparison of the functional and surgical hemidecorticate preparations, if used with caution, can provide a valuable means of assessing the functional significance of compensatory and other changes occurring during the postoperative recovery period in the surgical preparation.

Although the case for equivalence of functional and surgical hemidecortication must not be overstated we believe much can be learned from their conjoint use and that this is an area of enquiry which merits more attention than it has so far received. Worth mentioning in passing is the claim that the functional hemidecorticate is not the only preparation which might be used as a control for aspects of surgical hemidecorticate function. Plotkin & Russell[71] and Sechzer[97] have suggested that surgical split-brain animals in which sensory input is lateralised to one hemisphere might be seen as functioning in an effectively hemidecorticate state. Such an argument assumes a lack of extra-callosal communication between the hemispheres, however, and the use of split brain subjects to study hemidecorticate function should be approached with great caution, therefore.

4. A powerful argument for using the surgical hemidecorticate animal in the investigation of recovery of function is that, in anatomical terms, it has a human equivalent in many hemispherectomy procedures. Elsewhere in this volume work on recovery of function following hemispherectomy in humans is reviewed by Vargha-Khadem. As she observes, whilst some hemispherectomies have involved a very radical resection of one hemisphere, frequently these procedures might be more accurately described as hemidecortications. That hemidecorticate data is available not only from rats, cats, rabbits, dogs and monkeys, but also from humans provides a unique opportunity for neuroscientists to compare recovery of function across different species

and, in particular, to begin to assess the importance of cerebral asymmetry and language to the recovery process. We shall return to question of cerebral asymmetry below.

METHODOLOGICAL CONSIDERATIONS IN STUDYING HEMIDECORTICATION

Methods of Hemidecortication

Hemidecortication, although an extensive lesion, is relatively uncomplicated from a surgical point of view. Indeed, in the lissencephalic brain it presents fewer problems than more restricted neocortical extirpations because the lesion boundaries are much more clearly defined. Nevertheless, in practice complete hemidecortication is an ideal[91,92] and the possibility of some sparing of neocortcal tissue must be taken into account in interpreting hemidecorticate behaviour.

In detail, methods of hemidecortication vary from one laboratory to another but usually involve either direct aspiration of neocortical tissue[121] or removal of the pial blood supply to one hemineocortex as recommended by Woolsey[123]. Whilst the former method may carry a greater risk of direct subcortical damage, in practice there seems little to choose between the methods in terms of the extent and accuracy of the lesion.

Effects of Hemidecortication Elsewhere in the Brain

Hemidecortication causes secondary degenerative damage, of course, and this must also be taken into account in explaining hemidecorticate deficits and recovery from them. However, the nature and extent of this secondary damage has been extensively studied over the years and is now well documented[15,20,21,43,56,58,59,68,69,70,74,89, 108,109,110,111].

Given the extent of the intervention involved, removal of neocortex unilaterally has surprisingly benign effects on the rest of the brain. Expectedly many researchers [15,56,58,59,68,69,70,74,89,108,109,111] have found extensive retrograde changes in the thalamus affecting all five morphological groups of thalamic nuclei[78] ipsilateral to the lesion. There is evidence of degenerative damage due to surgical hemidecortication in other parts of the brain also[20,21,56,59,68,69,111] but there is some disagreement about the extent of this extra-thalamic degenerative damage. Most of the rest of the brain with which the cortex shares reciprocal connections, including the hippocampus, basal ganglia, brainstem, cerebellum and spinal cord appear to be relatively unaffected by hemidecortication[43].

Further evidence of the relatively confined effects of hemidecortication on other parts of the brain comes, firstly, from the observation that brain weight changes in operated animals can be attributed mainly to the surgically removed tissue[43]. Secondly, hemidecortication causes surprisingly little disruption of the overall electrical activity of the brain. Kennard and Nims[38] recorded both pre- and post-operative EEG patterns from six electrodes applied to the scalp above frontal, parietal and occipital areas in four hemidecorticated monkeys. In the few days immediately following the operation a general slowing and flattening of the EEG was noticed, but this was a transient pattern and, being independent of the locus of the lesion, was probably due to some aspect of the operative procedure. Within a week of operation this transient effect disappeared and no further abnormality of the EEG was noticed despite a three year follow up observation period for two of the subjects.

Behavioural Assessment of the Hemidecorticate

The kinds of behavioural analysis that have been undertaken with hemidecorticate rats can be divided into studies in which general behavioural assessments are made and studies in which a single behaviour is analyzed in some detail. An example of the first kind of study is the "test battery" model described by Kolb and Whishaw[45]. This test battery approach is based on neurological and neuropsychological procedures used with humans, in which a wide range of tests are given to a subject in order to gain an overall view of sensorimotor and cognitive status. In animals the tests are designed to be administered both quickly and easily and to provide insights into the effects of age at surgery, age since surgery, and lesion size. Any interesting differences found using this procedure can then be examined in more detail.

The test battery approach has been successful in revealing a surprising array of impairments in hemidecorticate animals, including changes in postural adjustments, turning behaviour, orientating to sensory stimuli, use of limbs in swimming, and claw cutting. An example of its use in examining changes of appearance is illustrative. Hemidecorticate rats may fail to cut their claws [114], or when they do cut them they will do so only on the ipsilateral-to-lesion side [45]. The impairments can be quite different in adult and neonatally lesioned animals. Neonatal hemidecorticate rats are much more likely to cut their claws than adult lesioned animals [114]. Simple changes in testing procedure can also be used to uncover interesting abnormalities in the animals. For example, adult hemidecorticate animals twist contralateral to the lesion when suspended by the tail, but when placed on a flat surface or in water, they turn ipsilateral to the lesion. Neonatal animals will turn ipsilateral on a surface but contralateral in water. The lateralized biases appear immediately postoperative in adult animals and are enduring, whereas in neonatally lesioned animals the biases take a number of postoperative days to emerge.

The importance of this test battery approach in research on recovery of function cannot be overemphasised. Whilst earlier in this chapter we counted substantial sparing of pathways in all sensory modalities as a major advantage of the hemidecorticate in studying recovery, this is not to say that hemidecortication does not engender sensory impairment. Equally it is clear that the hemidecorticate has motor impairments (see below). A battery of tests has the advantage over single function behavioural tests in allowing such impairments to be detected and their individual and conjoint influence on both impairment levels and recovery curves to be estimated.

The second type of hemidecorticate study, in which a systematic analysis is made of one, or only a few behaviours, has been valuable in developing animal models of human disorders, analyzing the neural basis of a behaviour, or analyzing chemical or other changes that may occur following brain damage or during recovery. Included among the problems that hemidecorticate preparations can be used to study, are those that involve distinguishing between the contributions of subcortical vs cortical structures. Many kinds of subcortical damage involve damage to subcortical processing systems as well as to fibres of passage from the neocortex. Whishaw and Kolb [116] have examined the relative contributions of the neocortex and the lateral hypothalamus to feeding by making hypothalamic lesions in one hemisphere and decortications in the other. The behaviours of the animals were then compared to animals with bilateral lesions in either structure. The study demonstrated, among other things, that motoric impairments in mouth movements and licking could be ascribed to damage to corticofugal fibres whereas changes in regulation of feeding and drinking per se could be ascribed to hypothalamic damage. Thus, the study demonstrated that some of the deficits associated with the "lateral hypothalamic syndrome" were motoric and could be ascribed to cortical rather than hypothalamic function. Clearly this must be taken into account in explaining any recovery from the consequences of lateral hypothalamic damage.

In the following pages we shall refer to several other hemidecorticate studies of recovery related issues in which the emphasis is on one particular behaviour or category of behaviours.

HEMIDECORTICATION, RECOVERY AND RELATED PROCESSES: SPECIFIC CONTEXTS

Cerebral Lateralization and Dominance

Prominent features of human cognitive function are cerebral lateralization and cerebral dominance. Lateralization refers to the fact that one hemisphere is much more important for one aspect of the behaviour than is the other. For example, spoken language is usually mainly controlled by one hemisphere. Dominance refers to the fact that one hemisphere in an entire population is much more likely to control a given function than is the other. Thus, the left hemisphere controls speech in most people. Any explanation of recovery of function following brain damage in humans must take due account of this aspect of human brain organisation.

Lateralization and dominance are much more difficult to demonstrate in non-human species and are especiallly rare in non-primates. There have been extensive searches for evidence of dominance in non-human animals in the hope that such evidence might give insights into the evolution of human dominance. As might be expected, a good deal of this work has taken place with rats, and hemidecorticate preparations have played a role in this research. That is because if dominance could be demonstrated in a hemidecorticate preparation, the finding would be unequivocal. If a behaviour survived left but not right hemidecortication, for example, then it would be clear that that hemisphere would be responsible for mediating the behaviour. At least part of the impetus for a search for dominance comes from anatomical findings. The neocortex in the right hemisphere is thicker[18], larger and heavier than the left when measured in fixed normal rat brains[42], and the cross sectional area of the neocortex is greater for the right than for the left hemisphere[41]. In addition, there are several neurochemical asymmetries (see Kolb et al[42]) and reports of asymmetrical changes in activity in response to middle cerebral artery injury[80].

Despite extensive investigation, however, there is no evidence of behavioural dominance in terms of runway performance, brightness discrimination or reversal learning[81,83,87,88] or in motor coordination, social behaviour, spatial learning, feeding behaviour, beam running, puzzle latches, hoarding, nest building, running wheel activity or aggressive behaviour[41]. In all these respects the performances of rats with left hemidecortications have been found to be equivalent to rats with right hemidecortications. These results, of course, do not address whether behaviour may be lateralized in individual rats. They simply argue for the absence of behavioural dominance despite the presence of anatomical dominance.

There is evidence that some behaviours may be lateralized in individual rats, however. Mittleman, Whishaw and Robbins[57] have demonstrated lateralization in hemidecorticate rats tested in a visual reaction time task. In this study rats were trained to hold their heads still in a feeder and then to orient to either left or right when a light in the appropriate visual field went on. The light came on at some variable interval between 0 and 1.5 seconds after the rats had positioned their heads. The orienting response was reinforced with a food pellet delivered at the stimulus light source. Once the rats were trained and baseline performance was established, they were retested after an eye patch had been placed on either the left or right eye. Following this the rats were hemidecorticated.

Preoperatively all the rats showed a response bias although the bias was to the left in some rats and to the right in others. The bias consisted of a fast reaction time to the presentation of a stimulus on one side. The response to the stimulus on the other side was slow early in the delay interval and became progressively faster as the interval progressed. That is, the rats behaved as if they attended only to the light on one side. They oriented to it immediately when it came on and only turned in the other direction as it became evident that it was not coming on. The eye that they used to attend to the light could be called their dominant eye, therefore. Moreover, that this was the dominant eye could be demonstrated by an eye patching procedure. If the non-dominant eye was patched, the animal's behaviour was unaffected. However, if the dominant eye was patched the behaviour changed. Response latencies were elevated and the animal's bias switched so that it now appeared to watch for the light only with the non-dominant eye. Thus normal rats, although displaying a reaction time response bias indicating that they had a dominant eye, could respond using the other eye.

Half the rats then received hemidecortications ipsilateral to their dominant eye and half received hemidecortications contralateral to their dominant eye. The non-dominant lesions did not change reaction times or response bias. Thus the lesions were as benign as an eye patch on the non-dominant eye. In contrast, hemidecortications contralateral to the dominant eye profoundly affected a rat's ability to make cued responses to either side of visual space and the deficit was enduring. In fact reaction times to stimuli presented to the dominant eye could not be collected because the rats behaved as if they never saw stimuli in that hemispace (i.e. they always oriented in the contralateral direction). Thus, whereas the rats could compensate when a patch was placed on the dominant eye, they were completely unable to compensate for the loss of their "dominant" hemisphere.

This study provides perhaps the first demonstration of a lateralized capacity for bilateral visuomotor integration at the neocortical level in the rat. What the results show is that problems can be presented to the nervous system in such a way that it is efficient for the nervous system to lateralize its solution. Clearly this may have relevance to the question of the evolution of lateralization. Should a problem of this sort become pervasive in the ecological niche of a species, not only might the animal evolve asymmetric neural changes to solve the problem efficiently, it might also evolve cerebral dominance, if that were adaptive. Although the rat does not display dominance, the lateralization that it does display may represent a necessary stage in the evolution of cerebral dominance.

In the more immediate context of what we can learn about recovery of function from studying hemidecortication the finding is also of importance. The work of Mittleman, Whishaw and Robbins[57] increases the relevance of studies of rats to the understanding of recovery and related proceses in humans. Moreover, by careful selection of test situations it is now possible to compare recovery from deficits in lateralized and non-lateralized cortical functions in the same species. Additionally, by employing hemidecortication in these studies it may be possible to examine the role of intact cortex as opposed to subcortical structures in recovery. At present this line of enquiry is in its very early stages but, in the opinion of the present authors, it promises important insights into the benefits and limitations lateralization and dominance may impose on recovery of function in the damaged brain.

Sensorimotor Neglect

It is well known that in humans, damage to one hemisphere can result in changes in the detection of stimuli in the contralateral to lesion hemispace[25,47]. Neglect is said to occur if stimuli in the contralateral hemispace are not detected even though they are intense. Neglect is usually transient. A more long lasting consequence of injury is called simultaneous extinction[29]. In this case, if stimuli are presented simultaneously to both sides of the body only the stimulus in the good hemispace is detected. The contralateral stimulus appears to be masked until the ipsilateral stimulus is removed. A less pronounced phenomena is called obscuration[4]. Here two equally intense stimuli are detected, but the stimulus in the affected hemispace is reported to be subjectively weaker than that in the unaffected hemispace.

Neglect and phenomena related to neglect have been investigated in hemidecorticate rats in both naturalistic[115,120] and formal tests[95]. The former, a study of food related interactions between rats provides a good example of neglect and recovery from neglect in hemidecorticated animals. In this paradigm one hungry rat, the victim, is given a food pellet and a second hungry rat, the robber, attempts to steal its food. The robber typically approaches the victim from behind, walks along its side, and attempts to wrest the piece of food from the victim's mouth. The victim avoids this by dodging away from the robber, first stepping with the contralateral rear foot and then stepping with the ipsilateral rear foot, thus reversing its position by about 170^0. The dodge leaves the robber inconveniently located at its starting position with respect to the victim. All the while, the victim holds the food in its paws and continues to eat[119]. This interaction provides an excellent model for the study of neglect[115,120]. The response of a hemidecorticate victim to the approach of the robber on either its good or bad side can be contrasted. Also, the hemidecorticate animal can be used as the robber and its success in using either its good or bad side can be contrasted. Behaviours can be measured as success or failure and more detailed measures of distance, speed, and direction of movement can be made.

A hemidecorticate rat displays no impairment in using its "good" side. It can dodge a rat that is approaching its ipsilateral-to-lesion side and it can use its ipsilateral-to-lesion side to wrest food from a victim. It is impaired when using its contralateral-to-lesion side, but the severity and duration of the impairment depends upon the behaviour in which it is engaged. A victim is initially unable to evade the robber that approaches it on its bad side. The robber is always successful in stealing the victim's food. The victim gradually recovers, however, and by about 20 to 60 days postoperatively it is as successful in dodging the robber as it was preoperatively. The victim's initial impairment is not simply caused by a motor deficit in turning. When paired with another rat that steals its food, it will circle in the direction to which it could not dodge in order to approach the other rat and steal its food back. Thus, its inability to detect the robber is an important initial component of its deficit in dodging. A hemidecorticate rat's neglect of the hemispace contralateral to its decortication is not absolute, however. It recovers the ability to steal food using its bad side more rapidly than it recovers the ability to dodge. For example, by about three days postoperatively, two hemidecorticate rats, with lesions in opposite hemispheres, can be placed side by side and observed to take turns stealing the food from each other while neither dodges.

The more subtle forms of neglect, including simultaneous extinction and obscuration, have been reported in rats hemidecorticated in adulthood and studied for as long as one year following surgery[16,82,95].

In Schallert and Whishaw's experiments[95] pieces of sticky tape of various sizes were placed on the radial aspect of each forelimb as stimuli or else bracelets tied with knots of various difficulty were placed around each wrist. For a few days following surgery, the rats displayed neglect and did not remove stimuli placed on the wrist contralateral to the lesion hemisphere. Once they recovered from this absolute neglect, and for about two weeks after this, they displayed simultaneous extinction. They would not remove a stimulus contralateral to the lesion as long as there was a stimulus on the ipsilateral limb. They improved still further until by about three months postoperatively they displayed obscuration. Now they treated a stimulus on the affected limb as being smaller than it actually was. Thereafter, the rats displayed almost complete recovery. When tested as long as three to twelve months after surgery they displayed no asymmetry and sometimes actually showed a bias in responding to the stimulus on the wrist contralateral to the lesion. Only when the testing environment was altered could a residual impairment be revealed. Asymmetry in animals tested at 12 months was readily "reinstated" by testing the rat in a partially open rather than closed cage. When the cage was closed the rats displayed no bias, when the cage was opened the rats immediately displayed a bias away from the limb contralateral to the lesion. In addition, this form of stress could set back recovery at each stage. For example, rats that were no longer showing neglect after about five days of postsurgical recovery displayed neglect when their cage was opened.

In view of the striking progression of "recovery" in adult operated animals, it might be expected that neonatal hemidecortications would produce little effect on somatosensory responses. This was not the case for animals operated on neonatal day 1[96]. Neonatal hemidecorticate animals showed a persistent sensorimotor asymmetry. With equivalent stimuli on both wrists, they consistently removed the ipsilateral-to-lesion stimulus first. Furthermore, by adjusting the size of the stimuli on each wrist, the difference in stimulus size required to reverse their response could be shown to be nearly twice that required in adult animals. In another way, the neonatal operates were more resistant than adults to the effects of the surgery. The neonatally operated rats appeared to be capable of processing stimuli from both sides of the body simultaneously and thus seemed spared of the condition of simultaneous extinction displayed by adult rats during their asymmetrical stage of recovery. Thus, it appears that the neural reorganization associated with neonatal hemidecortication is associated with more severe or less severe impairments than associated with adult lesions, depending upon the test used.

These studies of neglect provide a good example of the potential value of the hemidecorticate in recovery of function research. Neglect findings with hemidecorticate rats constitute an animal model of a common consequence of brain injury in humans. The model allows not only detailed investigation of the neural basis, stages and time course of recovery of function but also the effects upon it of age and potentially restorative interventions, for example, postoperative environmental enrichment[82].

Motor Responding

The investigation of motor responding in hemidecorticate animals has already provided some useful insights into age dependent effects of brain damage and this use of the preparation certainly merits further attention from those with an interest in recovery and related phenomena.

Loss of hopping and placing following cortical damage in dogs cats rabbits and rats was the subject of considerable study during the first half of the century[1,2,3,7,8,9,19,76,77]. More recently van Hof and his colleagues have used this particular motor impairment to investigate age dependent sparing of function following hemidecortication in rabbits[31,104,105]. In these studies the hopping reaction of the forelegs was tested by means of a conveyer belt moving at a speed of 2.5 cm/second, on which the rabbit was held in such a way that the experimenter's hand supported the animal and one of its forelegs. The other forepaw touched the surface of the conveyer belt and supported the body. The animal was held at right angles to the direction of movement of the belt. The hopping response contains a passive component in which the leg follows the conveyer belt and an active one in which the leg is lifted and returned to its standing position.

It was found that the effects of hemidecortication on this hopping response was crucially dependent upon the age at which surgery was carried out. Five groups of rabbits were hemidecorticated between 0-1, 2-3, 4-5, 6-7, and 12-13 weeks of age, respectively. After a two week postoperative recovery period their hopping reactions were tested weekly for a period of fifteen weeks. Whilst the hopping reaction developed normally in the groups operated on before the end of the 5th week of life this was not the case with those animals operated on from 6 weeks onwards. In an attempt to identify the basis of this sparing process Hobbelen, Gramsbergen and Van Hof[31] carried out a serial hemidecortication study. A left hemidecortication was carried out on 14 rabbits aged between 14 and 21 days. Expectedly, in view of the earlier finding, a normal monopedal lateral hopping reaction was present in both forelegs following this operation. After a further 13 weeks, when the animals were adult, a hemidecortication of the remaining hemisphere was carried out and, three days later the hopping reaction tested. In all animals the hopping response in the right foreleg, contralateral to the first hemidecortication, was found to have survived, indicating that the sparing of the hopping response in animals operated on before the age of 6-7 weeks in the earlier study, was not mediated by corticofugal connections from the undamaged hemineocortex. Consistent with this conclusion is the confirmation from van Hof's group[106] of Macht's earlier finding with cats[53] that the lost placing response can be temporarily reinstated by amphetamine. In this case the hopping reaction contralateral to the side of lesion in 11 hemidecorticated rabbits was found to be present two hours after a subcutaneous injection of 5mg/kg of d-l amphetamine sulphate although the effect had disappeared 24 hours after the injection.

Rats with hemidecortications also show some spasticity and loss of placing and contactual responses in the limb contralateral to the lesion[92]. A symptom of these impairments is readily apparent when they are picked up by the tail because they immediately adduct the contralateral forelimb to the body rather than extending it to make contact with a surface as is normal[45]. Despite this they appear to perform a variety of movements, including walking, grooming, eating, etc. quite normally. However, several studies show that hemidecorticate rats do display motor impairments when performing some tasks requiring skilled movements. These movements include cutting the claws by nibbling at them with the teeth[44,114], successfully placing the contralateral to lesion rear paw when walking a narrow beam and successfully holding the contralateral forepaw immobile when swimming[44]. Once again, these impairments are less pronounced following neonatal hemidecortications, especially if they are given at the earliest ages[44].

The use of ipsilateral and contralateral forelimbs in a skilled reaching task has also been examined following hemidecortications by Whishaw and Kolb[117]. Impairments in limb use have been assessed by two end point measures, limb preference and success in obtaining food. Hemidecortication significantly affects preference in that all rats will strongly prefer to use the limb ipsilateral to the hemidecortication. Nevertheless, use of this limb is impaired. Intact rats successfully obtain food on about 60% of reaches, whereas hemidecorticate rats obtain food using their "good" limb on only about 20 to 30 per cent of reaches. The source of the impairment in use of the good limb has not been investigated. Skilled reaching, however, does require preparatory adjustments to position the body, movements that balance the body while the limb is advanced, as well as use of the "bad limb" in aiding in holding the food. Thus, it is likely that impairments of the bad side of the body contribute to the impairment in use of the good limb.

Use of the limb contralateral to the lesion is more impaired than is use of the ipsilateral limb. If a bracelet is placed on the ipsilateral to the lesion limb, in order to force use of the contralateral limb, this impairment can be demonstrated. Most animals are unable to reach efficiently, although they do make some attempts. Surprisingly, for some of the animals the attempts are successful, although the posture and the reaching movements are clearly abnormal. It is possible that the successful reaches that the rats do make are not really independent limb movements, but are stepping movements, involving some coordination in movement of the two forelimbs. Whatever their source, that some rats are able to use the limb at all does suggest that innovative therapeutic training may produce further enhancement in limb use. Restriction of the good limb in human stroke patients is similarly used to induce them to make use of their bad limb. Physiotherapists, however, have the patient sit on their good hand. The residual capacity to make these movements appears to depend upon the caudate-putamen, since if is removed along with the neocortex, rats are no longer able to use the limb contralateral to the lesion.

If hemidecortication is performed neonatally, limb preference is still biased toward the limb ipsilateral to the lesion. Use of both limbs is improved over levels achieved by adult hemidecorticate rats, and use of the contralateral limb is worse than use of the ipsilateral limb. Again, there are individual differences in successful limb use, as some neonatal hemispherectomized rats appear almost normal in use of the limb contralateral to the lesion. Anatomical investigations of enhanced neonatal performance suggest that enhanced limb use may be supported by the aberrant ipsilateral corticospinal pathway first described by Hicks and D'Amato[30]. A detailed description of the anatomy and restorative influences of this pathway has been given by Castro[14].

Cognitive Function

Learning and memory clearly play an important role in the development and use of cognition. There is a good deal of evidence that learning can be divided into two general types. One kind involves learning motor responses, such as turning in a certain direction, or responding to a single salient cue, such as approaching or avoiding an illuminated beacon. The other kind of learning involves responding to cues only if they have a certain relationship to each other. Examples of this kind of learning would involve using a variety of ambient cues to travel to a given location in space or pressing a bar for food reinforcement in response to a tone only when the bar was illuminated. A variety of terms have been developed for these two kinds of learning and memory, including associative as opposed to contingency learning[92,93], taxon as opposed to locale learning[67] and simple as opposed to configural learning[99].

A common suggestion made with respect to the neural basis of the two kinds of learning has been that the former can be mediated subcortically whereas the latter is crucially dependent upon the cortex (for example see Russell[91,92]). More recently this distinction has been questioned[60]. However, it is widely accepted that the cortex has a differential importance in the two types of learning and, therefore, it might be expected that hemidecortication should have a greater effect in disrupting the latter as opposed to the former kind of learning. Often a learning task will engender significant elements of both types of learning, of course, making it difficult to interpret hemidecorticate deficits. It is also important to recognize that many learning tests may be confounded in that they have more than one solution, leading to the possibility that a normal animal may solve a task one way and a brain damaged animal may solve it another way. However, despite these methodological difficulties the objective of most surgical hemidecorticate studies has been to investigate hemidecorticate learning [81,87].

Quite a number of studies do show that surgical removal of a single cortex does not result in impairment in learning on simple associative tasks. For example, in an extensive series of studies of classical conditioning of the nictitating membrane in the rabbit hemidecorticates performed as well as controls and this continued even when an element of discrimination was superimposed on the conditioning schedule[61,62,63,64,65]. Similarly in simple appetitively reinforced instrumental tasks such as orienting to a stimulus[112], solving a double platform latch box problem[49], and in simple avoidance learning[81,87] hemidecortication failed to impair performance.

In contrast, a clear hemidecorticate deficit has been found in a range of species, in contingency learning tasks such as the Lashley Type 3 maze[103], the water maze [43], object and brightness discrimination[28,100], visual and auditory GO/NO-GO discrimination[92] and reversal[84] and simultaneous two-choice brightness discrimination[81,87].

There are discrepant findings within the literature, however. For example, some tests have revealed a hemidecorticate deficit in classical conditioning[26] whereas in the most complex cognitive process on which hemidecorticates have been tested, the formation of learning sets, no evidence of a hemidecorticate deficit has been found[28,87,100].

This has led to further consideration of the exact nature of the hemidecorticate's impairment in learning tasks. Russell[92] argued that it is in maintaining the inhibition of error responses that hemidecorticate rats are impaired. Thus, in Skinner box GO/NO-GO learning, the hemidecorticate has no difficulty in inhibiting errors when the end of the GO period is signalled but an impairment in maintaining that inhibition manifests itself in an accumulation of errors towards the end of the NO-GO period. Rose and Plotkin[87] subsequently extended this finding by demonstrating that in a light signalled simultaneous discrimination in a two-choice box it was only at higher criterion levels, where maintenance of error inhibition is crucial, that hemidecorticates showed a significant impairment. Moreover, there is some evidence relevant to this point from the functional hemidecorticate literature (see above) in that, following the elicitation of unilateral cortical spreading depression, rats show an increasing magnitude of impairment as the performance criterion is raised in both escape[72] and avoidance[94] learning situations.

The suggestion that the hemidecorticate brain is deficient in maintaining the inhibition of inappropriate responses has implications for a range of cognitive processes and has led to investigations of how recovery of the damaged inhibitory processes might be facilitated. Rose et al[84] recommended the use of hemi-decortication as a means of separating out the contributions of recovery and compensation (see above) to any environmental enrichment induced improvement in GO/NO-GO reversal learning following cortical injury. Whilst they found clear evidence of a hemidecorticate deficit on the GO/NO-GO reversal task, evidence of enrichment effects on error inhibition in lesioned animals was somewhat equivocal. However, in a subsequent study[85] using a DRL schedule, in which maintenance of response inhibition is directly tested, postoperative environmental enrichment caused a significant reduction in a hemidecorticate deficit when compared with standard housing of hemidecorticate controls. Moreover, the longer the DRL time out interval the more beneficial the enrichment effect. Further investigation is needed, of course. For example, it would be interesting to know whether the beneficial effect of postoperative environmental enrichment on hemidecorticate water maze perform-ance[121] was, in part, due to enrichment-induced enhancement of error inhibition. If remediation of the hemidecorticate deficit might be achieved by enhancing inhibitory processes this is also an area which lends itself to pharmacological enquiry.

Within the existing literature on the hemidecorticate learning deficit there are the beginnings of still other lines of enquiry into issues related to recovery of cognitive function following hemidecortication. For example, three reports[44,103,121] all suggest age dependent effects on the hemidecorticate learning deficit. Here also there are discrepant reports[104,105] but this category of hemidecorticate studies merit further investigation even so.

Neural Mechanisms

As we have noted earlier in this chapter, given the extent of the resection involved, surgical hemidecortication is remarkable in causing relatively little damage elsewhere in the brain. Degenerative damage to the subcortex is largely confined to the ipsilateral side of the thalamus and whilst the contralateral neocortex shows some shrinkage[44] and inevitable degeneration of some pathways[20,21] the limited EEG evidence available to us[38] suggests this causes very little disruption of normal electrical activity. Of course the brain, above all, is a dynamically interacting whole and it would be naive to pursue too far the argument that the non-lesioned hemineocortex is not influenced by the hemidecortication procedure. For example, Pritzel and Huston [75] have reported the appearance of afferents from the intact hemineocortex to underlying thalamus by postoperative day seven which, they have suggested, may dampen the ipsilateral to lesion turning bias seen following hemidecortication. However, function on the uninjured side of the brain appears to be sufficiently normal to use it as a control for the damaged side in studying neural mechanisms of recovery. In this respect the hemidecorticate affords the researcher a unique opportunity.

A particular value of this self-contained control facility may lie in investigating the neural mediation of interventions which overcome or reduce hemidecorticate behavioural impairments. For example, examination of the non-lesioned hemisphere may provide clues to why postoperative environmental enrichment has beneficial effects on adult hemidecorticate water maze performance[118,121] and Skinner box DRL performance[85]. Given the very clear effects of environmental enrichment on cerebral cortex in unoperated rats[79] there is good reason to expect at least some of these changes in non-lesioned cortex in the hemidecorticate. Moreover, if environmental enrichment can enhance the structure and efficiency of the unlesioned cortex of the hemidecorticate in the way it appears to with cortex in unoperated animals it is reasonable to expect that it might partially overcome hemidecorticate behavioural impairments. As yet there is no evidence that postoperative environmental enrichment has any effect on the intact hemineocortex in the adult hemidecorticate[121] but this has not yet been extensively researched and, in the opinion of the present authors, it is an area which merits further attention.

The study of the hemidecorticate brain may also help unravel the neural basis of the age dependent nature of lesion impairments and sparing of function. The changes that take place following neonatal hemidecortication are much different from those following adult lesions. Here, despite the lack of callosal projections, there is clear thickening of the unlesioned cortex[43,44] and increased dendritic arborization in layer II/III pyramidal cells of the somatosensory and motor cortex but not the visual or temporal cortex[40]. There is also development of the uncrossed corticospinal tract[14,30,46] and contralateral corticostriatal connections[40]. Despite this the weight of the remaining brain is much less than can be accounted for through the loss of the removed cortex. The ipsilateral medial anterior, ventral anterior and lateral geniculate nuclei are no longer present, and the gliosis and calcium deposits which follow hemidecortication of the adult animal are absent. Thus, there is a marked asymmetry in the appearance of the thalamus and some parts of the basal ganglia and brainstem.

The differences between the effects of neonatal and adult lesions are more striking the earlier the neonatal lesions, and the dividing line between obtaining adult vs neonatal effects appears to be around 10 days of age postnatally[44]. It is against this background that the differential degrees of impairment and sparing following hemidecortication in neonatal and adult animals must be viewed.

The hemidecorticate has yielded mixed results regarding neurochemical aspects of plasticity following injury. A number of studies have looked for changes in catecholamine and other transmitter substances following hemispherectomy. Castenada et al[13] reported no asymmetrical changes in dopamine or its metabolites in the extracellular tissue in freely moving animals either 3 days or 60 days after hemidecortication. Since the animals displayed a bias to circle ipsiversively immediately postoperatively but not on later tests, they were unable to correlate lateralised behavioural induced changes in dopamine or its metabolites. Nor were they able to confirm a number of reports of depressed striatal function in the early post-surgical period following cortical damage.

A good deal of inferential data suggest that noradrenaline is importantly involved in plasticity following brain injury. Increases in synaptosomal noradrenaline have been reported in brainstem and cerebellum following hemidecortication in adult rats[102]. As yet this change has not been related to change in behaviour. One behavioural study has suggested an important role for noradrenaline in infant and adult hemidecorticate rats[118]. Noradrenaline depletion did not affect compensation on a place navigation task in neonatally hemidecorticate rats nor affect improvements provided by subjecting rats to an enriched environment following hemidecortication. If adult rats depleted of noradrenaline were simply left in their home cages, however, their performance was worse than that of rats that only received surgery. This study suggested that noradrenaline is important for enhancing recovery from brain damage when other sources of compensation (neonatal injury, enriched environment) were absent.

SUMMARY AND FUTURE DIRECTIONS

As research on recovery of function following brain damage assumes a more prominent position within neuroscience there is an increasing demand for suitable test paradigms. We believe surgical hemidecortication in animals merits serious consideration in this context.

In the study of recovery of function and related phenomena the hemidecorticate has several valuable characteristics which we have discussed in some detail. Not least of these is that there is already an extensive literature relating to both anatomical and behavioural aspects of surgical hemidecortication in a range of different species. In many respects hemidecorticate deficits are already well understood and this makes much easier the analysis of mechanisms of post injury recovery. There are also related literatures on functional hemidecortication, induced by unilateral cortical spreading depression, and on the surgical split brain against which surgical hemidecorticate findings can be checked, although caution must be exercised in doing this.

The surgical hemidecorticate also affords a number of experimental advantages. It is a relatively straightforward lesion and one that is easily replicable even in lissencephalic brains. In sparing a significant proportion of the pathways of all sensory modalities it can also help in distinguishing the roles of recovery and sensory compensation in the aftermath of brain injury. Moreover, that the procedure leaves one hemineocortex relatively intact to some extent allows each subject to be used as its own control in carrying out both neural and behavioural analyses.

In the course of the chapter we have discussed several uses of hemidecortication in studying recovery and recovery related phenomena in which use has been made of these experimental advantages. However, we believe that the hemidecorticate has not yet been thoroughly exploited in this type of research. There is still much to be done by way of documenting recovery following hemidecortication. Also, existing lines of enquiry into neural changes in the intact hemineocortex during recovery, age dependent effects, and the potentially therapeutic role of environmental enrichment, merit further work. However, we should like to see an extension of research, for example, to examine the efficacy of pharmacological and other interventions in facilitating recovery, differential mechanisms of recovery following large and small lesions (by comparing hemidecortication with smaller unilateral extirpations), and lesion momentum effects (perhaps incorporating a functional hemidecorticate group).

We have no wish to make exaggerated claims for the hemidecorticate. The preparation is not without its complications and complexities as we have explained. However, it also has significant advantages and we believe these can be put to greater use than they have so far been in elucidating mechanisms of recovery of function following brain damage.

A final advantage of hemidecortication in animals, and one which should be stressed given the objectives of the present volume, is that it has a human analogy in some hemispherectomy procedures. The aim of bringing together those doing basic animal research and those whose research interest is more clinically orientated is obviously laudable. However, from a practical viewpoint such contact must depend, in part, on the existence of comparable research paradigms in humans and animals. Hemidecortication does provide a bridge between human and animal studies and a potentially valuable channel of communication between those engaged in these two areas of research.

REFERENCES

1. Bard, P., 1933, Studies on the cerebral cortex, *Arch. Neurol. Psychiat.*, **30**, 40-74.
2. Bard, P., 1937, Studies on the cortical representation of somatic sensibility, *The Harvey Lectures*, **33**, 143-169.
3. Bard, P., and Brooks, C.M., 1934, Localised cortical control of some postural reactions in the cat and rat together with evidence that small cortical remnants may function normally, *Res. Publ. Assoc. Res. Nerv. Ment. Dis.*, **13**, 107-157.
4. Benton, A.L. and Levin, H.S., 1972, An experimental study of "obscuration", *Neurology*, **22**, 1176-1181.
5. Blagowestschenskaja, W., 1929, Ausarbeitung der associativen Reflexe bei Welpen mit einer fehlenden Hemisphare, *Beitrage z Reflexologie d. Nervensystems u. Physiologie*, **3**, 333-377. (Cited by Tsang[103])
6. Bromiley, R.B., 1948, The development of conditioned responses in cats after unilateral decortication, *J. Comp. Physiol. Psychol.*, **41**, 155-164.
7. Brooks, C.M., and Peck, M.E., 1940, Effect of various lesions on development of placing and hopping reactions in rats, *J. Neurophysiol.*, **3**, 66-73.
8. Brooks, C.M. and Woolsey, C.N., 1936, Relation in rabbit of electrically excitable areas of cortex to placing and hopping reactions, *Amer. J. Physiol.*, **116**, 17-18.
9. Brooks, C.M., and Woolsey, C.N., 1940, Placing and hopping reactions in relation to the electrically excitable "motor" areas in the cerebral cortex of the rabbit, *Bull. John Hopkins Hosp.*, **67**, 41-60.
10. Bures, J., 1959, Reversable decortication and behaviour, in *The Central Nervous System and Behaviour*, M.A.B. Brazier, ed., pp. 207-248, Josiah Macy, Jr. Foundation, New York.
11. Bures, J., Buresova, O., and Krivanek, J., 1974, *The Mechanism and Applications of Leao's Spreading Depression of Electroencephalographic Activity*, Academic Press, New York.
12. Carville, C., and Duret, H., 1875, *Arch. Physiol.*, 2me ser., **2**, 352-491. (Cited by Tsang [103]. Full reference not given in this case).
13. Castenada, E., Whishaw, I.Q., and Robinson, T.E., 1992, Recovery from lateralized neocortical damage: dissociation between amphetamine-induced asymmetry in behavior and striatal dopamine neurotransmission in vivo, *Brain Research*, **571**, 248-259.

14. Castro, A.J., 1990, Plasticity in the motor system, in *The Cerebral Cortex of the Rat*, B. Kolb and R.C. Tees, eds., pp. 563-588, MIT Press, Cambridge Mass.

15. Clark, W.E. LeGros, and Russell, D.S., 1940, Atrophy of the thalamus in a case of aquired hemiplegia associated with diffuse porencephaly and sclerosis of the left cerebral hemisphere, *J. Neurol. Psychiat.*, **3**, 123-146.

16. Davey, M.J., Rose, F.D., Dell, P.A., and Love, S., 1988, Simultaneous extinction following hemidecortication and unilateral lesions of parietal cortex in the rat, *Med. Sci. Res.*, **16**, 1043-1044.

17. Demeedov, V.A., 1908, Conditioned Reflexes after Extirpation of the Anterior Halves of the Hemispheres in the Dog. Thesis, Petrograd. (Cited by Tsang [103]).

18. Diamond, M.C., Johnson, R.E., and Ingham, C.A., 1975, Morphological changes in the young, adult, and aging cerebral cortex, hippocampus and diencephalon, *Behav. Biology*, **14**, 163-174.

19. Dusser de Barrenne, J.G., and McCulloch, W.S., 1941, Suppression of motor response obtained from area 4 by stimulation of area 4S, *J.Neurophysiol.*, **4**, 311-323.

20. Ebner, F.F., amd Myers,R.E., 1965, Distribution of corpus callosum and anterior commissure in cat and racoon, *J. Comp. Neurol.*, **124**, 353-366.

21. Federova, K.P., 1971, Features distinguishing commissural connections of different areas of the cat visual cortex, *Arkhiv. Anatomii. Gistologii. i Embriologii*, **61**, 107-113.

22. Finger, S., and Almli, C.R., 1988, Margaret Kennard and her "principle" in historical perspective, in *Brain Injury and Recovery Theoretical and Controversial Issues*, S. Finger, T.E.LeVere, C.R.Almli and D.G.Stein, eds., pp. 117-132, Plenum, New York.

23. Foursikov, D.S., 1925, The effect of extirpation of the cortex of one hemisphere in the dog, *Russian J. Physiol.*, **8**, 1-2. (Cited by Tsang [103]).

24. Foursikov, D.S., 1925, The effect of extirpation of the cortex of one hemisphere (third communication). Generalisation and the development of conditioned reflexes to tactile stimuli, *Russian J. Physiol.*, **8**, 5-6. (Cited by Tsang [103]).

25. Friedland, R.P., and Weinstein, E.A., 1977, Hemi-inattention and hemisphere specialisation: introduction and historical review, *Advances in Neurology*, **28**, 1-31.

26. Girden, E., Mettler, F.A., Finch, G., and Culler, E., 1936, Conditioned responses in a decorticate dog to acoustic, thermal and tactile stimulation, *J.Comp. Psychol.*, **36**, 367-385.

27. Goltz, F., 1881, *Uber die Verrichtungen des Grosshirns*, Bonn. (Cited by Tsang[103])

28. Harlow, H.F., 1949, The formation of learning sets, *Psychol. Rev.*, **56**, 51-65.

29. Heilman, K.M., and Watson, R.T., 1977, The neglect syndrome. A unilateral defect of the orienting response, in *Lateralization in the Nervous System*, S. Harnad, R. W. Doty, J.Jaynes, L. Goldstein, and G. Krauthamer, eds., pp. 285-302, Academic Press, New York.

30. Hicks, S.P., and D'Amato, C.J., 1975, Motor-sensory cortex-corticospinal system and developing locomotion and placing in rats, *Amer. J. Anat.*, **143**, 1-42.

31. Hobbelen, J.F., Gramsbergen, A. and Van Hof, M.W., 1988, The hopping response after two stage cortical ablation in young and adult rabbits, *Behav. Brain Res.*, **31**, 97-102.

32. Hunter, W.S., 1930, A consideration of Lashley's theory of equipotentiality of cerebral action, *J. Gen. Psychol.*, **3**, 455-488.

33. Irle, E., 1987, Lesion size and recovery of function: some new perspectives, *Brain Res. Rev.*, **12**, 307-320.

34. Karplus, J.P., and Kreidl, A., 1914, Ueber total extirpation einer und beider Grosshirnhemispharen an Affen (Macacus Rhesus), *Arch. f. Anat. u Physiol.*, pp. 155-212. (Cited by White et al[122]).

35. Kellogg, W.N., 1948, Conditioning involving the two body sides after hemidecortication, *Amer. Psychol.*, **3**, 237.

36. Kellogg, W.N., 1949, Locomotor and other disturbances following hemidecortication in the dog, *J. Comp. Physiol. Psychol.*, **42**, 506-516.

37. Kellogg, W.N., and Bashore, W.D., 1950, The influence of hemidecortication upon bilateral avoidance conditioning in dogs, *J. Comp. Physiol. Psychol.*, **43**, 49-61.

38. Kennard, M.A., and Nims, L.F., 1942, Effect on electroencephalogram of lesions of cerebral cortex and basal ganglia in Macac Mulatta, *J. Neurophysiol.*, **5**, 335-348.

39. Klassowski, B., 1929, Die technik der operation, die morphogenetischen und einiger functionelle folgen der entfernung einer hemisphare in den ersten lebenstagen des hundes, *Bietrage z. Reflexologie u. Physiologie d. Nervensystems. Bd.*, **3**, 326-332. (Cited by Tsang [103]).

40. Kolb, B., Gibb, R., and van der Kooy, D., 1992, Cortical and striatal structure and connectivity are altered by neonatal hemidecortication in rats, *J. Comp. Neurol.* In press.

41. Kolb, B., Macintosh, A., Whishaw I.Q., and Sutherland, R.J., 1984, Evidence for anatomical but not functional asymmetry in the hemidecorticate rat, *Behav. Neurosci.*, **98**, 44-58.

42. Kolb, B., Sutherland, R.J., Nonneman, A.J., and Whishaw, I.Q., 1982, Asymmetry in the cerebral hemispheres of the rat, mouse, rabbit and cat: The right hemisphere is larger, *Exper. Neurol.*, **78**, 348-359.

43. Kolb, B., Sutherland, R.J., and Whishaw, I.Q., 1983, Abnormalities in cortical and subcortical morphology after neonatal neocortical lesions in rats, *Exper. Neurol.*, **79**, 223-244.

44. Kolb, B., and Tomie, J., 1988, Recovery from early cortical damage in rats. IV. Effects of hemidecortication at 1, 5, or 10 days of age on cerebral anatomy and behaviour, *Behav. Brain Res.*, **28**, 259-274.

45. Kolb, B., and Whishaw, I.Q., 1985, An observer's view of locomotor asymmetry in the rat, *Behav. Toxicol. Teratol.*, **7**, 71-78.

46. Kolb, B., and Whishaw, I.Q., 1989, Plasticity in the neocortex: Mechanisms underlying recovery from early brain damage, *Progress in Neurobiol.*, **32**, 235-276.

47. Kolb, B., and Whishaw, I.Q., 1990, *Fundamentals of Human Neuropsychology*, W.H.Freeman & Co., New York. (Third edition)

48. Kourdrin, A.N., 1911, Conditioned reflexes in the dog after extirpation of the posterior halves of the hemispheres. Thesis, Petrograd. (Cited by Tsang[103]).

49. Lashley, K.S., 1920, Studies of cerebral function in learning, *Psychobiology*, **2**, 55-128.

50. Leao, A.A.P., 1944, Spreading depression of activity in the cerebral cortex, *J. Neurophysiol.*, **7**, 359-390.

51. LeVere, T.E., 1980. Recovery of function after brain damage: A theory of the behavioural deficit, *Physiol. Psychol.*, **8**, 297-308.

52. LeVere, T.E., 1988, Neural system imbalances and the consequences of large brain injuries, in *Brain Injury and Recovery. Theoretical and Controversial Issues*, S. Finger, T. E.LeVere, C.R. Almli & D.G. Stein, eds., pp 15-28, Plenum, New York.

53. Macht, M. B., 1950, Effects of d-amphetamine on hemidecorticate, decorticate and decerebrate cats, *Amer. J. Physiol.*, **163**, 731-732.

54. Magnus, R., 1921, Korperstellung und labarynthreflexe beim affen, *Arch. Ges. Physiol.*, **193**, 396. (Cited by White et al[122]).

55. Marshall, W.H., 1959, Spreading cortical depression of leao, *Physiol. Rev.*, **39**, 239-279.

56. Mettler, F.A., 1943, Extensive unilateral cerebral removals in the primate: Physiologic effects and resultant degeneration, *J. Comp. Neurol.*, **79**, 185-245.

57. Mittleman, G., Whishaw, I.Q., and Robbins, T.W., 1988, Cortical lateralization of function in rats in a visual reaction time task, *Behav. Brain Res.*, **31**, 29-36.

58. Murphy Combs, C., 1949, Fibre and cell degeneration in the albino rat brain after hemidecortication, *J. Comp. Neurol.*, **90**, 373-401.

59. Murphy Combs, C., 1951, The distribution and temporal course of fibre degeneration after experimental lesions in the rat brain, *J.Comp. Neurol.*, **94**, 123-175.

60. Oakley, D.A., 1979, Cerebral cortex and adaptive behaviour, in *Brain, Behaviour and Evolution*, D.A. Oakley and H.C. Plotkin, eds., pp. 154-188, Methuen, London.

61. Oakley, D.A., and Russell, I.S., 1968, Mass action and Pavlovian conditioning, *Psychonom. Sci.*, **12**, 91-92.

62. Oakley, D.A., and Russell, I.S., 1972, Neocortical lesions and Pavlovian conditioning, *Physiol.Behav.*, **8**, 915-926.

63. Oakley, D.A., and Russell, I.S., 1973, Acquisition, differentiation and reversal of conditioning in partially decorticate rabbits, *I.R.C.S. Med. Sci.*, **1**, 56.

64. Oakley, D.A., and Russell, I.S., 1974, Pavlovian discrimination learning in decorticate and hemidecorticate rabbits, *I.R.C.S. Med. Sci.*, **2**, 1065.

65. Oakley, D.A., and Russell, I.S., 1974, Retention of Pavlovian conditioning from the hemidecorticate to the decorticate state, *I.R.C.S. Med. Sci.*, **2**, 1067.

66. Ochs, S., 1962, The nature of spreading depression in neural networks., *Int. Rev. Neurobiol.*, **4**, 1-69.

67. O'Keefe, J., and Nadel, L., 1978, *The Hippocampus as a Cognitive Map*, Clarendon Press, Oxford.

68. Papez, J.W., 1938, Thalamic connections in the hemidecorticate dog, *J. Comp. Neurol.*, **69**, 103-121.

69. Peacock, J.H., and Murphy Combs, C., 1965, Retrograde cell degeneration in diencephalic and other structures after hemidecortication in rhesus monkeys, *Exp. Neurol.*, **11**, 367-399.

70. Peacock, J.H., and Murphy Combs, C., 1965, Retrograde cell degeneration in adult cat after hemidecortication, *J. Comp. Neurol.*, **125**, 329-336.

71. Plotkin, H.C., and Russell, I.S., 1969, The hemidecorticate learning deficit: evidence for a quantitative impairment, *Physiol. Behav.*, **4**, 49-55.

72. Plotkin, H.C., and Russell, I.S., 1969, Unilateral cortical spreading depression and escape learning, *Physiol. Bohemoslov.*, **18**, 395-399.

73. Poltyrev, S.S., and Alexjev, W., 1936, Uber die moglichkeit der bildung bedingte reflexe bei hunden mit extirpierter hirnrinde von der hemisphare

gegenuberliegenden koperoberflache aus, *Z.Biol.*, **97**, 207-305. (Cited by Bromiley[6]).

74. Powell, T.P.S., 1952, Residual neurons in the human thalamus following hemidecortication, *Brain*, **75**, 571-583.

75. Pritzel, M., and Huston, J.P., 1981, Unilateral ablation of telencephalon induces appearance of contralateral cortical and subcortical projections to the thalamic nuclei, *Behav. Brain Res.*, **3**, 43-54.

76. Rademaker, G.G.J., 1927, On the physiology of reflex standing, *Versl. Vergad. K. Acad. Wet. Med.*, **36**, 635-649.

77. Rademaker, G.G.J., 1931, *Das Stephen*, J. Springer, Berlin.

78. Ranson, S.W., and Clark, S.L., 1959, *The Anatomy of the Nervous System*, W.B. Saunders Company, Philadelphia. (Tenth edition)

79. Renner, M.J., and Rosenweig, M.R., 1987, *Enriched and Impoverished Environments, Effects on Brain and Behaviour*, Springer-Verlag, New York.

80. Robinson, R.G., 1979, Differential behavioural and biochemical effects of right and left hemispheric infarction in the rat, *Science*, **205**, 707-710.

81. Rose, F.D., 1975, Learning in the Surgical Hemidecorticate Rat, Doctoral Dissertation, University of London.

82. Rose. F.D., Davey, M.J., Love, S., and Dell, P.A., 1987, Environmental enrichment and recovery from contralateral sensory neglect in rats with large unilateral neocortical lesions, *Behav. Brain Res.*, **24**, 195-202.

83. Rose, F.D, Dell, P.A., Davey, M.J., and Love,S., 1987, Hemidecortication in the rat as a model for investigating recovery from brain injury, *Med. Sci. Res.*, **15**, 157-158.

84. Rose, F.D., Dell, P.A., Love, S., and Davey, M.J., 1988, Environmental enrichment and recovery from a complex GO NO-GO reversal deficit in rats following large neocortical lesions, *Behav. Brain Res.*, **31**, 37-45.

85. Rose, F.D., Love, S., Dell, P.A., and Davey, M.J., 1988, Environmental attenuation of DRL performance in the rat following hemidecortication, *Med. Sci. Res.*, **16**, 563-564.

86. Rose F.D., Morgan, S., Oakley, D.A., and Plotkin, H.C., 1980, Learning in surgical and functional hemidecorticate rats: A preliminary study of compensation, *Behav. Brain Res.*, **1**, 93-99.

87. Rose, F.D., and Plotkin, H.C., 1977,. Surgical hemidecortication and learning in the rat, *Behav. Biol.*, **19**, 172-188.

88. Rose, F.D., and Plotkin, H.C., 1978, Brightness preference in surgical hemidecorticate rats, *Brain Res.*, **157**, 142-146.

89. Rose, J.E., and Woolsey, C., 1943, Thalamo cortical relations in the rabbit, *Bull. J. Hopkins Hosp.*, **73**, 65-128.

90. Rosenthal, I.S., 1936, Conditioned reflexes in dogs lacking one cerebral hemisphere, *Arch.Sc.Biol.St Petersbburg*, **42**, 287. (Cited by Bromiley [6]).

91. Russell, I.S., 1966, Animal learning and memory, in *Aspects of Learning and Memory*, D. Richter, ed., pp 121-171, Heinemann, London.

92. Russell, I.S., 1969, Cortical mechanisms and learning, in *Animal Discrimination Learning*, R. Gilbert and N.S. Sutherland, eds., pp. 335-356, Academic Press, London.

93. Russell, I.S., 1971, Neurological basis of complex learning, *Brit. Med. Bull.*, **27**, 278-285.

94. Russell, I.S., and Plotkin, H.C., 1972, Interhemispheric relations and learning in the functional split brain rat, in *Cerebral Interhemispheric Relations*, J. Bernacch and F. Podovinsky, eds., pp. 299-319, Slovak Academic Press, Bratislava.

95. Schallert, T., and Whishaw, I.Q., 1984, Bilateral cutaneous stimulation of the somatosensory system in hemidecorticate rats, *Behav. Neurosci.*, **98**, 518-540.

96. Schallert, T. and Whishaw, I.Q., 1985, Neonatal hemidecortication and bilateral cutaneous stimulation in rats, *Develop. Psychobiol.*, **18**, 501-514.

97. Sechzer, J.A., 1970, Prolonged learning and split-brain cats, *Science*, **169**, 889-892.

98. Soltmann, O., 1876, Experimentalle studien uber die functionenden grosshirns der neugeborenen, *Jahrb. Kinderheilkd.*, **9**, 106-148. (Cited by Finger and Almli[22])

99. Sutherland, R.J., and Rudy, J.W., 1989, Configural asssociation theory: The role of the hippocampal formation in learning, memory and amnesia, *Psychobiol.*, **17**, 129-144.

100. Thompson, V.E., and Bucy, P.E., 1969, Learning after cerebral hemidecortication in monkeys, *Physiol Behav.*, **4**, 455-459.

101. Toropov, N.K., 1908, Visual Conditioned Reflexes in the Dog after Extirpation of the Occipital Lobes. Thesis, Petrograd. (Cited by Tsang[103]).

102. Toyama, M., and Satake, M., 1981, Increased concentration and accelerated synaptosomal uptake of noradrenaline in the central nervous tissues of neonatally hemispherectomized adult rats, *Brain Res.*, **208**, 447-450.

103. Tsang, Y., 1937, Maze learning in rats hemidecorticated in infancy, *J. Comp. Psychol.*, **24**, 221-248.

104. Van Hof, M.W., De Vos Korthals, W. H., and Hobbelen, J.F., 1988, The effects of early and late hemidecortication on vision and locomotion in the rabbit, in *Post-Lesion Neural Plasticity*, H. Flohr, ed., pp. 157-163, Springer-Verlag, Berlin.

105. Van Hof, M.W., Hobbelen, J.F., and De Vos-Korthals, W.H., 1987, Motor behaviour and visual discrimination after neonatal and adult hemidecortication in the rabbit, *Behav. Brain Res.*, **25**, 247-253.

106. Van Hof, M.W., Hobbelin, J.F., and Gramsbergen, A., 1990, The effects of brain lesions on the hopping reaction in newborn and adult rabbits: A model for studying age dependent recovery, *Acta. Neurobiol. Exp.*, **50**, 135-139.

107. Vulpian, A., 1866, *Lecons dur la Physiologie Generale et Comparee du Systeme Nerveux*, Balliere, Paris. (Cited by Finger and Almli [22]).

108. Walker, A.E., 1935, The retrograde cell degeneration in the thalamus of macacus rhesus following hemidecortication, *J. Comp. Neurol.*, **62**, 407-419.

109. Walker, A.E., 1938, The thalamus of the chimpanzee. II. Its nuclear structure normal and following hemidecortication, *J. Comp. Neurol.*, **69**, 487-507.

110. Walker, A.E., 1938, *The Primate Thalamus*, University of Chicago Press, Chicago.

111. Waller, W.H., 1938, The thalamus of the cat after hemidecortication, *J. Anat.*, **72**, 475.

112. Wenzel, B.M., Tschirgi, R.D., and Taylor, J.L., 1962, Effects of early postnatal hemidecortication on spatial discrimination in cats, *Exp. Neurol.*, **6**, 332-339.

113. Whatmore, G.B. and Kleitman, N., 1946, The role of sensory and motor cortical projections in escape and avoidance conditioning in dogs, *Amer. J. Physiol.*, **146**, 282-292.

114. Whishaw, I.Q., 1983, Cortical control of claw cutting in the rat, *Behav. Neurosci.*, **97**, 370-380.

115. Whishaw, I.Q., 1988, Food wrenching and dodging: use of action patterns for the analysis of sensorimotor and social behaviour in the rat. *J. Neurosci Methods.*, **2134**, 169-178.

116. Whishaw, I.Q., and Kolb, B., 1984, We should deemphasise the importance of the role that we give amines in the LH syndrome, *Appetite*, **5**, 272-276.

117. Whishaw, I.Q., and Kolb, B., 1988, Sparing of skilled forelimb reaching and corticospinal projections after neonatal motor cortex removal or hemidecortication in the rat: support for the Kennard doctrine, *Brain Res.*, **451**, 97-114.

118. Whishaw, I.Q., Sutherland, R.J., and Kolb, B., 1986, Effects of neonatal forebrain noradrenaline depletion on recovery from brain damage: Performance on a spatial navigation task as a function of age at surgery and postsurgery housing, *Behav. Neural Biol.*, **46**, 285-307.

119. Whishaw, I.Q., and Tomie, J., 1987, Food wrestling and dodging: strategies used by rats (Rattus norvegicus) for obtaining and protecting food from conspecifics, *J. Comp. Psychol.*, **101**, 202-209.

120. Whishaw, I.Q., and Tomie, J., 1988, Food wrenching and dodging: a neuroethological test of cortical and dopaminergic contributions to sensorimotor behaviour in the rat, *Behav. Neurosci.*, **102**, 110-123.

121. Whishaw, I.Q., Zaborowski, J.A., and Kolb, B., 1984, Postsurgical enrichment aids adult hemidecorticate rats on a spatial navigation task, *Behav. Neural Biol.*, **42**, 183-190.

122. White, R.J., Schreiner, L.H., Hughes, R.A., MacCarty, C.S., and Grindlay, J.H., 1959, Physiologic consequences of total hemispherectomy in the monkey, *Neurology*, **9**, 149-159.

123. Woolsey, C.N., 1970, Quoted by Meyer, P.M. and Meyer, D.R., 1971, Neurosurgical procedures with special reference to aspiration lesions, in *Methods in Psychobiology*, R.D. Myers, ed., Volume 1, pp. 91-130, Academic Press, London.

A REVIEW OF COGNITIVE OUTCOME AFTER

HEMIDECORTICATION IN HUMANS

Faraneh Vargha-Khadem
Institute of Child Health and Hospital for Sick Children
Great Ormond Street, London, England

and

Charles E Polkey
The Neurosurgical Unit
Maudsley Hospital, London, England

INTRODUCTION

The surgical procedure of hemispherectomy was originally described by Dandy[8] and then independently by L'Hermitte[22] as a radical treatment for malignant gliomas within a cerebral hemisphere. The procedure was first applied for relief from intractable epilepsy in a patient with infantile hemiplegia by McKenzie[26] and gradually thereafter it came into use as one possible treatment for certain severe forms of epilepsy and behaviour disorder[2,20,23,46]. Although the surgical procedure is still commonly referred to in the neurosurgical literature as hemispherectomy, the actual resections as currently performed are more correctly referred to as hemidecortications. With the elimination of some of the long-term complications of hemidecortication through modified surgical procedures[1,34,42], and with the introduction of new imaging techniques for guiding patient selection[6], hemidecortication has gained widespread acceptance today as a treatment for severe epilepsy[13] arising from such diverse conditions as Sturge-Weber-Dimitri disease[30], hemimegalencephaly[18], infantile hemiplegia, and "Rasmussen's Encephalitis"[33,35].

The first three aetiological conditions listed above involve congenital or perinatal pathology of one cerebral hemisphere. Patients suffering from such conditions are diagnosed during infancy or early childhood, and most commonly their seizure disorder develops in the presence of hemiplegia and other severe functional losses, such as hemianasthesia, hemianopia, as well as cognitive and behavioural dysfunctions. Under these circumstances, i.e. with hemispheric dysfunction already severe, hemidecortication adds virtually no cost to the patients' neurological or cognitive status; indeed, long-term improvements in cognitive status are sometimes reported[4], these being attributable to arrest of seizures, elimination of anticonvulsant medications, or both.

Recovery from Brain Damage, Edited by F.D. Rose and
D.A. Johnson, Plenum Press, New York, 1992

In contrast to the three aetiological conditions just listed, "Rasmussen's encephalitis" is an acquired brain disease that can occur at any time during childhood, from one year of age[29] through adolescence (i.e. age 14-15 years). In this disease, intractable epilepsy develops in the absence of any other neurological signs, and only after a period of uncontrollable seizures of from six months to two years or more, does hemiplegia and other evidence of unilateral hemispheric disorders appear. Therefore, if onset of seizures occurs late in development and the time between onset and operation is short, the intial cost of hemidecortication to the patients' neurological and cognitive status can be substantial. Even under these circumstances, however, the benefits to quality of life from relief of chronic seizures (which, if unabated, would ultimately lead to severe hemispheric dysfunction) are sometimes judged to outweigh the initial costs of hemidecortication.

The majority of studies assessing functional outcome after hemidecortication have involved patients with congenital or perinatal pathology who underwent the radical surgical procedure during adolescence or adulthood. These patients thus had long histories of seizures and hemispheric disorders often dating from birth or the first two years of life onward[3,25,46]. When surgical cases with "Rasmussen's encephalitis" have been studied, their results have not been separately analysed with respect to the age at seizure onset, thereby leaving open the question of the importance of this variable in determining functional outcome[41]. In the present review an attempt will be made to address this question. Other variables that need to be taken into account for a complete understanding of cognitive outcome after any type of damage sustained by the immature brain are hemispheric side of damage, elapsed time since damage (i.e. the recovery period), the task used to evaluate the cognitive effects of damage, and the developmental stage of the function at the time of damage[47]. Whenever possible, these issues also will be addressed. The specific domains of cognitive function to be examined in this review include intelligence, memory, language, and visuo-perceptual processes, based on studies carried out during the past twenty years. Discussion of cognitive outcome will be preceded by a brief description of the hemidecortication procedure.

THE SURGICAL PROCEDURE OF HEMISPHERECTOMY (HEMIDECORTICATION)

Hemidecortication involves the removal of most of one cerebral hemisphere, including the insular cortex and variable portions of the basal ganglia. Standard hemidecortication results in the creation of a massive cavity in continuity with the ventricular system. Although the effectiveness of the standard operation for arresting seizures is well established[34,46], there is an unacceptably high risk (33%) of serious late complications due to hydrocephalus and haemosiderosis[42]. To reduce this risk, three modifications of the standard procedure have been introduced: subtotal hemispherectomy; functional hemispherectomy[34], and Adam's modified hemispherectomy[1].

Subtotal hemispherectomy refers to the removal of between two-thirds and four-fifths of the cortex of the affected hemisphere. The block of hemisphere remaining is usually decided on neurophysiological or anatomical grounds. Depending on the extent of removal, the remaining cortical tissue may be functionally intact. The presence of an intact block of the damaged hemisphere acting as a buttress appears to protect the patient from the late complications of haemosiderosis and hydrocephalus[32].

Functional hemispherectomy[33,34,37,42] consists of the removal of the central cortical region, including the parasagittal tissue and cingulate gyrus. A temporal lobectomy, including amygdala and hippocampus, is also carried out to complete the functional hemidecortication. The remaining portions of the frontal lobe and parieto-occipital lobes are then disconnected from the brain stem and the opposite hemisphere by transection of the white matter connections. This procedure isolates the frontal and parieto-occipital poles from the rest of the brain while protecting the blood vessels that serve these regions.

Complete hemispherectomy using Adam's modification[1] refers to special precautions taken to avoid long-term complications after a standard hemidecortication has been performed. The convexity dura on the operated side is sutured down to the falx, tentorium, and the floor of the anterior and middle cerebral fossae. This results in the cavity being filled with extradural fluid rather than the subdural fluid that accumulates following a standard hemidecortication. Any residual subdural accumulation is isolated from the ventricular system through the insertion of a muscle plug in the foramen of Monro. The author also emphasises the importance of meticulous hemostasis.

Compared to classical hemidecortication, the functional operation and Adam's modification lead to similar rates of seizure relief, whereas subtotal hemidecortication lowers the seizure relief rate by 10-15%. The long-term follow-up results have been impressive and very few late complications reported[4,16,34,45].

Villemure et al.[45] contrasted surgical outcome as a function of type of hemidecortication in their populations of patients with Rasmussen's encephalitis. Of the group given the standard operation (N = 8), 37.5% remained seizure-free and 87.5% had none or less than two seizures per year since surgery. In the functional hemidecortication group (N = 10), 6% remained seizure-free and 90% had none or less than two seizures per year. Across the two groups, the follow-up period ranged from 8 months to 36 years, with a median follow-up of 9 years. Even more impressive results were reported by Honavar et al.[16] on their sample of patients (N = 10) with Rasmussen's encephalitis who underwent either subtotal hemidecortication or Adam's modified procedure. Eight patients were seizure-free and one showed much reduced seizures. The remaining patient continued seizing and subsequently died. Follow-up periods in this sample ranged from less than 1 year to 12 years.

COGNITIVE OUTCOME FOLLOWING HEMIDECORTICATION

Intelligence

Diverse factors, such as age at onset of seizures, duration of preoperative illness, degree of postoperative seizure control, side of pathology, and elapsed time since hemidecortication (i.e. recovery period), could play a role in determining intellectual outcome. Studies involving eight or more patients with congenital or perinatal disease leading to surgery during later childhood or adolescence report a high proportion of cases (varying from 40 to 70% across the various studies) showing a 10-point or greater improvement in intelligence quotients following hemidecortication[4,23,44]. A far smaller proportion (10-25%) are reported to show a 10-point or greater decline.

In contrast to the foregoing studies, improvement in postoperative intellectual ability occurred infrequently in the only previous study to report on a sizeable series of patients with Rasmussen's encephalitis[41]. In that study, only two children in nine were described as intellectually improved after hemidecortication (though one of these gained as much as 30 points); the others remained constant. Similarly, in our own (unpublished) series of nine patients with Rasmussen's disease (Table 1), only one patient showed an improvement of 10 points or more in overall intellectual level after hemidecortication (Table 2). In six of the nine cases intellectual levels remained virtually the same as before, while in the remaining two cases, postoperative scores fell at least 10 points below preoperative levels.

It should be noted that, in the several studies referred to, none of the patients, including those who exhibited postoperative improvement, had an IQ level above 85 (except for the one greatly improved patient with Rasmussen's disease, who ultimately attained a score of 103). Most often the patients' IQs remained far below normal, averaging in the 60s in each of the several series. (In the published series of hemidecortication, irrespective of the underlying disease processes, average postoperative IQ was 67, range 45-85, eliminating the one exceptional case). Because hemidecortication in the two aetiological groups (i.e. Rasmussen's disease vs. infantile hemiplegia with seizures) resulted in the same average intelligence score postoperatively, the two groups differ not only in the proportion of cases exhibiting postoperative intellectual improvement but also, necessarily, in the average amount of postoperative intellectual decline that they sustained following seizure onset. Thus, children with severe perinatal seizure disorder generally exhibit a greater overall reduction (or developmental arrest) of intellectual ability than do children with late onset of seizures. Further, early seizure onset adversely affects the potential for development of the intellectual functions of both hemispheres[4]. By contrast, if seizures first occur in later stages of development, the initial loss of intellectual skills is predominantly in those served by the directly affected hemisphere, and only later does the impairment spread to include the functions served by the other hemisphere.

Table 1. Details of Cases with Rasmussen's Encephalitis

Patient	Sex	Hemisphere Removed	Seizure Onset	Age at Operation	Age at Testing
1	F	Left	12.10	15.04	16.11
2	F	Left	6.00	17.07	20.02
3	M	Left	4.03	8.09	15.00
4	F	Left	2.00	6.10	10.05
5	F	Right	9.00	5.09	16.11
6	M	Right	6.02	6.08	11.03
7	F	Right	5.11	10.01	16.06
8	M	Right	4.06	7.00	7.11
9	F	Right	4.00	5.08	7.00

(All ages in years and months)

An example of preoperative intellectual decline and postoperative outcome in a child with Rasmussen's encephalitis is illustrated in Fig. 1. This child had acquired left hemisphere disease at the age of six and had her IQ measured for the first time at the age of 10.5 and then aperiodically until the age of 20. Initially, only verbal IQ appears to have been affected, performance IQ falling within the normal range. By the age of 14, however, this child's performance IQ, above 90 at first testing, had dropped more than 10 points, and then continued to drop further during the next two years to a low of 77. Hemidecortication, which was performed when the child was 17.5, resulted in an abrupt rise of a few points in both measures, but this improvement was short-lived, presumably because of the unfortunate recurrence of epilepsy several months later. This child (AL) was the only patient in the series to suffer recurrence of seizures following surgery, although even in this case they were substantially reduced in severity and frequency.

Table 2. Preoperative and postoperative IQ scores for the hemidecorticated cases described in Table 1.

Patient	Hemisphere Removed	Preoperative			Postoperative		
		FSIQ	VIQ	PIQ	FSIQ	VIQ	PIQ
1	Left	45	-	-	66	55	80
2	Left	69	66	77	68	64	77
3	Left	65	74	60	68	69	70
4	Left	<45	54	<45	48	57	48
5	Right	>70	>82	>62	77	80	75
6	Right	105	108	101	80	94	71
7	Right	79	92	69	55	68	49
8	Right	87	87	96	85	98	73
9	Right	-	-	-	50	60	48

FSIQ - Full Scale IQ; VIQ - Verbal IQ; PIQ - Performance IQ

Memory

There is a dearth of information about memory function in patients who have undergone hemidecortication. Gott[14] reported on verbal and nonverbal memory ability in three such patients (one with left hemidecortication and two with right) who were examined between four and ten years postoperatively. All three patients suffered from acquired disorders (two cases of malignant tumours and one case of encephalitis).

On the Wechsler Memory Scale, which mainly measures verbal short-term memory and processing ability, all three patients were seriously impaired. Their memory quotients, which ranged from 49 to 77, were from 13 to 28 points less than their verbal IQs (range, 63 to 105), indicating that their verbal memory and processing abilities fell substantially below predictions derived from IQ. Similar results were obtained on a test of memory for designs[15], leading Gott[14] to conclude that two cooperating hemispheres are needed for normal short-term memory, verbal and nonverbal alike.

Somewhat different conclusions were reached by Ogden[27,28], who studied verbal and nonverbal memory function in two adult patients who had had infantile hemiplegia with seizures and had undergone left hemidecortication during late adolescence. Memory function was assessed three times in each patient during long-term follow-up, extending from four to sixteen years postoperatively in one case and from fifteen to twenty-seven years postoperatively in the other. The patient with the shorter recovery period obtained memory quotients ranging from 66 to 80, with the score on each occasion being essentially the same as verbal IQ, which ranged from 74 to 82.

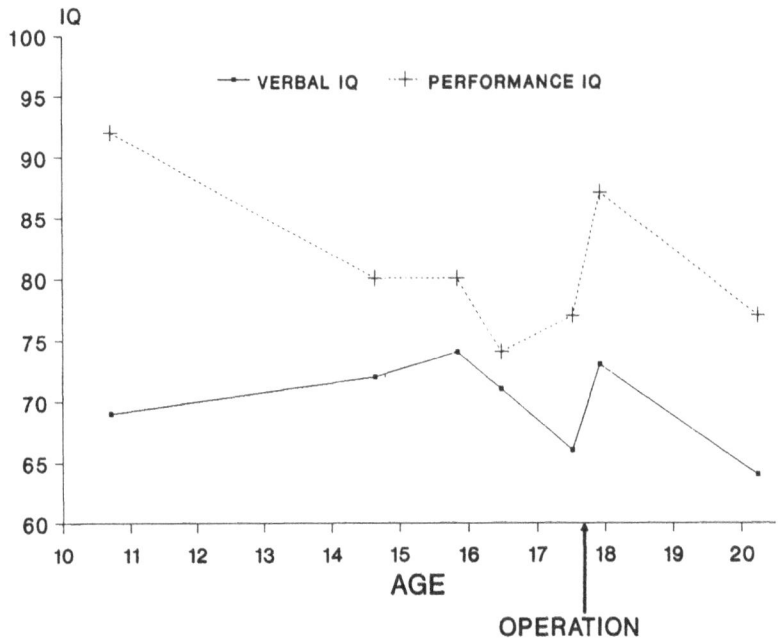

Figure 1. Verbal and Performance IQ at various ages before and after surgery in case AL.

However, the patient with the longer recovery period showed a different pattern. The memory quotient of 97 measured at fifteen years follow-up was consistent with the verbal IQ at that time which was also 97, but subsequent memory quotients, measured at 22 and 27 years follow-up, were 19 and 25 points higher than the verbal IQ, which remained roughly constant throughout follow-up. While familiarity with the test may account for some of the improvement, it is unlikely to explain all of it. Support for this conclusion is provided by the finding that the patient's nonverbal memory, which was also tested repeatedly during follow-up, failed to show improvement. In fact, whereas both patients' scores on the verbal memory subtests of the Wechsler Memory Scale rose over the follow-up period, their short-term memory for complex visuo-spatial information (Rey and Taylor Complex Figure Tests) deteriorated, with all their recall scores falling below the 10th percentile for normal adults[27].

In our own series of nine surgical patients with Rasmussen's disease, memory quotients on the Wechsler Memory Scale were calculated using Taylor's children stories[17] together with an age correction for those over the age of 20 years as suggested by Taylor (personal communication, 1981). All patients were evaluated once postoperatively, with the follow-up period for the group ranging from about 1 to 6½ years (Table 1). As indicated in Table 3, their memory quotients ranged from 57 to 86. The average MQ of the patients with right hemidecortication was higher than that of the patients with left hemidecortication (means of 77 and 61.5 respectively), but the difference was not statistically significant ($X^2 = 2.08$; P = 0.15). Two patients with left and one with right hemidecortication had memory quotients higher than their verbal IQs (range, 3 to 11 points), whereas the remaining patients (two with left and three with right hemidecortications) obtained memory quotients below their verbal IQs (range 7 to 14 points). Since none of the discrepancies between memory quotient and verbal IQ exceeded 14 points, the patients' memory scores appeared to be consistent with predictions derived from their intelligence levels.

Language

Much of the research on language function in hemidecorticated patients has arisen out of the controversy over the hypothesis of hemispheric equipotentiality. Since there have been no reported cases of chronic loss of speech (i.e. mutism) following

Table 3. Memory quotients for the hemidecorticated cases described in Table 1.

Patient	Hemisphere Removed	Memory Quotient	MQ vs VIQ Differential
1	Left	62	(+) 7
2	Left	57	(-) 7
3	Left	61	(-) 8
4	Left	66	(+)11
5	Right	83	(+) 3
6	Right	80	(-) 14
7	Right	60	(-) 8
8	Right	86	(-) 12
9	Right	-	-

MQ - Memory Quotient; VIQ - Verbal IQ

(+) MQ > VIQ
(-) MQ < VIQ

decortication of hemisphere[3,25], it is clear that either isolated hemisphere has sufficient capacity to subserve at least the gross aspects of speech and language function, particularly if the surgical procedure occurs during childhood[27,39,40]. Traditionally, this degree of equipotentiality of the two cerebral hemispheres has been attributed to the 'plasticity' of the immature nervous system[21]. Brain plasticity allowing right hemisphere mediation of speech and language function appears to operate along a continuum, with maximum reorganisation occurring when the injury is sustained before the age of five or six years[36], but with some potential for reorganisation continuing through the middle childhood years, becoming progressively restricted as age at insult increases.

Since the majority of patients comprising the larger series of hemidecorticated patients (e.g. 25, 46) suffered early seizure onset associated with congenital or perinatal pathology, and none of the patients were investigated longitudinally prior to surgery, the relation between degree of language reorganisation and age at onset of injury in these series cannot be examined in any detail. With the hemidecortication procedure becoming more prevalent for treatment of acquired seizure disorder in patients who have had normal brain development up to some stage during childhood, it will gradually become possible to examine the role of age at onset of the disorder in determining language outcome after hemidecortication, provided that the variable of elapsed time since seizure onset is controlled for.

During the past twenty years, a number of studies have uncovered deficits in selective aspects of language processing after left as compared with right hemidecorticatioyn. Areas of language performance investigated have included: auditory vocabulary[50], auditory language comprehension[27,48], use of pronouns in narrative discourse[24], syntactical comprehension[9,10,12,27], production and judgement of morphological markers[43] and reading and writing[11,14,27,31].

The majority of the above studies have focused largely on the laterality of the surgical removal, contrasting the performance of either pairs of patients or small groups of patients with left vs right hemidecortications. This has necessitated ignoring or pooling of data across many other variables, such as age at initial insult or disorder, age at hemidecortication, elapsed time since initial insult or disorder, elapsed time since surgery and aetiology, among others.

Despite these deficiencies, it can be concluded from the studies of hemidecorticated patients in combination with those on callosotomized (split-brain) patients[48,49,50,51], that: (a) the isolated right hemisphere has a basic visual and auditory lexicon consisting of concrete and high-frequency words; (b) the isolated right hemisphere can recognise, comprehend, and produce words from this lexicon through both speech and writing; and (c) in contrast to these domains of ability, the isolated right hemisphere has difficulty in comprehending abstract, low-frequency, and low-imagery words, manipulating subtleties of grammatical structure, and analysing words according to their phonetic features.

In the domain of syntactical competence, particular attention has been paid to receptive grammar and comprehension of sentences marked by active/passive distinctions. Specifically, left hemidecorticated patients are reported[9,10,12] to be impaired in the comprehension of passive negative constructions (e.g. the truck was not hit by the car). For these sentences to be interpreted correctly, the normal subject-verb-object (SVO) sequence must be disregarded and replaced through a decoding strategy with the reverse sequence. Accurate comprehension of such sentences thus requires syntactic rather than pragmatic knowledge. Dennis and Kohn[10] conclude that after left hemidecortication, patients are unable to adopt a reversal strategy, and as a result they misinterpret negative passive sentences. The impaired performance of left hemidecorticated patients is not restricted to comprehension of passive structures, but extends to production and judgement of morphological markers and indeed to global comprehension of grammar[43]. These patients are impaired in the various aspects of syntax in relation not only to normal subjects and control groups with less extensive brain damage, but also to right hemidecorticated patients with intellectual abilities comparable to theirs.

This selective impairment after left hemidecortication does not seem to vary with aetiology. Virtually the same results are found in small groups of hemidecorticated patients with diagnosis of Rasmussen's encephalitis as in those with congenital or perinatal pathology. Thus, in our own (unpublished) series of hemidecorticated patients, performance on the Test for Reception of Grammar[5] was far more severely impaired in those with left sided removals than in those with right. In addition, the patients with left hemidecortications made their first errors on the test significantly earlier than those with right (L mean = 34.00; SD= 3.56; R mean = 53.00; SD = 13.94; X^2 = 6.05; P<0.01).

A test of morphological production yielded similar results[43]. Patients were shown a drawing (Figure 2) and asked to complete a sentence read to them by saying a word containing an appropriate inflection (e.g. This snake is thinner than this one. But this one is the ......). The test consisted of two subtests, with one subtest requiring the subject to provide an inflected real word and the other requiring an inflected nonword (e.g. These creatures are very brout. But this creature is the ......"broutest").

The results for each patient are shown in Table 4. Relative to the right hemidecorticated group (N=3), the left hemidecorticated group (N=4) was significantly impaired on the nonword subtest (L mean = 9.25; SD = 2.87; R mean = 17.0; SD= 1.73; X^2= 4.66; P<0.03). On the word subtest, the difference between the two groups fell just short of significance (L mean = 16.0; SD = 1.82; R mean = 18.33; SD = 0.57; X^2 = 3.36; P = 0.06).

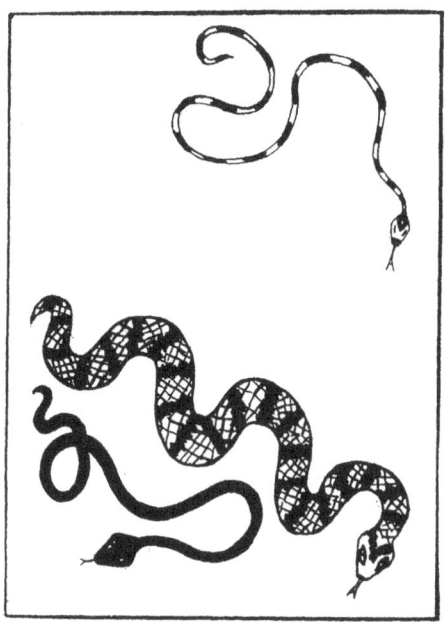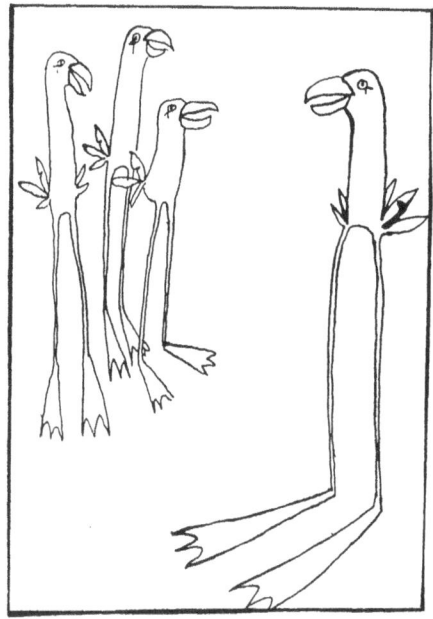

Figure 2. Drawings accompanying one of the words (Left) and nonwords (Right) in the Morphological Production Task.

Visual Perception

Compared to the interest focused on the language function of hemidecorticated patients, relatively little attention has been paid to their visual perception. Three case studies of hemidecorticated patients with right hemisphere disease acquired at ages, five[7], six, and twenty eight,[14] found, contrary to expectation, no gross deficits on many visual tasks sensitive to right hemisphere function, such as spatial orientation, visuospatial construction and face perception. An exception to these negative findings is the case reported by Sergent and Villemure[38]. This patient, who underwent hemidecortication at age 13 following seizure onset at age 5, was found to be densely prosapagnosic when tested at age 33, despite having normal or only mildly impaired intellectual and cognitive functions. This is the only hemidecorticated patient with prosopagnosia that has been reported to date.

Table 4. Scores (percent correct) on the Morphological Production Test of the first seven hemidecorticated patients described in Table 1.

Patient	Hemisphere Removed	Age at Testing	Morphological Production %	
			Words	Non-words
1	Left	16.11	75	45
2	Left	20.03	90	30
3	Left	15.00	85	45
4	Left	10.05	70	65
5	Right	16.11	90	75
6	Right	11.03	95	90
7	Right	16.06	90	90

Because the cases with right hemidecortication examined by Damasio et al.[7], and Gott[14] showed no gross visuoperceptual deficits despite having acquired brain damage relatively late, it might be predicted that cases with congenital or perinatal brain damage would be even less likely to demonstrate such deficits. In fact, the opposite was found in a study of eight patients with infantile hemiplegia who underwent hemidecortication (four left and four right) for relief of seizures during late childhood or early adulthood[19]. Although the four patients with right hemidecortication were unimpaired or only mildly impaired relative to the four with left hemidecortication on the Weinstein/Semmes Personal Orientation test, the Porteus Maze Test, and the WISC Maze subtest, the former group showed a pronounced deficit on the Money Road-Map test and a map-reading test of extrapersonal orientation. The authors concluded that either hemisphere can mediate simple visuospatial functions, but when task demands increase, the selective visuospatial disability of the isolated left hemisphere becomes evident.

Yet, a similar pattern of results, i.e. no impairment on simple visuospatial tasks but pronounced impairment on more demanding ones, was reported by Ogden[28] in two patients with infantile hemiplegia and seizures who underwent left hemidecortication during adolescence. Both patients were tested after long recovery periods of 16 and 28 years, respectively. Ogden's data address the intriguing question of the fate of visual functions normally dependent on the right hemisphere in the face of a shift of language function to that hemisphere. The abilities and disabilities shown by the two patients led Ogden[28] to suggest that an isolated right hemisphere that has reorganised to subserve speech and language following early damage to the left hemisphere is capable of mediating only low level visuospatial processes. As with the isolated left hemisphere, according to Ogden, the isolated right hemisphere also fails to develop higher order visuospatial functions.

The difficulty with this as a general formulation of course is that Dennis and Kohn's[10] patients with left hemidecortications failed to show the same visuospatial impairment, despite similar aetiology and age at onset of seizures. This discrepancy in the effects of early onset left hemisphere disease, like that referred to earlier regarding the effects of late onset right hemisphere disease, has yet to be accounted for satisfactorily.

SUMMARY

This review of the effects of hemidecortication in humans has been limited to studies of cognitive outcome published during the last 20 years. More directly than in the case of split-brain patients, the patients reviewed here attest to the remarkable ability of a single hemisphere, whether left or right, to support at least at modest levels a wide range of cognitive functions - from visual perception, through memory and intellectual processes, to language and even speech. In some cases, as has been indicated, the surgical removal of a diseased hemisphere has resulted in improvement of cognitive function. This positive outcome has occurred more frequently in patients with early (i.e. congenital or perinatal) onset of seizure disorders than in those with late onset (e.g. Rasmussen's disease). But even for the latter patients, the cognitive costs of the surgery per se have rarely been severe. And in both types of case, the incidence of either complete or substantial postoperative relief from intractable seizures has been high, ranging around 80-90%.

Although the therapeutic efficacy and small cognitive costs of the surgery are now quite well established, little is known yet regarding the specific cognitive defects that arise from the loss of one as opposed to the other cerebral hemisphere. Intelligence levels have been found to be equally low, averaging in the mid-60s and almost never rising above 100 in patients with either left or right hemidecortications, and memory quotients have most often appeared to fall in line with the IQ scores, again without clear evidence of any difference in the effects of left and right removals. Even in the case of visual spatial perception, considered to be a hallmark of right hemisphere function, the evidence is unclear, one study reporting selective impairment on difficult visuospatial tasks in right hemispherectomised patients, but another not. Only in regard to language processes is there a consensus regarding the differential effects of left and right hemidecortication, and here the differences are apparent only in the relatively subtler aspects of language. Thus, the isolated right hemisphere is at a significant disadvantage compared with the left in the comprehension of abstract, low frequency words, in phonetic feature analysis, and in the subtleties of grammar, such as the comprehension of passive negative constructions and the correct use of morphological markers in unfamiliar contexts (e.g. application of comparative and superlative forms of an adjective to nonwords).

Several cautions must be raised in interpreting the foregoing findings. First, cognitive outcome after hemidecortication is almost always assessed after a longstanding disease process has affected the functional organization of not only one hemisphere but both. Second, the effect of the disease process on the 'intact' hemisphere is likely to be highly complex, involving both interference with that hemisphere's functions by the seizure disorder (and, presumably, the anticonvulsant medication) as well as forced reorganization of its functions due to the functional failure of the diseased hemisphere. Adding to the complexity is the likelihood that the interference and the forced reorganization will not affect all systems of the 'intact' hemisphere equally; the ones affected will depend in part on the nature, locus, and severity of the pathology. Third, as already indicated, a host of temporal variables, including age at onset, age at surgery, and age at testing, will influence the extent of both the interference and the forced reorganization. Finally, uncontrolled experiential variables are certain to affect any reorganization of cognitive function as well as its recovery. To unravel the effects of these numerous variables, case studies alone are obviously inadequate. Attempts must be made to gather series of cases so that the consequences of these diverse factors can be directly assessed.

ACKNOWLEDGEMENTS

We thank Elizabeth Isaacs and Kate Watkins for their assistance in investigating our series of patients with hemidecortication, and Lynne Salmon for typing this manuscript. The operation of patient 4 in our series (see Tables 1 to 4) was performed by Mr. Sam Galbraith, Southern General Hospital, Glasgow, and that on patient 6, by Mr. C.B.T. Adams, The Radcliffe Infirmary, Oxford; we are indebted to both neurosurgeons for making their patients available to us. Elizabeth Beardsworth (recently deceased) had generously provided us with some of the preoperative IQ data illustrated in Figure 1. Finally, we thank all nine of our patients (and their families) for permitting us to study them. The investigation was supported by project grants from the Medical Research Council to the first author.

REFERENCES

1. Adams, C.B.T., 1983, Hemispherectomy - a modification, *J. of Neurol. Neurosurg. and Psychiat.*, **46**, 617-619.
2. Ameli, N.O., 1980, Hemispherectomy for the treatment of epilepsy and behaviour disturbance, *Le Journal Canadien des Sciences Neurologiques*, **7**, 33-38.
3. Basser, L.S., 1962, Hemiplegia of early onset and the faculty of speech with special reference to the effects of hemispherectomy, *Brain*, **38**, 239-258.
4. Beardsworth, E.D. and Adams, C.B.T., 1988, Modified hemispherectomy for epilepsy: early results in 10 cases, *British J. of Neurosurg.*, **2**, 73-84.
5. Bishop, D.V.M., 1982, *TROG: Test for Reception of Grammar*, Thomas Leach, Abingdon Oxon (For the Medical Research Council).
6. Chugani, H.T., Shewmon, D.A., Peacock, W.J., Shields, W.D., Mazziotta, J.C. and Phelps, M.E., 1988, Surgical treatment of intractable neonatal-onset seizures: the role of positron emission tomography, *Neurology*, **38**, 1178-1188.
7. Damasio, A.R., Lima, A. and Damasio, H., 1975, Nervous function after right hemispherectomy, *Neurology*, **25**, 89-93.
8. Dandy, W.E., 1928, Removal of right cerebral hemisphere for certain tumours with hemiplegia, *J. Amer. Med. Assoc.*, **90**, 823.
9. Dennis, M., 1980, Capacity and strategy for syntactic comprehension after left or right hemidecortication, *Brain and Lang.*, **10**, 287-317.
10. Dennis, M. and Kohn, B., 1975, Comprehension of syntax in infantile hemiplegics after cerebral hemidecortication: left hemisphere superiority, *Brain and Lang.*, **2**, 472-482.
11. Dennis, M., Lovett, M. and Wiegel-Crump, C.A., 1981, Written language acquisition after left or right decortication in infancy, *Brain and Lang.*, **12**, 54-91.

12. Dennis, M. and Whitaker, H.A., 1976, Language acquisition following hemidecortication: linguistic superiority of the left over the right hemisphere, *Brain and Lang.*, **3**, 404-433.

13. Goodman, R., 1986, Hemispherectomy and its alternatives in the treatment of intractable epilepsy in patients with infantile hemiplegia, *Dev. Med. Child Neurol.*, **28**, 251-258.

14. Gott, P.S., 1973, Cognitive abilities following right and left hemispherectomy, *Cortex*, **9**, 266-274.

15. Graham, F.K. and Kendall, B.S., 1960, Memory-for-designs test, *Percep. Mot. Skills*, **11**, 147-188.

16. Honavar, M., Janota, I. and Polkey, C.E., 1992, Rasmussen's Encephalitis in surgery for epilepsy, *Dev. Med. Child Neurol.*, **34**, 3-14.

17. Kimura, D. and McGlone, J., 1979, Children's stories for testing LTM, in *Neuropsychological Test Manual*, D. Kimura and J. McGlone, eds., DK Consultants, London.

18. King, M., Stephenson, J.B.P., Ziervogel, M., Doyle, D. and Galbraith, S., 1985, Hemimegancephaly - A Case for Hemispherectomy? *Neuropaediatrics*, **16**, 46-55.

19. Kohn, B. and Dennis, M., 1974, Selective impairments of visuo-spatial abilities in infantile hemiplegics after right cerebral hemidecortication, *Neuropsychologia*, **12**, 505-512.

20. Krynauw, R.A., 1950, Infantile hemiplegia treated by removing one cerebral hemisphere, *J. Neurol., Neurosurg. and Psychiatry*, **13**, 243-267.

21. Lenneberg, H., 1967, *Biological Foundations of Language*, Wiley, New York.

22. L'hermitte, J., 1928, L'ablation complete de l'hemisphere droit dans les cas de tumeur cerebrale localisée compliquée d'hemiplegie: la decerebration suprathalamique unilaterale chez l'homme, *L'Encephale*, **23**, 314-323.

23. Lindsay, J., Ounsted, C., and Richards, P., 1987, Hemispherectomy for childhood epilepsy: a 36 year study, *Develop. Med. and Child Neurol.*, **29**, 592-600.

24. Lovett, M.W., Dennis, M. and Newman, J.E., 1986, Making reference: the cohesive use of pronouns in the narrative discourse of hemidecorticate adolescents, *Brain and Lang.*, **29**, 224-251.

25. McFie, J., 1961, The effects of hemispherectomy on intellectual function in cases of infantile hemiplegia, *J. Neurol., Neurosurg. and Psychiatry*, **24**, 240-249.

26. McKenzie, K.G., 1938, The present status of a patient who has a right cerebral hemisphere removed, *J. Amer. Med. Assoc.*, **111**, 168.

27. Ogden, J.A., 1988, Language and memory functions after long recovery periods in left hemispherectomised subjects, *Neuropsychologia*, **26**, 645-659.

28. Ogden, J.A., 1989, Visuo-spatial and other 'right hemispheric' functions after long recovery periods in left hemispherectomised subjects, *Neuropsychologia*, **27**, 765-776.

29. Oguni, H., Andermann, F. and Rasmussen, T., 1991, The natural history of the syndrome of chronic encephalitis and epilepsy: a study of the MNI series of 48 cases, in *Chronic Encephalitis and Epilepsy: Rasmussen Syndrome*. Frederick Andermann, ed., pp. 7-35, Butterworth-Heinemann, Stoneham, Massachusetts.

30. Oluwole Ogunmekan, A., Hwang, P.A. and Hoffman, H.J., 1989, Sturge-Weber-Dimitri disease: role of hemispherectomy in prognosis, *Can. J. Neurol. Sciences*, **16**, 78-80.

31. Patterson, K., Vargha-Khadem, F. and Polkey, C.E., 1989, Reading with one hemisphere, *Brain*, **112**, 39-63.

32. Rasmussen, T., 1975, Surgery for epilepsy arising in regions other than the frontal or temporal lobes, in D. P.Purpura, K .K. Perry, and R. D. Walter, R.D., eds., *Advances in Neurology*, **8**, 207-226, Raven Press, New York.

33. Rasmussen, T., 1978, Further observations on the syndrome of chronic encephalitis and epilepsy, *Applied Neurophysiol.*, **41**, 1-12.

34. Rasmussen, T., 1983, Hemispherectomy for seizures revisited, *Can. J. Neurol. Science*, **10**, 71-78.

35. Rasmussen, T., and McCann, W., 1968, Clinical studies of patients with focal epilepsy due to chronic encephalitis, *Trans. Amer. Neurol. Association*, **93**, 89-94.

36. Rasmussen, T. and Milner, B., 1977, The role of early left brain injury in determining lateralisation of cerebral speech functions, *Annals N. Y. Acad. Sci.*, **299**, 355-369.

37. Rasmussen, T. & Villemure, J.G., 1989, Cerebral hemispherectomy for seizures with hemiplegia, *Cleveland Clinical Journal of Medicine*, **56**, (supplementary part of 1), 562-568.

38. Sergent, J. and Villemure, J.G., 1989, Prosopagnosia in a right hemispherectomised patient, *Brain*, **112**, 975-995.

39. Smith, A., 1974, Dominant and nondominant hemispherectomy, in *Hemisphere Disconnection and Cerebral Function*, M. Kinsbourne and W.L. Smith, eds., pp. 5-33, Springfield, Illinois: Thomas.

40. Smith, A. and Sugar, O., 1975, Development of above-normal language and intelligence twenty one years after left hemispherectomy, *Neurology*, **25**, 813-818.

41. Taylor, L.B., 1991, Neuropsychologic assessment of patients with encephalitis, in *Chronic Encephalitis and Epilepsy: Rasmussen Syndrome*, Frederick Andermann, eds., pp. 111-124, Butterworth-Heinemann, Stoneham, Massachusetts.

42. Tinuper, P., Andermann, F., Villemure, J.G., Rasmussen, T., and Quesney, L.P., 1988, Functional hemispherectomy for treatment of epilepsy associated with hemiplegia: rationale, indications, results, and comparison with callosotomy, *Ann. Neurol.*, **24**, 27-34.

43. Vargha-Khadem, F., Isaacs, E.B., Papaleloudi, H., Polkey, C.E. and Wilson, J., 1991, Development of language in six hemispherectomised patients, *Brain*, **114**, 473-495.

44. Verity, C.M., Strauss, E.H., Moyes, P.B., Wada, J.A., Dunn, H.G. and La Pointe, J.S., 1982, long-term follow-up after cerebral hemispherectomy: neurophysiological, radiologic and psychological findings, *Neurology*, **32**, 629-639.

45. Villemure, J.G., Andermann, F. and Rasmussen, T., 1991, Hemispherectomy for the treatment of epilepsy due to chronic encephalitis, in *Chronic Encephalitis and Epilepsy: Rasmussen Syndrome*, Frederick Andermann, ed., pp. 235-241, Butterworth-Heinemann, Stoneham, Massachusetts.

46. Wilson, P.J.E., 1970, Cerebral hemispherectomy for infantile hemiplegia: a report of 50 cases, *Brain*, **93**, 147-180.

47. Woods, B.T. and Teuber, H.L., 1973, Early onset of complementary specialisation of cerebral hemispheres in man, *Trans. Amer. Neurol. Association*, **98**, 113-117.

48. Zaidel, E., 1977, Unilateral auditory language comprehension on the Token Test following cerebral commissurotomy and hemispherectomy, *Neuropsychologia*, **15**, 1-17.

49. Zaidel, E., 1978, Lexical organisation in the right hemisphere, in *Cerebral Correlates of Conscious Experience*, P.A. Buser and A. Rougeul-Buser, eds., pp. 177-197, North Holland, Amsterdam and Oxford.

50. Zaidel, E., 1978, Auditory language comprehension in the right hemisphere following cerebral commissurotomy and hemispherectomy: a comparison with child language and aphasia, in *Language Acquisition and Language Breakdown: Parallels and Divergencies*, A. Caramazza and E.B. Zurif, eds., pp. 229-275, Johns Hopkins University Press, Baltimore and London.

51. Zaidel, E., 1980, The split and half brains as models of congenital language disability, in *The Neurological Basis of Language Disorders in Children: Methods and Directions for Research*, NINCES Monograph No. 22. C.L. Ludlow and M.E. Doran-Quine, eds., pp. 55-86, Bethesda, M.D.: U.S. Department of Health, Education and Welfare, Public Health Service, National Insititutes of Health, National Institutes of Communicative Disorders and Stroke.

COMPENSATORY MECHANISMS - NEURAL AND BEHAVIOURAL:

EVIDENCE FROM PRENATAL DAMAGE TO THE FOREBRAIN COMMISSURES

M A Jeeves

Psychological Laboratory
University of St. Andrews
College Gate
St. Andrews, Scotland

INTRODUCTION

In the ten years since I last reviewed this topic[18], focussing in particular on how it may add to our understanding of recovery from early brain injury, there have been several significant developments. These make it timely to reassess earlier views on compensatory mechanisms, neural and behavioural, in callosal agenesis. First, in the last ten years new emphases have developed in our thinking about the diversity of functions subsumed by the forebrain commissures[20,56]. An earlier concentration on the integrative functions of these commissures has been enlarged by a fresh recognition of their likely inhibitory[56] and facilitatory[33] roles (see Table 1). Second, a series of replications of earlier studies carried out on additional cases of callosal agenesis have enabled a re-evaluation of the earlier findings, many of which were based on single cases. This more recent work has helped to eliminate the unwanted effects of possible artefacts resulting from associated abnormalities in callosal agenesis, making possible a greater confidence that the deficits noted in earlier reports are specifically attributable to the failure of the forebrain commissures to develop. Third, investigations have been extended into new domains so that the overall neuro-psychological profile of callosal agenesis has become more comprehensive and well documented. Thus reports have appeared of studies of language[8,28,49,50], memory[3] and stereo perception[21] in callosal agenesis, as well as detailed and careful analyses of bimanual motor performance[28,29]. Fourth, the work of Innocenti and his co-workers[12,13,14] on the exhuberant growth of callosal fibres in early life and their subsequent reduction in number has been published. Fifth, the increasing availability of new imaging techniques, in particular MRI, has afforded a much more detailed knowledge of brain structures in callosal agenesis patients. In particular they have made possible a better assessment of whether the dysgenesis is total or partial; and most importantly of whether or not the anterior commissure is present. Finally, in some cases single patients have been studied for periods extending up to thirty years. This has made possible the monitoring of neural and/or behavioural compensations occurring later in life. A better indication is thus now available of the limits of hypothesised compensatory mechanisms.

Recovery from Brain Damage, Edited by F.D. Rose and
D.A. Johnson, Plenum Press, New York, 1992

Table 1. Hemispheric Interactions Mediated through the Forebrain Commissures.

Integration		ensures sharing of lateralized sensory input and coordination of bilaterally controlled motor output
Inhibition	(1)	ensures the development of topographic sensation and precise motor control by suppressing the contribution from uncrossed ipsilateral pathways
	(2)	ensures hemispheric independence, thus allowing implementation of modularity of representation and processing in the normal brain
Facilitation	(1)	in the intact cortex, the corpus callosum exerts a facilitatory, or modulating, influence on the neural activity of both hemispheres
	(2)	this modulatory action may actively participate in the functional reorganization that takes place after brain injury

THE DIVERSITY OF FUNCTIONS OF THE FOREBRAIN COMMISSURES

The Integrative Role of the Forebrain Commissures

Sperry's work with split-brain animals and patients (e.g. 48) convincingly demonstrated the importance of the major forebrain commissures for integrating activity in the two cerebral hemispheres and for transferring information from one hemisphere to the other. Almost all of the early work whether on split-brain patients or on animals was done on adults. There were occasional early attempts to examine the effects of early neonatal callosal sections in animals (e.g. 23) and these have since been extended by, for example, Ptito and his co-workers[43].

The convincing demonstration by Sperry and his colleagues of the vital importance of intact forebrain commissures for many psychological functions naturally raised the question of how it is that people born without the major commissure nevertheless, at times, appear to grow up apparently normal. This is not entirely surprising because it remains the case that the surgical split-brain patients also appear normal in brief social interactions. It is only careful testing which lays bare the deficits which, once identified, become so dramatic, so we might well expect a similar picture would apply in the case of these "experiments of nature", who, after all, have a pre- and post-natal lifetime to develop appropriate compensatory mechanisms for the missing forebrain commissures.

The special relevance for understanding this integrative function, in the context of recovery of function, is that it may help us to discover what we can learn from callosal agenesis patients about the extent to which other pathways can take over the functions of the missing corpus callosum, and in some cases of the anterior commissure also. That raises a further question. If other pathways do appear to take over, then which pathways are they and how do they achieve their compensatory role? Thus, specifically, in the present context we need to raise and address the question of the limits to the functions of the anterior commissure when it is present[44]; to raise the question of the plasticity within the corpus callosum when there is early partial damage to it; we need to raise the question of the limits to the transfer functions of the sub-cortical pathways, noting in particular the series of studies in the past decade by Justine Sergent[45,46] which suggest the possibility of interhemispheric transfer in the classical split-brain patients of a kind not previously observed. Finally, it raises the question of the possibility of intrahemispheric integration and the extent to which this can replace interhemispheric integration through the corpus callosum.

The Inhibitory Role of the Forebrain Commissures

As far back as the 1962 John's Hopkins conference on cerebral asymmetries the neurophysiologist Richard Jung[30], in his discussion of the early results of a series of studies of hemispheric specialisation, had noted that, in his judgement, most, if not all, of the reported findings could only come about as a result of the inhibitory role of the forebrain commissures. The same view has been reiterated in a different context by Berlucchi[l] who points out how the local inhibitory inter-neurones are activated by the callosal input. In a behavioural context it was Dennis[7] who, after studying two acallosal patients, had argued that the course of normal development involves the progressive suppression of crossed sensory and motor projections. The acquisition of fine distal motor control she argued involves the progressive inhibition of motor pathways other than crossed pyramidal ones. In this context the notion of inhibition is extended to a somewhat looser conceptualisation in terms of suppression. Dennis[8] followed this up by further studies of callosal agenesis patients in which she argued that agenesis results in an inability to suppress the ipsilateral component of an auditory stimulus when there is spectral temporal overlap of stimuli.

Preilowski[42] had also noted this role of the callosum when he attributed a lowered quality in speed and performance in split-brain patients when performing a bimanual coordination task in part to a lack of callosal inhibition. Zaidel[56] suggested that:

> "Some problems may require facile interhemispheric integration, while others may call for a unique hemisphere processing style and *may actually be inhibited by the other hemisphere*" (p 448 - my italics).

He believes that the corpus callosum is a complex dynamic channel of both facilitatory and inhibitory codes". Others who have made use of this notion of an inhibitory or suppressive role for the corpus callosum include Moscovitch[38] who argued that the corpus callosum plays a crucial role in establishing hemispheric asymmetry since each hemisphere exerts an inhibitory influence on the other and in this way prevents the dual establishment of specialised functions in both hemispheres. Subsequent research has failed to support this hypothesis[24,36].

Facilitation

In addition to the facilitatory function proposed by Zaidel[56] referred to above we also have the discussion of this putative role for the forebrain commissures by Lassonde[33]. Her argument is that the corpus callosum may play an important role in the activation of each cerebral hemisphere and thus that, in this sense, it has an important facilitatory role.

In a task requiring acallosals and matched IQ normals to make a same/different judgment of pairs of visual stimuli (letters, numbers, colours, or forms) Lassonde[33] found that acallosals were able to effect interhemispheric comparisons and that their

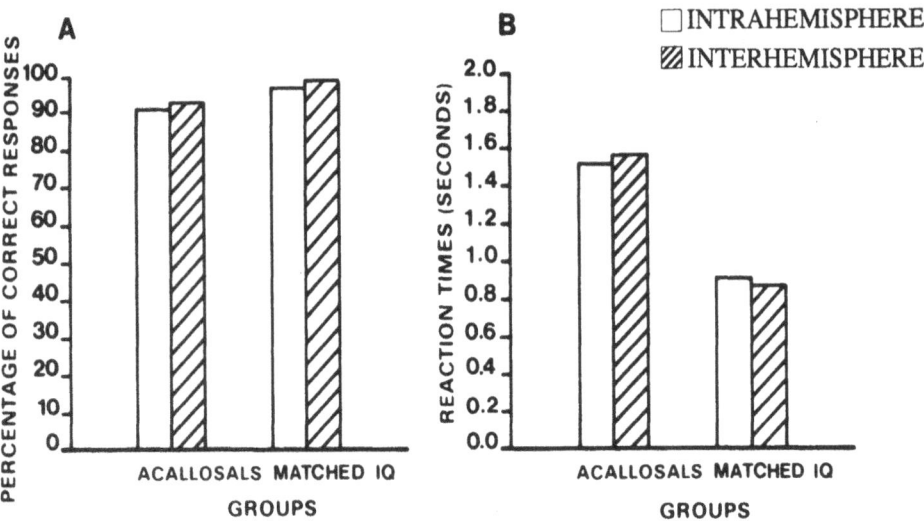

Figure 1. Percentages of correct responses (A) and mean reaction times (B) obtained from acallosals and matched IQ subjects (n = 6) on an intra- and interhemispheric discrimination task. (Taken from reference 33)

accuracy level making both inter and intra hemispheric judgments did not differ from matched IQ controls (see Figure 1). However a different result emerged when reaction times were compared.

As Figure 1 also shows the acallosals required twice as much time to respond as the control groups. Lassonde believes that the corpus callosum participates in the bilateral activation of those regions specifically implicated in the specific neural activity required by her tasks. She argues that in the absence of the corpus callosum neural activity in the regions concerned may be reduced and hence the delayed responsiveness. She cites further evidence in support[33].

EXTENDING AND CONSOLIDATING THE NEUROPSYCHOLOGICAL PROFILE IN CALLOSAL AGENESIS

Recent Studies Extending the Profile

1) – Language Studies: Dennis[8] reported a study of a 27 year old female with callosal agenesis and summed up her results by identifying difficulties which this patient had with :

> "syntactic comprehension, pragmatic use and understanding and metalinguistic knowledge, despite good capacity for phonological and lexical semantic processing".

Three more recent studies[25,49,50] have extended Dennis' findings confirming some aspects and pointing to additional language deficits in callosal agenesis. In our 1987 study[25], in one of our patients we confirmed the syntactic-pragmatic deficit reported by Dennis but demonstrated that the patients language deficits were not restricted to this (see Table 2). We also identified difficulty in retrieving words from rhyming cues and pointed to a possible phonological deficit. In two further cases[49,50] we studied children of average intelligence both of whom displayed difficulties in the production and recognition of rhyme. Overall the pattern of skills found in these two acallosal children turned out to be comparable to that seen in some cases of developmental phonological dyslexia. This raised the possibility that the corpus callosum may be essential for the normal development of a phonological reading route[50] and that whatever compensatory mechanisms had occurred in the course of development in these acallosal patients were insufficient to make possible entirely normal language abilities.

Table 2. Summary of results on tests of language used by Dennis[8] on Dennis's patient DS and two further acallosal patients. (Taken from reference 25)

	D.S.	B.F.	K.C.
Visual naming	—	—	—
Cued retrieval	× (Rhyme)	× (Rhyme)	× (Rhyme)
Fluency	×	—	×
Sentence construction	—	—	×
Sentence repetition	×	×[a]	×
Active-Passive			
AA	—	—	×
PA	—	—	—
AN	×	—	×
PN	×	—	—

Note. × = deficit; — = no deficit
[a] One type only.

The tentative conclusions that are possible from these studies of language in acallosals suggest that the only language impairment which has been consistently observed (to date in five acallosals) is in the production and recognition of rhyme. This raises the question of the possible involvement of both hemispheres in language processing in normals but in which the contribution of each hemisphere differs[55]. According to this way of thinking it is possible that the left hemisphere has the exclusive domain of phonological processing and the right hemisphere a conative function and that these two must be combined, presumably through the forebrain commissures, for fully efficient language processing. When the callosum is absent and no adequate compensatory route is available it results in a residual phonological deficit as seen in acallosals[50]. Further studies are in hand and will help to indicate whether this is a general feature of acallosals or not.

2) – Motor Performance: The clumsiness of some acallosals noted in the older neurological text-books was observed under more controlled conditions by us in the early 1960's[16,22]. At that time we administered a series of simple tasks requiring bimanual coordination. These included stringing wooden beads onto a lace and winding a string onto a stick. The tasks were required to be completed as quickly as possible. Performance was markedly worse than that of matched normal controls. Dennis[7] subsequently reported that acallosals had difficulties on tasks requiring fine motor control. In his studies of the Californian splitbrain patients, Preilowski[42] had demonstrated the importance of the anterior parts of the corpus callosum in performing a task requiring bimanual coordination without visual feedback (see Figure 2). When the visual feedback was available the partial commissurotomy patients were

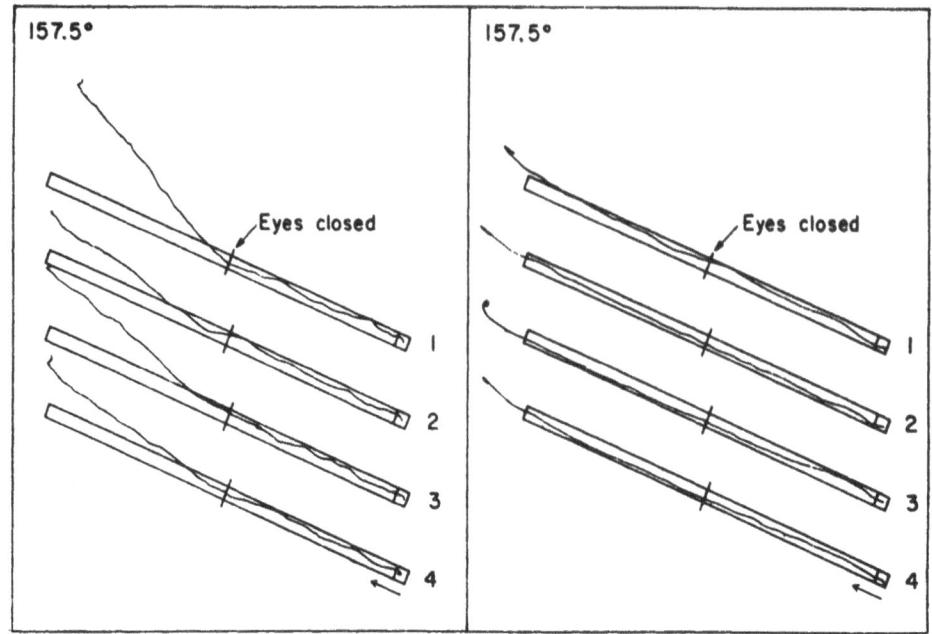

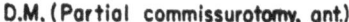

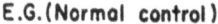

Figure 2. Sample of performance of a partial commissurotomy patient (DM) in whom the anterior commissure and the anterior two thirds of the corpus callosum had been sectioned in a single operation, and of a normal control (LG) when visual feedback was eliminated after crossing the halfway mark. The numbers indicate consecutive trials. (Taken from reference 42).

able to do the task, though somewhat slower than normal controls. When Preilowski's task was administered to adult acallosals and a child acallosal[28,29] it was found that acallosals were able to do the task after extended practice but their peak level of performance did not reach that of matched normal controls. Moreover, when visual feedback was withdrawn they experienced the same problems as the commissurotomy patients studied by Preilowski[28] (see Figure 3).

The conclusion from these series of studies was that acallosals exhibit a substantial deficit in bimanual coordination. It was also evident that on the simpler tasks administered in 1964[22] and 1965[16] the same patients when tested at intervals over a period of 25 years showed no improvement in the course of development when compared with normal controls. The most likely explanation offered for these results was the enhanced development of ipsilateral motor pathways and the lack, during development, of normal callosal inhibition. This will be expanded later when we discuss compensatory mechanisms.

It was noted that on a further task studying visuo-motor control acallosals[26] showed a deficit when compared with normals. In this study the patients were required to reach out and grasp a variety of objects which had been briefly exposed in front of them and to the left or right of a fixation point for less than 200 msec. It was found that whilst they were able to reach out and point to where an object had been with an accuracy comparable with normals, nevertheless when required to grasp these objects their performance fell far below that of the normals. This was interpreted in terms of the enhanced development of ipsilateral motor control pathways and the failure, due to the absence of callosal inhibition, to inhibit these as they competed with the crossed pathways responsible for fine distal control (see Figure 4).

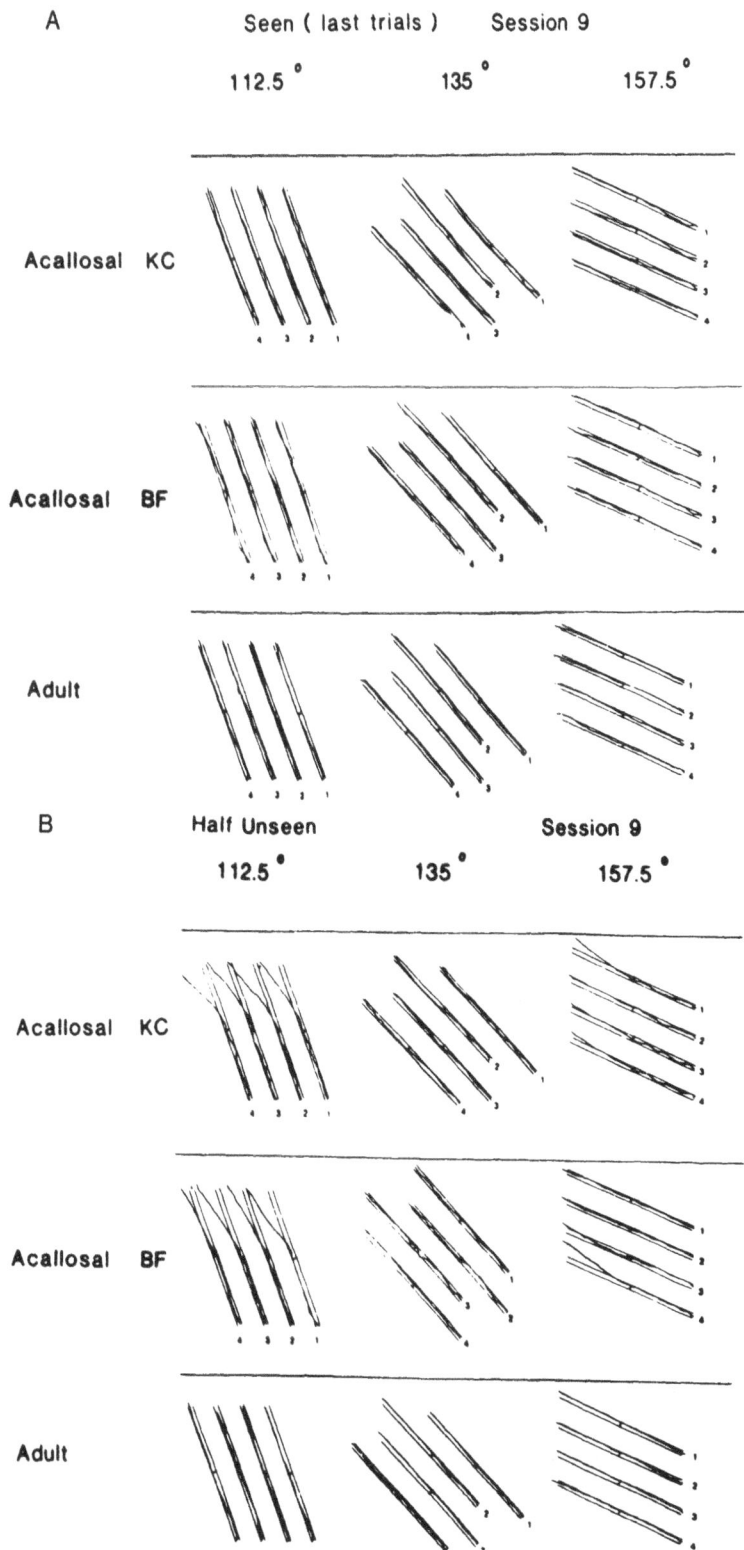

Figure 3. Examples of performance of two acallosals and a typical adult control (top) with visual feedback throughout, and (bottom) when visual feedback was withdrawn at the mid-point. (Taken from reference 28)

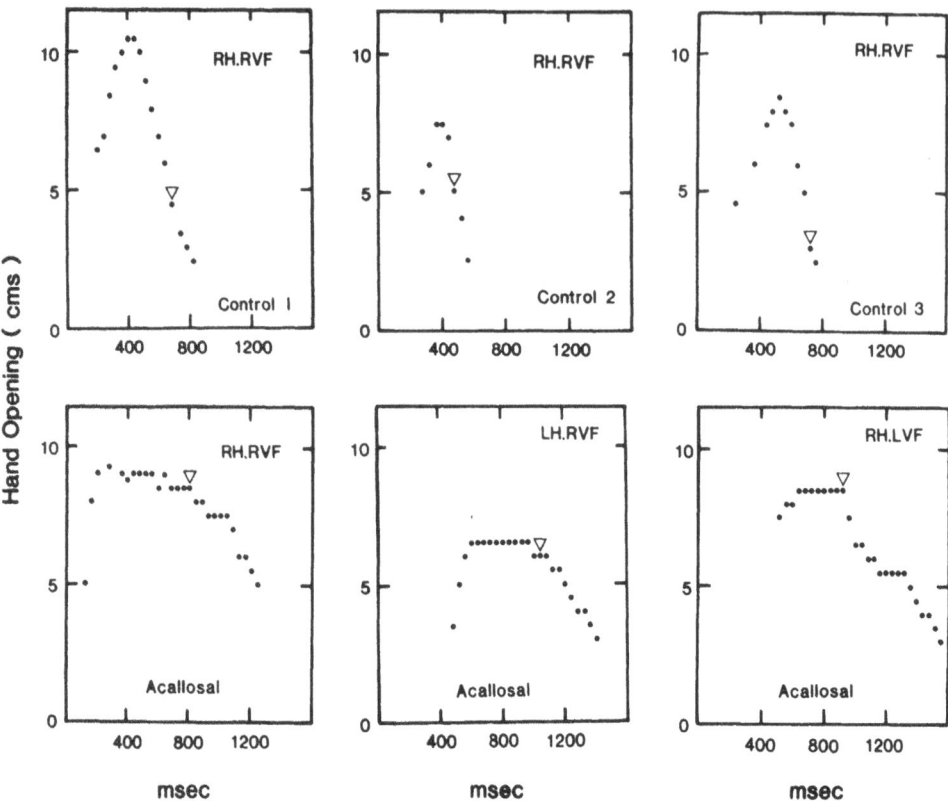

Figure 4. Finger-thumb separation (measured from record) plotted against time in an object-grasping task. Upper three graphs; control subjects. Lower three graphs; adult acallosals. (Taken from reference 26.

3) – Stereoperception: In 1979 I reported a preliminary study of mid-line stereopsis in acallosals[17] using an adaptation of the method devised by Mitchell and Blakemore[37] (see Figure 5 and the attached legend for further details). Results indicated that the patients had difficulty in judging depth on the vertical meridian. In these studies, however, only 20 trials were given and this we judged to be an insecure basis on which to base a firm conclusion as to their abilities in mid-line stereopsis. Subsequently Lassonde[33] administered a different stereoscopic task. This consisted of judging the distance between pairs of familiar objects differing only in their colours, for example yellow or green and occasionally in size. The objects were placed either side of a fixation point one to the left, the other to the right with a distance of approximately 1° between each other (central condition) or at 4.5° both to the right or to the left of the fixation point (intra periphery condition) or at 4° of visual angle, one to the right the other to the left of the central fixation point (inter periphery condition). Lassonde reported impairments in both inter and intra peripheral conditions as well as centrally (see Figure 6). She postulated that the corpus callosum functions not only to relay input from each eye to the small group of binocular neurones but that it also exerts a facilitatory influence on binocular cells. In a second study she used random dot stereo grams which appeared either in front of or in the same plane as the central fixation point. She found both inter- and intra-hemispheric deficits which increased around liminal conditions. These results, she believed, were consistent with her first experimental results.

Most recently[21] we have reported a detailed investigation of mid-line stereopsis in acallosals and partial commissurotomy patients. In our study the patients underwent extensive testing over a two day period completing 400 trials in all. These results

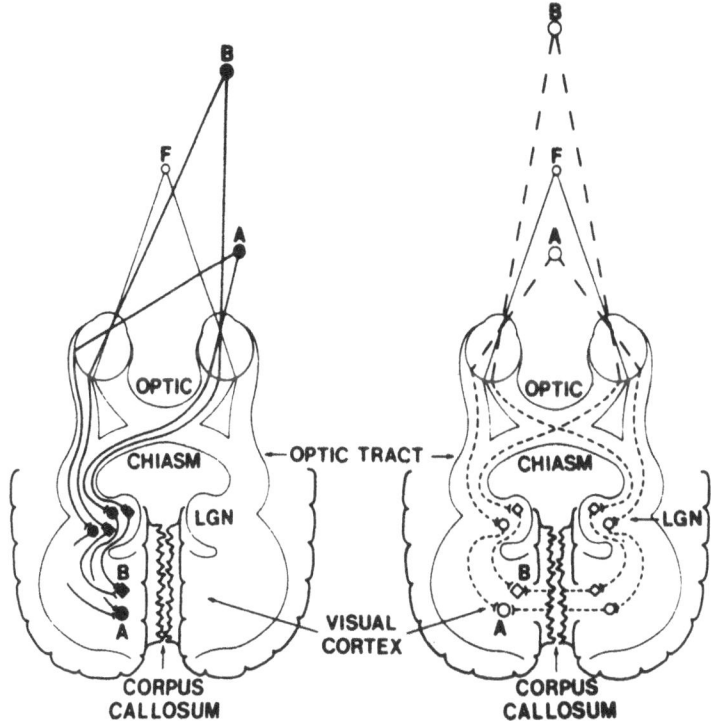

Figure 5. Depicts the possible neural system for binocular depth perception in a split-brain human. On the left is the arrangement of neurones enabling a split-brain (or acallosal?) patient to recognize the depth of a the peripheral objects A and B, relative to the fixation point F. On the right objects A and B lie directly in the midline and therefore, their images fall on the temporal or nasal retina, respectively, in both eyes. The binocular cells A and B in the cortex receive one of their inputs from a fibre from the opposite visual cortex, crossing in the corpus callosum. Section (or absence) of the commissure has severed this link and binocular integration (in the surgical patient) is impossible. (Taken from reference 37).

indicated quite specific difficulties experienced by acallosals in judging depth based on uncrossed disparities. We concluded from these studies and those of others that acallosals have a deficit in mid-line stereopsis, that there may in addition to the interhemispheric deficit be an intrahemispheric one, and that the reason for the deficit is a lack of normal interhemispheric integration through the splenium of the corpus callosum. At this point the importance of the anterior commissure becomes significant. The possibility of compensation through the anterior commissure[51,52] is discussed later in this chapter.

4) – Memory: Clark and Geffen[3] reviewed studies published up to that time which had looked at memory impairments supposedly associated with callosal damage. They showed convincingly that in every case where there was a memory impairment there was also extra callosal damage, most often to the fornix or the mamiliary bodies. Where extra callosal damage was either absent or minimal no significant memory impairment was evident.

This 1989 picture by Clark and Geffen has to be revised in the light of a more recent study by Geffen et al[10]. In this study they used an auditory verbal learning test. One acallosal patient aged 8 showed after a 20 minute delay that his recall of previously learned words was well below that of a control group thus demonstrating significant forgetting. He also showed a deficient ability to retrieve stored memory and a deficient ability to lay down permanent memory traces. A second patient, aged 12 years, also showed impairment on the acquisition of words over five learning trials.

Both subjects therefore showed deficient memory performance and this raised the question of whether the corpus callosum is implicated in the efficient consolidation of memory traces. It raised further the question, when the corpus callosum is absent have alternative compensatory mechanisms adequate for these tasks failed to develop? We should note that these results so far are on only two acallosal patients. Further studies are clearly required before firm conclusions can be drawn. We may, however, tentatively conclude that due to the absence of the corpus callosum memory consolidation processes do not occur with their normal efficiency.

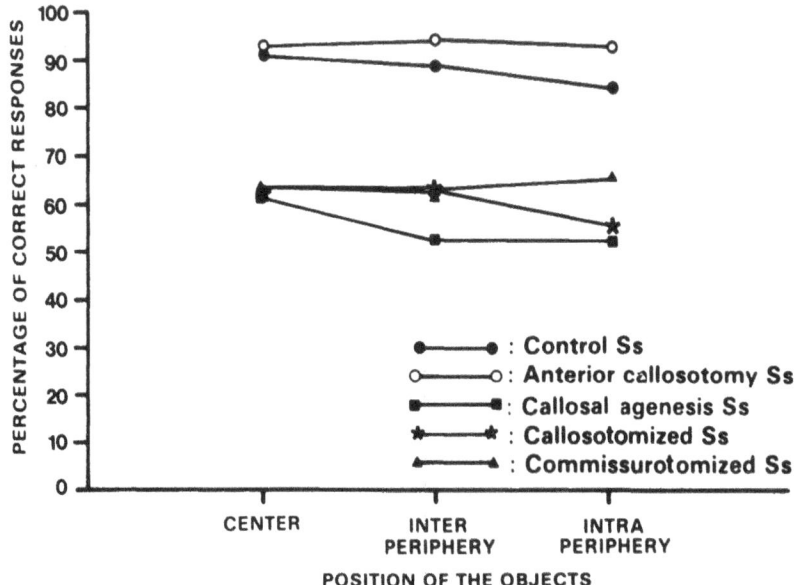

Figure 6. Lassonde's[33] data indicates that callosal agenesis patients like the callosotomized and commissurotomized patients were less able to make accurate depth judgements than their matched controls, regardless of the position of the stimuli. Thus deficits were observed in the <u>intra</u>periphery condition as well as the <u>inter</u>periphery condition and this Lassonde attributes to the absence of the <u>facilitatory</u> influence normally exerted through the corpus callosum.

The Neuropsychological Profile of Callosal Agenesis

Chiarello[2] reviewed 29 cases of callosal agenesis and identified as the most frequent and robust deficits: (1) lengthened interhemispheric transfer times[4]; (2) slowing on tasks requiring bimanual visual coordination; (3) reduced transfer in form board and stylus maze learning; (4) the presence of unintentional finger movements; (5) deficits in cross tactile discrimination.

In the light of the more recent findings reviewed above we could add four further deficits: (1) a failure of accurate bimanual motor coordination in the absence of visual feedback; (2) deficits in some aspects of stereoperception; (3) reduced language competence especially when handling certain syntactic structures and performing rhyming tasks; (4) reduced efficiency in the consolidation of memory traces.

The most obvious thing about those patients with callosal agenesis, who, as far as is known do not have any other associated brain abnormalities, is their apparent normality. This applies as we noted earlier to the classical split-brain patients of Sperry and his colleagues. However, whilst the split-brain patients in whom the callosum had been sectioned in adulthood revealed, on careful examination, a whole variety of deficits in the interhemispheric transmission and transfer of information, similar deficits do not in general occur in patients with callosal agenesis. The most notable exceptions are stereoperception and cross-tactile localisation. The question therefore arises, what kinds of alternative neural networks have developed in the course of normal development which enable seemingly normal interhemispheric integration to occur although it is absent in surgical split-brain patients. A number of possibilities have been proposed[2]. We will first describe them briefly and then assess the probability that they are in fact operating in callosal agenesis.

1.   The bilateral representation of function. In 1960 Saul and Sperry[45] having examined one acallosal patient reported that the amytal test revealed bilateral representation of language. He suggested that a general bilateral representation of function in acallosals would be an effective adaptation to partially overcome the normal interhemispheric communication through the corpus callosum. Thus the necessity to tap into the opposite hemisphere through the corpus callosum was obviated by the bilateral representation of function in the two hemispheres. Since that time a series of studies have steadily accumulated evidence against this hypothesis[24]. Rather the evidence points in favour of normal hemispheric specialisation in callosal agenesis. This applies to verbal behaviour[24], visuospatial behaviour[35], spatial motor tasks[35] and motor dominance[28]. The possibility, of course, remains that whilst there is hemispheric specialisation in acallosals it is less extreme than in normals: a topic worthy of further investigation.

2.   An enhanced role for the anterior commissure in interhemispheric transfer. Even with MRI pictures it often still remains difficult to decide conclusively whether or not the anterior commissure is present in acallosals. One possibility is that when it is present it may be enlarged in acallosals compared with normals but as yet there is little evidence to give strong support to this claim and it requires further investigation. It is certainly the case that in some acallosals the anterior commissure as well as the corpus callosum is absent. There is one report[9] of an acallosal who read letters presented in the left visual field whilst having no difficulty with right visual field presentations. Unfortunately no MRI studies were available on this patient to verify or otherwise the presence of the anterior commissure.

   It remains the case that when it is present the anterior commissure may take over at least some of the functions normally performed by the corpus callosum. It is noteworthy that a distinction needs to be made between transmitting spatial information which seems unlikely in view of the termination of the fibres passing through the anterior commissure, and the carrying of pattern information which seems plausible in view of the fact that the temporal lobes are cross connected through the anterior commissure. This view is further strengthened by the work of Martin[34] and Meerwaldt[35] suggesting that acallosals cannot transfer spatial information.

   It is probable that the presence of the anterior commissure accounts in part at least for the competence that remains in stereo-perception. This view is strengthened through work with animals. For example Cowey[5] and Hamilton and Vermeire[11] with monkeys and Timney with cats[51,52]. There remains the further possibility that there is some sub-cortical transfer particularly of some forms of visual information. A series of studies by Justine Sergent supports this view[46,47]. Her evidence is based on careful re-testing of some of the Californian split-brain patients.

Thus evidence has accumulated that some forms of interhemispheric communication can still occur in the absence of the cerebral commissures. This includes both lower-level visual perceptual information[53] and higher-level linguistic and non-linguistic information[6,30,39,45,47]. In these studies the stimulus set sizes were small and the stimuli were normally verbalizable. This raises the possibility of the comparisons being done by crosscueing rather than by subcortical visual transfer. More recent work by Jeffrey Clarke (unpublished PhD thesis 1991) who carried out further studies on some of the Californian split brain patients showed that in at least one of them, NG, sensory information was transferring through subcortical visual pathways. It would certainly seem that the human subcortical visual pathways are sensitive to both rudimentary visual characteristics such as movement, stimulus position, and line orientation, as well as to simple high contrast patterns[40,41,53,54].

3. The enhanced development of ipsilateral sensory and motor pathways. This possibility has been suggested by several workers[19,33]. It would help to explain the success that is achieved by acallosal patients on tasks such as tactile discrimination whilst they still fail on fine tactile localisation or on fine motor control tasks. Moreover, there is evidence to suggest that acallosals readily revert to the use of these enhanced developed ipsilateral pathways when more distal processes are not sufficient to perform the task. It also helps to explain the observed performance on our reaching and grasping task[27] as well as on Preilowski's bimanual coordination task[28]. The studies by Laget[31,32] on evoked potentials from stimulation of the wrist give further support to the enhanced development and elaboration of ipsilateral pathways. Laget observed that in normals there was a strong contralateral scalp response to stimulation of the wrist but little or no ipsilateral response. In acallosals, however, there was a strong ipsilateral evoked response presumed to come through the ipsilateral pathways.

It is likely that bimanual coordination and the transfer of sensori-motor information mobilise jointly the ipsilateral and contralateral pathways. The evidence reviewed earlier suggests that whilst such an arrangement may confer benefits it may also impose limitations. The latter presumably arise because the enhanced development of ipsilateral sensory and motor pathways, in the absence of the transcallosal inhibition[20,42,56] normally mediated through the corpus callosum, allows competition between the contra and ipsilateral pathways with a consequent reduced overall level of performance measured in terms of accuracy or speed or both[42]. Such a formulation is consistent with the finding of a bilateral representation of the hand area of the monkey, area S2, which is not completely abolished after callosal transection.

4. Language deficits. Work in this area is limited[7,25,49,50] but it does appear that there are specific difficulties with phonology in the acallosals so far tested. It has been speculated that this may be due to the tasks used requiring both hemispheres to cooperate. Where this is not possible it would seem that the alternative pathways of the anterior commissure or of the sub-cortical pathways do not provide adequate compensation.

5. The importance of early exuberant growth of callosal fibres. Why should the adult surgically split-brain patient not benefit from the mechanisms described above to the same degree as the brain in which the callosum fails to develop? There are a number of possible reasons. Firstly, the general widely accepted assumption that cerebral plasticity is linked to the extent of the functional maturity of the lesioned structure at the time of the insult. Secondly, many cortical connections[14,15] undergo a

stage of exhuberant growth before synaptic stabilisation occurs in late adolescence. When damage occurs during the formative stage connections which would otherwise have been eliminated during the critical period of axon retraction and synaptic elimination may persist. Thirdly, it is possible that agenesis or early damage could extend the normal period of cerebral plasticity. Thus the decreasing availability of exhuberant connections in adulthood[12,13] would limit the possibilities of neural compensation to a greater extent than when this occurs prenatally as in callosal agenesis or early post-natally.

CONCLUSIONS

With the development and increasing availability of new brain scanning devices more cases of callosal agenesis are coming to light and at the same time there is less uncertainty about the status of other parts of the brain and especially of the anterior commissure. At the same time new techniques are being applied to extending and mapping the neuropsychological profile of these fascinating "experiments of nature". The result is that, it is now clear that there are deficits, both cognitive and behavioural which are not easily attributable solely to the lack of interhemispheric integration due to the absence of the corpus callosum. Rather there are deficits which are more likely to be due to the absence of the benefits normally conferred by interhemispheric inhibition and facilitation through the corpus callosum. Whilst interhemispheric integration may be in part taken over by the anterior commissure (when present) and/or by subcortical pathways, these latter structures seem less likely to compensate for absent or reduced interhemispheric inhibition and/or facilitation.

It remains the case that the enhanced development and functioning of the ipsilateral pathways, sensory and motor, are likely to constitute a major aspect of the neural compensatory mechanisms in callosal agenesis. These, together with the enhanced use of the anterior commissure (when present) and/or subcortical pathways, enable patients to present with apparent normality until subjected to detailed testing aimed at limiting initial sensory input to one hemisphere or which load bimanual coordination processes to their limit. In addition deficits can be detected in language, memory, stereoperception, motor coordination and bilateral tactile integration.

REFERENCES

1. Berlucchi, G., and Antonini, A., 1990, The role of the corpus callosum in the representation of the visual field in cortical areas, in C. Trevarthen, ed. *Brain Circuits and Functions of the Mind, Essays in honour of Roger W. Sperry*, pp 129-139, CUP, Cambridge.
2. Chiarello, C., 1980, A house divided? Cognitive functioning with callosal agenesis, *Brain and Lang.*, 11, 128-158.
3. Clark, C.R., and Geffen, G.M., 1989, Corpus callosum surgery and recent memory. A review, *Brain*, 112, 165-175.
4. Clarke, J.M., and Zaidel, E., 1989, Simple reaction times to lateralized light flashes: Varieties of interhemispheric communication routes, *Brain*, 112, 849-870.
5. Cowey A., 1985, Disturbances of stereopsis by brain damage, in D. Ingle, ed., *Brain Mechanisms and Spatial Vision*, NATO Advanced Study Institute Series, Martimas Nijhoff, The Hague.
6. Cronin-Golomb, A., 1986, Subcortical transfer of cognitive information in

subjects with complete forebrain commissurotomy, *Cortex*, **22**, 499-519.

7. Dennis, M., 1976, Impaired sensory and motor differentiation with corpus callosum agenesis: a lack of callosal inhibition during ontogeny. *Neuropsychologia*, **14**, 455-469.

8. Dennis, M., 1981, Language in a congenitally acallosal brain, *Brain and Lang.*, **12**, 33-53.

9. Donoso, A., and Santander, M., 1982, Hemialexia y afasia hemianoptica en agenesia del curepo calloso, *Rev Chilena Neuropsiquiatria*, **20**, 137-144.

10. Geffen, G.M., Forrester, G.M., Jones, D.L., and Simpson, D.A., 1992, Auditory verbal learning and memory in cases of callosal agenesis, in M. Lassonde, and M.A. Jeeves, eds., *Callosal Agenesis: The Natural Split Brain*, Plenum, New York. (in press)

11. Hamilton, C.R., and Vermeire, B.A., 1986, Localisation of visual functions with partially split-brain monkeys, in F. Lepore, M. Ptito, and H.H. Jasper, eds., *Two Hemispheres - One Brain*, pp. 315-333. Alan R. Liss Inc., New York.

12. Innocenti, G.M., 1981, Growth and reshaping of axons in the establishment of visual callosal connections, *Science*, **212**, 824-827.

13. Innocenti, G.M., 1986, The general organization of callosal connections in the cerebral cortex, in E.G. Jones, and A.A. Peters, eds., *Cerebral Cortex*, Plenum Press, New York.

14. Innocenti, G.M., 1986, What is so special about callosal connections, in F. Lepore, M. Ptito, H.H. Jasper, eds., *Two Hemispheres - One Brain: Functions of the Corpus Callosum*, pp. 75-81, Alan R. Liss, New York.

15. Innocenti, G.M., and Caminiti, R., 1980, Postnatal shaping of callosal connections from sensory areas, *Exp Brain Res.*, **38**, 381-394.

16. Jeeves, M.A., 1965, Psychological studies of three cases of congenital agenesis of the corpus callosum, in E.G. Ettlinger, ed., *Functions of the Corpus Callosum*, pp 7394, CIBA Foundation Study Groups, Vol 20, Churchill, London.

17. Jeeves, M.A., 1979, Some limits to interhemispheric integration in cases of callosal agenesis and partial commissurotomy, in I.S. Russell, M.W. Van Hof, and G. Berlucchi, eds., *Structure and Function of the Cerebral Commissures*, pp 449-474, Macmillan, London.

18. Jeeves, M.A., 1981, Age related effects of agenesis and partial sectioning of the neocortical commissures, in M.W. van Hof, and G. Mohn, eds. *Functional Recovery from Brain Damage*, pp 31-52, Elsevier, Amsterdam, North Holland.

19. Jeeves, M.A., 1986, Callosal agenesis: neuronal and developmental adaptations, in F. Lepore, M. Ptito, H.H. Jasper, eds., *Two Hemispheres - One Brain*, pp 403-421, Alan R. Liss Inc., New York.

20. Jeeves, M.A., 1991, Hemispheric Interactions, in *Encyclopedia of Human Biology*, Vol 4, pp. 129-134, Academic Press, San Diego.

21. Jeeves, M.A., 1991, Stereoperception in callosal agenesis and partial callosotomy, *Neuropsychologia*, **29**, 19-34.

22. Jeeves, M.A., and Rajalakshmi, R., 1964, Psychological studies of a case of congenital agenesis of the corpus callosum, *Neuropsychologia*, **2**, 247-252.

23. Jeeves, M.A., and Wilson, A.F., 1969, Tactile transfer in neonatal callosal section in the cat. *Psychon Sci*, **16**, 235-237.

24. Jeeves, M.A., and Milner, A.D., 1987, Specificity and plasticity in interhemispheric integration: evidence from callosal agenesis, in D. Ottoson, ed., *Duality and Unity of the Brain - Unified Functioning and*

Specialization of the Hemispheres, pp. 416-441, Macmillan, London.

25. Jeeves, M.A., and Temple, C.M., 1987, A further study of language function in callosal agenesis, *Brain and Lang.*, **32**, 325-335.

26. Jeeves, M.A., and Silver, P.H., 1988, The formation of finger grip during prehension in an acallosal patient, *Neuropsychologia*, **26**, 153-159.

27. Jeeves, M.A., and Silver, P.H., 1988, Interhemispheric transfer of spatial tactile information in callosal agenesis and partial commissurotomy, *Cortex*, **24**, 601-604.

28. Jeeves M.A., Silver, P.H., and Jacobson, I., 1988, Bimanual coordination in callosal agenesis and partial commissurotomy, *Neuropsychologia*, **26**, 833-850.

29. Jeeves M.A., Silver, P.H., and Milne, A.B., 1988, Role of the corpus callosum in the development of a bimanual motor skill, *Develop. Neuropsychol.*, **4**, 305-323.

30. Jung, R., 1962, Summary of the conference, in Moutcastle, V., ed., *Interhemispheric Relations and Cerebral Dominance*, pp 274-275, John Hopkins, Baltimore.

31. Laget, P., Raimbault J., d'Allest, A.M., Flores-Guevara, R., Mariani, J., and Thieriot-Prevost, G., 1976, La maturation des potentiels evoques somesthesiqiues (PES) chez l'homme, *Electroencephalogr Clin. Neurophysiol.*, **40**, 499-515.

32. Laget, P., d'Allest, A.M., Fihey, R., and Lortholary, O., 1977, L'interet des potentials evoques somesthesiques homolateraux dans les agenesies du corps calleux, *Rev. Electroencephalogr. Neurophysiol. Clin.*, **7**, 498-502.

33. Lassonde, M., 1986, The facilitatory influence of the corpus callosum on intrahemispheric processing, in F. Lepore, M. Ptito, H.H. Jasper, eds., *Two Hemispheres - One Brain: Functions of the Corpus Callosum*, pp. 385-401, Alan R. Liss, New York.

34. Martin, A., 1985, A qualitative limitation on visual transfer via the anterior commissure, *Brain*, **108**, 43-63.

35. Meerwaldt, J.D., 1983, Disturbance of spatial perception in a patient with agenesis of the corpus callosum, *Neuropsychologia*, **21**, 161-165.

36. Milner, A.D., and Jeeves, M.A., 1981, The functions of the corpus callosum in infancy and adulthood, *Behav. Brain Sci.*, **4**, 30-31.

37. Mitchell, D.E., and Blakemore, C., 1970, Binocular depth perception and the corpus callosum, *Vision Res.*, **10**, 49-54.

38. Moscovitch, M., 1977, The development of lateralization of language functions and its relation to cognitive and linguistic development: a review and some theoretical speculations, in S.J. Segalowitz, F.A. Gruber, eds., *Language Development and Neurological Theory*, pp. 193-211, Academic Press, New York.

39. Myers, J.J., and Sperry, R.W., 1985, Interhemispheric communication after section of the forebrain commissures, *Cortex*, **21**, 249-260.

40. Perenin, M.T., 1978, Visual function within the hemianopic field following early cerebral hemidecortification in man - II. Pattern discrimination, *Neuropsychologia*, **16**, 697-708.

41. Perenin, M.T., and Jeannerod, M., 1978, Visual function within the hemianopic field following early cerebral hemidecortication in man - I. Spatial localization, *Neuropsychologia*, **16**, 1-13.

42. Preilowski, B.F.P., 1972, Possible contributions of the anterior forebrain commissures to bilateral motor coordination, *Neuropsychologia*, **10**, 267-277.

43. Ptito, M., Lepore F., Lassonde M., Dion C., and Miceli, D., 1986, Neural mechanisms for stereopsis in cats, in F. Lepore, M. Ptito, and H.H. Jasper, *Two Hemispheres One Brain*, eds., pp. 335-350, Alan R. Liss Inc., New York.

44. Risse, G.L., Le Doux, J., Springer, S.P., Wilson, D.H., Gazzaniga, M.S., 1978, The anterior commissure in man: functional variation in a multisensory system, *Neuropsychologia*, **16**, 23-31.

45. Saul, R., and Sperry, R.W., 1968, Absence of commissurotomy symptoms with agenesis of the corpus callosum, *Neurology*, **18**, 307.

46. Sergent, J., 1986, Subcortical coordination of hemisphere activity in commissurotomized patients, *Brain*, **109**, 357-369.

47. Sergent, J., 1990, Furtive incursions into bicameral minds: Integrative and coordinating role of subcortical structures, *Brain*, **113**, 537-568.

48. Sperry, R.W., 1990, see *Brain Circuits and Functions of the Mind*. C. Trevarthen, ed., Essays in honour of Roger W. Sperry, CUP, Cambridge.

49. Temple, C.M., Jeeves M.A., and Vilarroya, O.O., 1989, Ten pen men- Explicit phonological processing in two children with callosal agenesis, *Brain and Lang.*, **37**, 548-564.

50. Temple, C.M., Jeeves M.A., and Vilarroya, O.O., 1990, Reading in callosal agenesis, *Brain and Lang.*, **39**, 235-253.

51. Timney, B., Elberger, A.J., and Vandewater, M.L., 1985, Binocular depth perception in the cat following early corpus callosum section, *Exp. Brain Res.*, **60**, 19-26.

52. Timney, B., and Lansdown, G., 1988, Binocular depth perception, visual acuity and visual fields in cats following neonatal section of the optic chiasm, *Exp. Brain Res.*, 207.

53. Trevarthen, C., and Sperry, R.W., 1973, Perceptual unity of the ambient visual field in human commissurotomy patients, *Brain*, **96**, 547-570.

54. Weiskrantz, L., 1986, *Blindsight: A Case Study and Implications*, Oxford Oxford University Press.

55. Zaidel, E., 1976, Language, dichotic listening and the disconnected hemispheres, in D.O. Walter, L. Rogers, and J.M. Finzi-Fried, eds., *Conference on Human Brain Function*, pp. 103-110. Brain Information Service/BRI Publications Office: UCLA.

56. Zaidel, E., 1986, Callosal dynamics and right hemisphere language, in F. Lepore, M. Ptito, and H.H. Jasper, eds., *Two Hemispheres - One Brain: Functions of the Corpus Callosum*, pp 435-459, Alan R. Liss, New York.

MECHANISMS UNDERLYING RECOVERY FROM CORTICAL INJURY:

REFLECTIONS ON PROGRESS AND DIRECTIONS FOR THE FUTURE

Bryan Kolb

Department of Psychology
University of Lethbridge
Lethbridge, Canada

INTRODUCTION

Perhaps the most perplexing and significant question facing neuropsychological investigations in the "Decade of the Brain" is the issue of how to repair the injured nervous system. This question is not only theoretically interesting but it also takes on particular importance for at least two practical and socially-relevant reasons. First, improvements in medical facilities and in safety devices, such as automobile seat belts, have led to a marked increase in the survival of people with head injuries. Thus, as we approach the twenty-first century there are increasing numbers of people who have sustained, and survived, significant brain damage. Indeed, it has been suggested that brain injuries may represent a "silent epidemic" of Western civilizations in which on the order of 0.25% of the population suffers a closed injury *each year*. This number is cumulative so that the chances of sustaining a closed head injury over a lifetime would be in the order of 1/20. This is a nontrivial social issue when we consider the billions of dollars needed for the treatment and maintenance of people with head injuries. Second, the proportion of the population that is living to old age is increasing and thus a greater proportion of the population can be expected to suffer diseases and other disorders related to the aging brain, including the normal degenerative process of aging.

Neuropsychological studies play an especially important role in the study of recovery from brain damage for it is the behavioural changes that represent the primary social challenge associated with brain injury. Over the past twenty years there have been important advances in neuropsychological knowledge regarding recovery from brain injury and the goal of this chapter will be to reflect upon some aspects of our progress. I will begin by outlining the 'rules' that appear to constrain brain and behavioural relationships in recovery of function. With these rules in mind, I shall next consider what I believe to be the principal unsolved problems that currently face the neuropsychological study of behavioural recovery. Finally, I will suggest directions to pursue and to avoid in the future.

Recovery from Brain Damage, Edited by F.D. Rose and
D.A. Johnson, Plenum Press, New York, 1992

RULES UNDERLYING RECOVERY

An important first step in understanding the mechanisms underlying recovery is to determine the regularities of both anatomical and behavioural change following brain injury. To this end, I have identified three basic rules: the rules of time, size, and reaction.

The Rule of Time

Time is crucial in several ways. First, there is the amount of time since the injury. It is well known, for example, that people with anterior left hemisphere strokes show an initial loss of various language functions, followed by marked improvement over time. Similarly, it can be shown experimentally that laboratory animals exhibit a slow improvement in the performance of both cognitive and motor tasks after cortical injury. For example, rats with motor or prefrontal injuries show an initial loss of the ability to use the forepaw to reach for food, which improves over time (Figure 1).

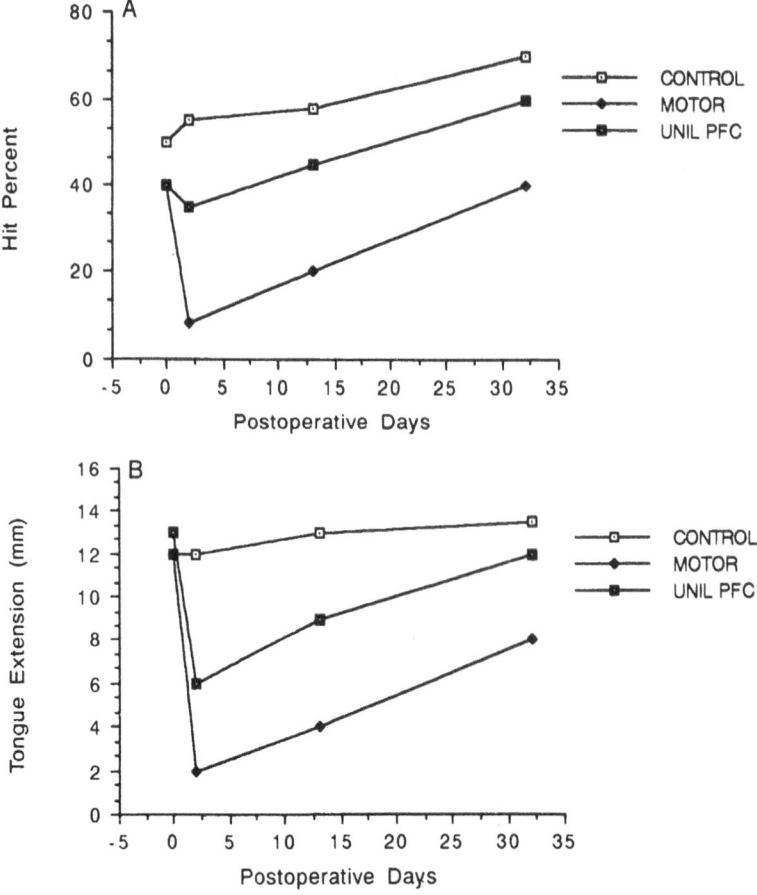

Figure 1. Examples of recovery of behaviour over time. Recovery of reaching for food by rats. Data are expressed as per cent accuracy in reaching through bars for small pieces of chicken feed. Recovery of ability to stick out the tongue to lick soft food from a ruler.

Although the causes of the behavioural improvements after cerebral injury have been a source of controversy for nearly a century, it is clear that postinjury behavioural changes are correlated with a series of cellular and molecular events that have a strict temporal sequence[35] (Figure 2). At least some of the behavioural changes must be directly related to the postlesion changes in the brain, although this has yet to be demonstrated. Nonetheless, it is likely that the failure to see significant recovery beyond a certain time after the injury is due, in part, either to the occurrence of certain physiological events or to the completion of others. An intriguing aspect of the lesion-induced physiological changes is that they may interfere with recovery by preventing the nervous system from regrowing injured regions in the same manner that it originally grew them during development. Indeed, Nieto-Sampedro & Cotman[35] have argued that the key to establishing neural regeneration may be found in the strict temporal order of anatomical and physiological events observed during development. Cotman suggests that interventions that are likely to prove successful in ameliorating behavioural loss after injury are going to be those that allow the nervous system to repeat the original developmental sequence of events in the nervous system. This may mean that several different neurological interventions will be required to ensure that each stage in regrowth occurs at the correct time.

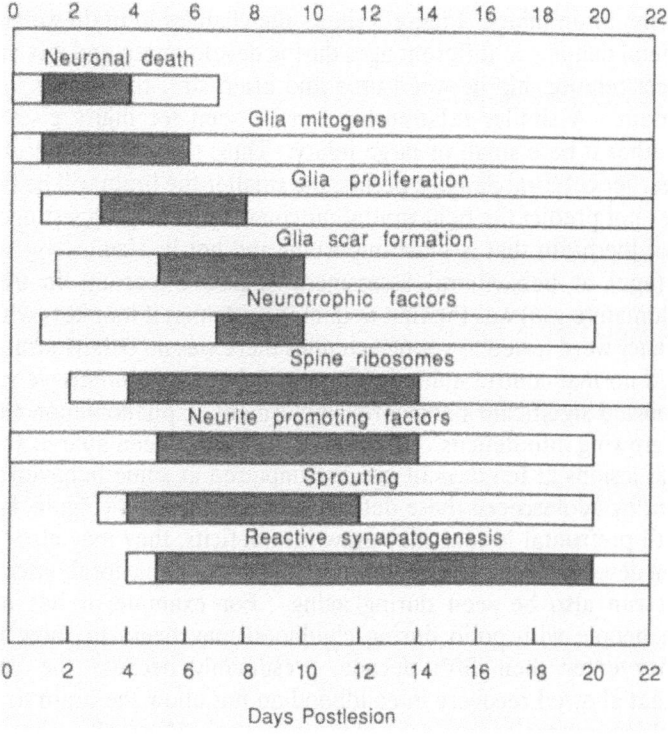

Figure 2. Time course of events following CNS injury. The beginning of the bars indicates the time postlesion when the event is initiated. The intensity of the shading parallels the intensity of phenomenon indicated by the bar. (After Nieto-Sampedro & Cotman[35]).

A second aspect of time is the age of the organism when the brain is injured. Thus, damage to a given area of the brain at different times in life may lead to markedly different behavioural symptoms. This was first suggested in the 1800s[5] but the idea is usually credited to Kennard[14] who showed that removal of the motor cortex in infant monkeys produced less behavioural impairment than similar injury in adulthood. Perhaps the most dramatic illustration of this phenomenon can be seen in the effects of early cortical injury on language. If the speech zones of the left hemisphere are injured in the first year or two of life, there is a shift of language to the right hemisphere and language development is surprisingly normal. This contrasts to the serious compromise of language functions if the same speech zones are injured in adulthood. Although it has been tempting to conclude from such observations that if one is going to have brain damage one should have it early, the relationship of age to brain injury is not quite so straight forward as it might appear. For instance, in our studies of rats with bilateral injury to the motor, prefrontal, parietal, visual, or temporal cortex we have been impressed by the consistent observation that cortical injury in the first 5 days of life is associated with far more severe behavioral loss than is similar injury at 7-10 days of life[28]. Cortical injury later, say at 20 days of life, is again associated with more severe behavioural loss, which is more or less equivalent to that observed in adulthood (e.g. 27). The crucial point is that there may be special times during life that the brain is especially able to compensate for injury. This is important for it implies that there is something different about the brain's reaction to injury at particular times in life. Whatever this difference might be may provide a key to mechanisms underlying optimal recovery. Curiously, however, the gross anatomical changes in the brain do not correlate well with the apparent 'windows of opportunity' for recovery from brain injury. Figure 3 shows the changes in brain weight following frontal or parietal damage at different ages during development and it is apparent that there is a direct relationship between time and brain size: the earlier the injury the smaller the brain. A similar relationship can be seen for injury elsewhere in the cerebrum, whether it be a small or large injury. Thus, there appears to be a general rule that the earlier cerebral damage occurs, the smaller the brain will be in adulthood. Brain size does not predict the behavioural outcome, however, suggesting that it is the organization of the brain that is most important and not its size.

Time (age) at behavioural assessment is also important to understanding recovery. Goldman (e.g. 8) was the first to demonstrate that if monkeys with prefrontal damage in infancy were tested as young juveniles there was no behavioural loss relative to age-matched normal control animals whereas if the same animals were tested later in life they showed significant behavioral impairment, a phenomenon that could be described as "growing into deficits". In contrast, we[20] have been able to show that rats with prefrontal lesions at ten days of age are impaired at some behavioral tasks very early in life but by adolescence these deficits have disappeared (Figure 4). Thus, just as animals with prefrontal lesions may grow into deficits, they may also "grow out of deficits" during development. The apparent variability of behavioral outcome with age at assessment can also be seen during aging. For example, it has now become apparent that people with polio during childhood may begin to show neurological deficits as they enter their fifth decade, presumably because the compensatory mechanisms that allowed recovery in childhood do not allow the brain to compensate for the normal losses usually experienced during aging[9]. A parallel phenomenon can also be seen in the aging boxer who begins to show neurological symptoms long after retirement. The brain was able to compensate for the injuries during the boxing career but is left unable to cope with the later neuronal loss that normally occurs with aging.

A final aspect of time is the effect of experience on recovery from brain injury. Thus there is now good evidence that environmental events can significantly ameliorate the effects of cortical injury (see Will, this volume). These effects have been shown experimentally in studies in which animals housed in complex changing environments have reductions in the severity and extent of behavioural loss following neocortical injuries (e.g. 15, 18). Similarly, clinical investigations have begun to demonstrate improvement in at least some cognitive abilities in people with head injuries as a result of cognitive therapies and other environmental manipulations[37]. What remains unknown, however, are answers to questions such as how these therapies work, what factors best predict who will best benefit from the therapies, and when is the optimal

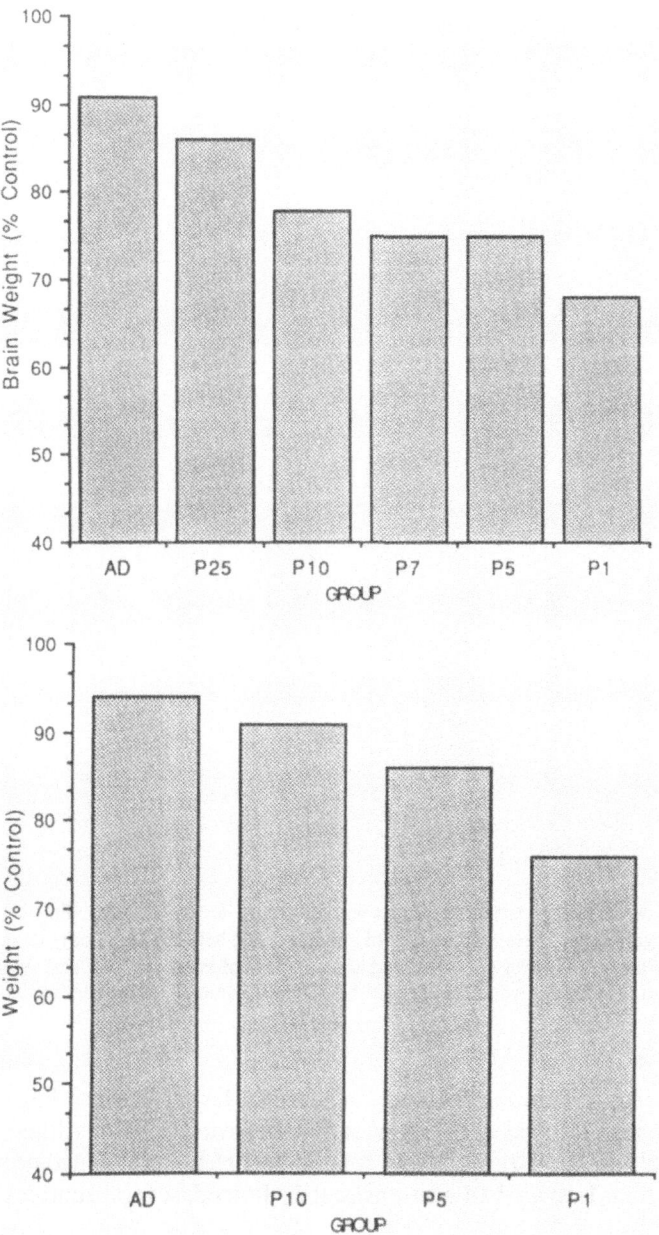

Figure 3. Relative adult brain weight of animals with prefrontal (top) or posterior parietal (bottom) lesions at different ages. Abbreviations: AD = adult lesion, P25 = postnatal day 25 lesion, P10 = postnatal day 10 lesion, P7 = postnatal day 7 lesion, P5 = postnatal day 5 lesion, P1 = postnatal day 1 lesion.

time for particular postinjury experiences to be implemented. Further, although experience may influence some behaviours following brain injury, this influence is clearly task-dependent and interacts with factors such as age at injury and sex (e.g. 15).

The Rule of Size

Lashley did the most extensive studies on the relationship between cortical lesion size and the subsequent behavioral outcome and he reached the conclusion that

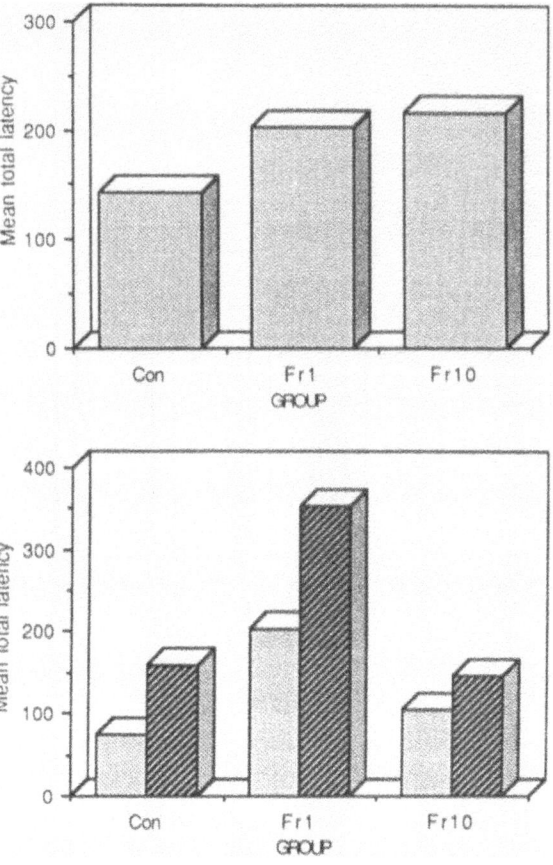

Figure 4. Morris water task performance of rats with prefrontal lesions at 1 day (Fr1) or 10 days (Fr10) of age. The top figure summarizes performance of animals tested between 19-22 days of age. The bottom figure summarizes the behaviour of animals tested at 56-59 days of age. The light bars summarize animals previously tested at 19-22 days while the stippled bars indicate animals tested for the first time at 56-59 days.

there was a direct relationship between neocortical lesion size and behavioral loss[32]. That is, the larger the lesion the greater the behavioral loss. Although Lashley's general rule still holds, size is clearly related to behavioural outcome in far more complex ways than Lashley had ever envisaged. Indeed, several subrules can now be identified.

My colleague, Ian Whishaw, and I first began to investigate the role of lesion size in recovery by studying the behavioural capacity of the decorticated rat (for a review, see 40). Two particularly important conclusions relevant to studies of recovery of function can be drawn from these studies. First, although these animals clearly have chronic and severe behavioural loss, there is little doubt that they have significantly more behavioural capacity than was previously recognized. Studies of recovery from neocortical lesions therefore must consider the chronic behaviour of decorticated rats before reaching conclusions about the role of residual cortex in recovery. For example, if decorticate rats show recovery on a particular behaviour and perform qualitatively like rats with smaller lesions, it is difficult to argue that the behavioural recovery is being mediated by changes in the remaining cortex. Second, rats with neonatal decortications show virtually no sparing of function relative to adult decorticates[26, 41]. This suggests that the Kennard effect requires the presence of residual neocortex for sparing to occur, although it may not be sufficient for this sparing.

We have shown that the absence of cortex precludes much recovery and sparing of function, but it is by no means clear how much cortex is required for any appreciable recovery to occur. With this idea in mind we removed all of the neocortex, except the sensorimotor representation of the face area, in newborn rats[42]. When the animals were assessed on a battery of motor tests it was evident that the only behavioural capacities upon which the animals performed better than decorticate rats were those related to the use of the face and tongue. When this tissue was subsequently removed the animals lost this capacity with no appreciable deterioration of other motor capacities. These results suggested that the mere presence of residual neocortex is not sufficient for sparing of function: either the amount or the location of the remaining tissue also must be important. This remains to be studied systematically.

Another aspect of lesion size revolves around the issue of unilateral versus bilateral injury. This can be considered in several ways. First, studies showing a positive relationship between the growth of anomalous projections and restitution of function have all used unilateral injuries in their studies. For example, in their seminal studies, Hicks & D'Amato[11] made unilateral motor cortex lesions and showed that sparing of motor behaviours was correlated with the presence of an abnormal ipsilateral cortico-spinal projection from the normal hemisphere. Analogous anatomical findings have also been shown in sensory systems (e.g. 3). In contrast, however, although bilateral cortical injuries may be associated with extensive abnormal connections, these connections are often negatively correlated with behavioural outcome: those animals with the most abnormal connections have the poorest behavioural outcomes (e.g 22).

Second, it appears that even a very small injury to one hemisphere is sufficient to interfere with the expected sparing and recovery from neonatal injury. For instance, my colleagues and I were able to demonstrate that neonatal hemidecortication allowed significant sparing of certain behavioural functions[25] and that this behavioural sparing was correlated with the presence of an increase in cortical thickness in the remaining hemisphere. The behavioural sparing and enhanced cortical thickness are, however, crucially dependent upon the integrity of the remaining hemisphere. Thus, even a small stab wound to the intact hemisphere at the time of hemidecortication attenuates the behavioural sparing and completely blocks the increase in cortical thickness (Figure 5). There is a clinical correlate of this observation as even small lesions of the right hemisphere appear to be capable of blocking the shift of speech from the left to the right hemisphere in children with perinatal injuries to the speech zones of the left hemisphere, resulting in severe and persisting language deficits[39].

Another aspect of size is important here: the increase in cortical thickness in the intact hemisphere only occurs when there is virtually complete removal of the damaged hemisphere[24, 31]. For example, removal of even 50% of the cortical mantle in one hemisphere appears to have no effect upon the contralateral hemisphere[31]. The mechanism underlying these observations is unknown but I believe that this aspect of lesion size may be relevant to the surgical treatment of children with various encephalopathies. In particular, the importance of large cerebral removals in stimulating growth in the contralateral hemisphere may provide a basis for the clinical observation that children given hemispherectomies for disorders such as Rasmussen's encephalitis may have better outcomes than those given more restricted cortical resections.

Lesion size may also be important in understanding apparent contradictions in the behavioural, anatomical, and neurochemical results of different studies. In particular, it appears that there is far better recovery if part of a functional system is spared by a cortical injury. For instance, it has become apparent in our studies of the effects of neonatal prefrontal injuries in rats that sparing of many behaviours is only present if part of the prefrontal cortex is left undamaged[16]. Similarly, Marshall[34] has

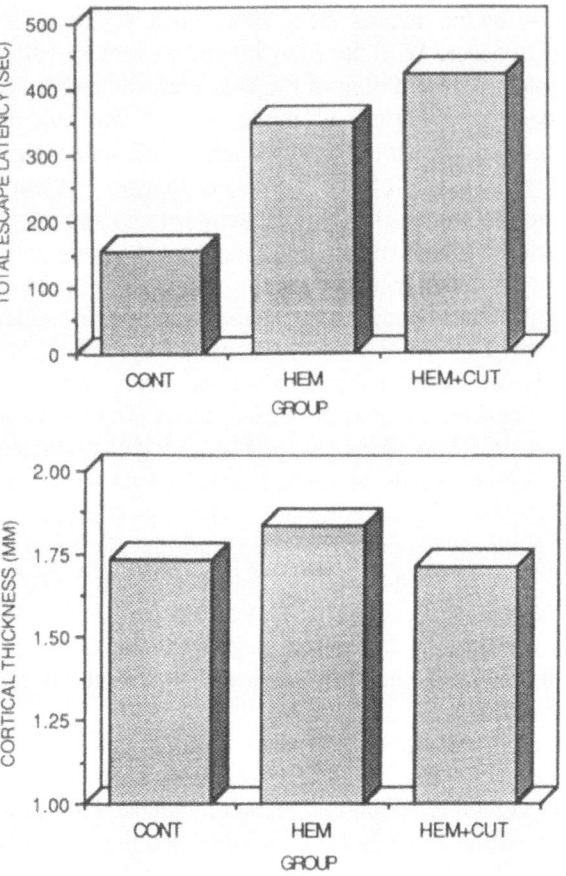

Figure 5. Top: Morris water task performance of animals given neonatal hemidecortications (HEM) or neonatal hemidecortications and small contralateral cortical stab wounds (HEM+CUT). The HEM+CUT group is significantly poorer at the task (p<.05). Bottom: Cortical thickness of rats tested in the water task. The HEM group is significantly thicker than the other two groups (p<.05).

concluded that there must be at least 5-10% sparing of a neural area affected by a lesion if there is to be a functionally significant neurochemical response and Nieto-Sampedro & Cotman[35] have emphasized that reactive sprouting only occurs when part of an existing neural pathway remains after injury. I should note, however, that even animals with large lesions will show some postoperative change in behaviour over time, possibly because animals develop new behavioural strategies to solve their problems (for a discussion of this issue, see 33).

There is one final, and counterintuitive, way in which size may be associated with recovery. It is a common clinical observation, especially in people with head injuries leading to the development of epilepsy, that rather small lesions may be associated with far worse behavioural outcomes than larger injuries[12]. This may be explained in several ways. First, it is a truism that "bad brain is far worse than no brain". Thus, the presence of abnormal brain may be associated with a worse outcome than expected because the bad brain interferes with the normal activity of the remaining brain. Epilepsy is a common example of such interference. Second, closed head injuries in particular may be associated with what has been described as disconnection syndromes[7]. Thus, head injuries that lead to damage to the white matter may functionally disconnect otherwise normal tissue, leading to unexpectedly severe behavioural symptoms from rather small injuries (see 29 for a more extensive discussion).

The Rule of Reactive Change

When damaged, the brain changes in various ways that contribute both to the occurrence of recovery as well as to its failure to appear. However, the brain's reaction to injury is unlikely to be a special response designed to repair itself but instead reflects the action of processes that are normally active for other reasons. These processes include normal developmental changes occurring from infancy through to old age, changes underlying plasticity required for learning and memory, and processes related to maintaining efficient functioning of neurons. I shall consider these changes under the headings of glial reaction, axonal reaction, and dendritic reaction.

A.   The glial reaction: The response of central nervous system glia to injury stands at the centre of the problem of recovery of function since, paradoxically, glia clearly play both a positive and a negative role in the control of regenerative events[35]. Figure 6 illustrates the normal relationship between glia and neurons in which there is a reciprocal interaction between them, with glia possibly functioning in some sort of supportive role. However, once neurons die, astrocytes actively produce trophic factors, such as laminin, which appear to induce sprouting of axonal and possibly dendritic elements (e.g. 36). Furthermore, astrocytes appear to have a positive feedback relationship with noradrenergic (NA) neurons such that the NA terminals pick up some factor produced by the glia, which in turn stimulates the NA cells to increase the release of noradrenaline. Since astrocytes have NA receptors, astrocytes that are distal from the site of cell death can then be induced to increase the production of trophic substances[1]. Finally, glia isolate the CNS from undesirable external influences by forming the glia limitans and contributing to the blood brain barrier. Unfortunately, this latter property also serves to interfere with neuron regeneration as glial scarring prevents sprouting or regenerating axons from gaining access to intact neurons in the region of injury (see figure 6). Thus, the glial response to injury may both help and hinder the brain and an understanding of the role of glia in brain plasticity is clearly important to understanding processes underlying recovery. To date, however, little is known about the relationship between glial reactions and subsequent behavioural recovery. Recently, we have noticed a curious relationship between glial development and sparing from early cortical injury, which may provide some clue to the role of glia in behavioural recovery. Figure 7 summarizes the normal postnatal development of several features of the neocortex, showing that the major glial (ie, astrocyte) development in the cortex begins around day 7 and continues to about day 15. Figure 7 also shows that there is no sparing of function resulting from neocortical injury in the first few days of life but after about day 7 there is significant sparing of function that declines after day 15. It is apparent from Figure 7 that the occurrence of sparing is correlated with the development of glia in the cortex. It is possible that the absence of glia in the first few days of life is at least partly responsible for the miserable behavioural outcome and that if the brain is damaged during the peak time of glial birth in the cortex the glia function in some way to promote behavioural recovery. I will return to this possibility below.

B.   The axonal reaction: It is generally believed that when central nervous system axons are damaged they do not regrow and although there is some recent evidence suggesting that under certain circumstances there may actually be axonal regrowth[6, 13], axonal regrowth is certainly rare. In contrast to damaged axons, however, there is considerable evidence that undamaged axons can exhibit sprouting of their terminal arborization in response to the death and retraction of competing projections. This axonal reaction is frequently referred to as reactive synaptogenesis[2] since the increased terminal arborization leads to the formation of new synapses. Perhaps the best exemplar of this axonal reaction is seen in the hippocampal formation when there is a disconnection of one of the normal afferents (see Figure 6). Thus, when space is

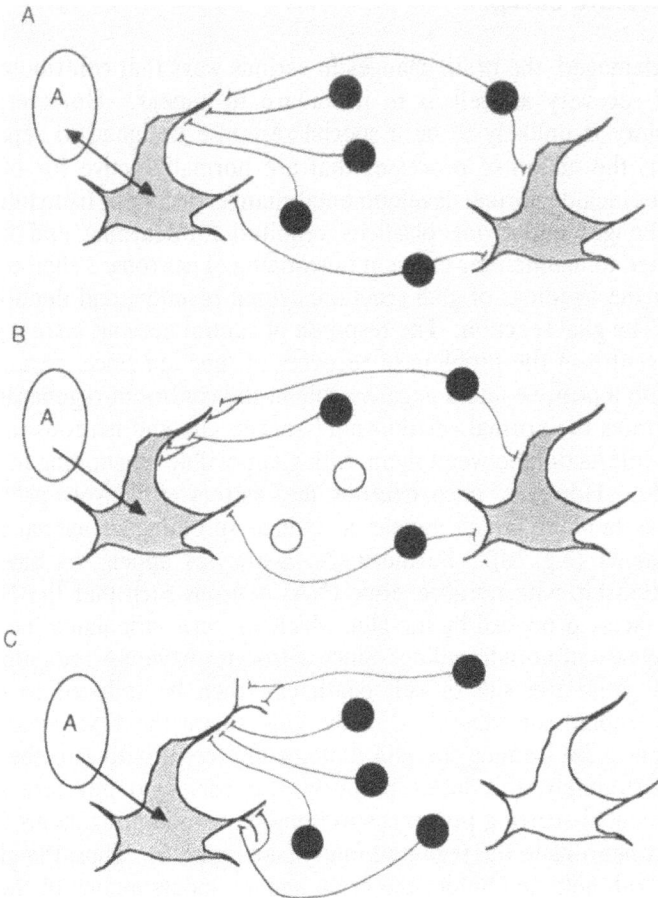

Figure 6. Hypothetical schematic model of neuron-glia intercommunication and the CNS response to injury. A. In the normal CNS (A) the neurons exchange signals on their metabolic state (arrow). Interneurons (black circles) have connections to two pyramidal neurons (grey). B. Injury to afferent interneurons (unshaded circles) alters the neuron-glia signal balance as glia produce an increased amount of neurotrophic substances. Remaining afferents (black circles) sprout new terminal branches to take up space vacated by the damaged neurons (unshaded circles). C. Injury to adjacent neurons of the same type (unshaded) leads to sprouting of new terminals from afferents deprived of their normal target and dendrites of the target cells.

vacated by degenerating hippocampal afferents, there is sprouting of axonal terminations of the remaining inputs, which could be responsible for behavioural recovery. Unfortunately, there is currently no behavioural evidence supporting the hypothesis that recovery is supported by the axonal sprouting, although the absence of this evidence is hardly evidence that such a process does not occur.

    C.   The dendritic reaction: Dendrites also show plasticity in response to brain injury and until recently it was generally assumed that the principal dendritic reaction was the loss of terminal branches in response to the loss of afferents. However, we now have shown that dendritic growth may be a more common reaction to cortical injury than was previously believed. We began by correlating the behavioural performance of rats with prefrontal lesions on the day of birth, 10 days of age, or in adulthood, with the extent of dendritic arborization of layer II/III pyramidal cells in parietal cortex. Unexpectedly, we found that: first, prefrontal lesions in adult rats produced a reliable increase in dendritic branching[17]; second, prefrontal lesions at

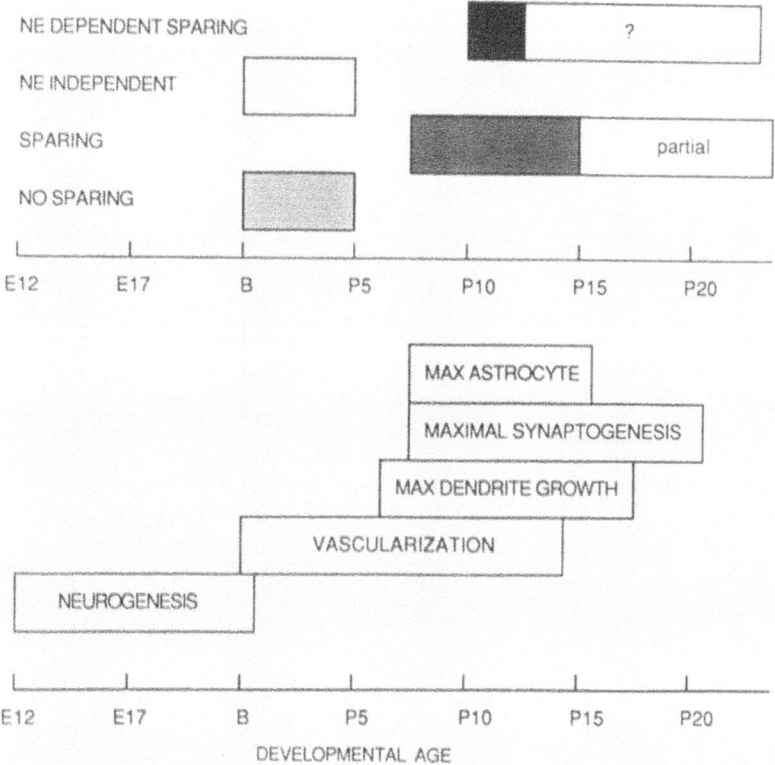

Figure 7. Time course of events during development of the neocortex. The boxes in the bottom portion indicate the period of maximum development of neurons (neurogenesis), blood vessels (vascularization), dendritic growth, synapse formation, and astrocyte formation. The boxes in the upper portion indicate the developmental periods during which there is or is not behavioral sparing after cortical lesions as well as the periods during which noradrenaline depletion blocks or does not effect sparing. The abscissa indicates developmental age, beginning at embryonic day 12 and continuing until postnatal day 25.

day 1 versus day 10 had a differential effect on dendritic branching[18]; and third, there was a striking correlation between behaviour and the extent of dendritic branching (Figure 8). In particular, we found that the animals with day 10 lesions had the most extensive dendritic branching and showed impressive behavioural sparing whereas the day 1 animals had the least dendritic branching and they performed miserably at the same behavioural tasks. We have now observed parallel results in animals with hemidecortications[21], cingulate lesions[30], and visual cortex lesions[19]. Furthermore, we have shown that there is a significant improvement in the performance of a variety of behavioural tasks following frontal cortical removal in adult animals and it is plausible to suggest that the increase in dendritic arbor in the adult animals may provide a basis for at least some of this improvement. Thus, we now believe that the dendritic reaction to injury may be widespread and may consistently correlate with behavioural outcome. Our next task is to determine what this dendritic response actually means to the operation of the brain and what factors might control the response. It would be especially interesting to know whether the dendritic and axonal reactions to cerebral injury are correlated. Furthermore, it would be interesting to determine the relationship between glial activity and dendritic branching. It may be that the production of trophic factors by glia might facilitate the increase in dendritic branching.

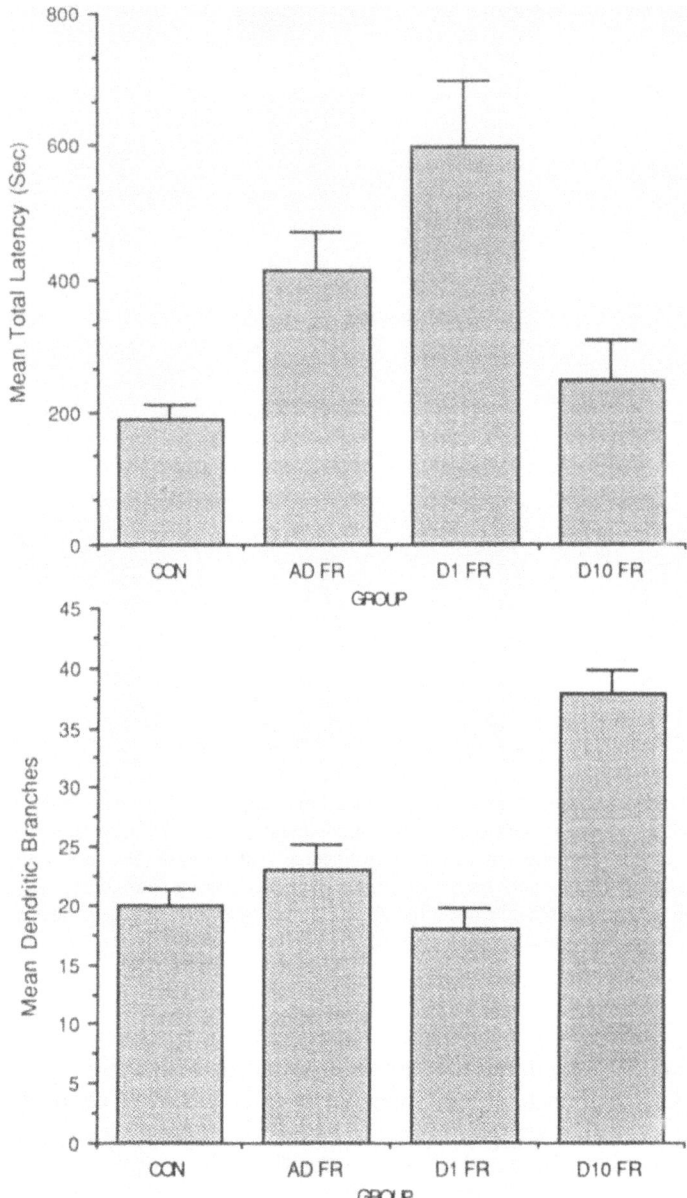

Figure 8. Summary of behavioural performance in the Morris water task (top) and extent of dendritic branching in parietal layer II/III pyramidal cells (bottom) in rats with frontal lesions in adulthood (AD FR), on the day of birth (D1 FR), or at 10 days of age (D10 FR). Rats with day 10 lesions show sparing of function, which is correlated with an increase in dendritic branching. Rats with day 1 lesions show an enhanced behavioural deficit and a reduction in dendritic branching relative to adult operates.

We have been impressed with one additional finding related to dendritic reactivity: there are limits to the extent of dendritic change. Our first hint of this came when Whishaw and I studied the effect of unilateral motor cortex injury on dendritic branching proximal to the injury. In the course of this study we trained some animals to use their paw contralateral to the injury in hopes of enhancing behavioural recovery. To our chagrin we failed to influence recovery rate with the training. However, when we examined the brains we discovered three things. First, the motor cortex lesion led to an increase in dendritic branching proximal to the lesion (Figure 9), much as we had seen previously for animals with prefrontal lesions in adulthood. Second, training normal animals to reach with one paw led to an increase in dendritic branching, much as had been described earlier by Greenough et al[10]. Third, training did not increase dendritic branching in the lesion animals. We have now obtained similar results in other experiments (e.g. 17) so that it appears that there may be limits to the brain's ability to change. That is, if the brain changes in response to the injury it may not be capable of further change in response to other factors such as experiences. Indeed, this limit to change is reminiscent of the fact that the injured brain may not be able to respond normally to the processes related to aging, which was discussed earlier.

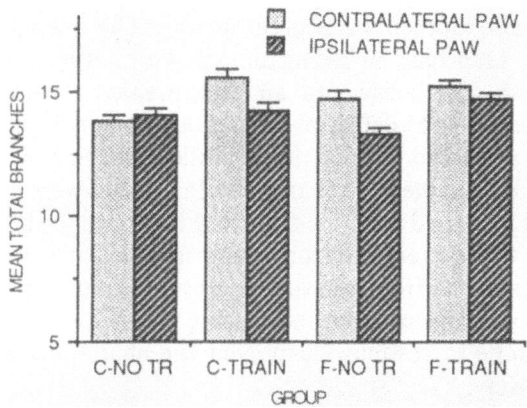

Figure 9. The effect of unilateral motor cortex lesions and training upon dendritic branching. Normal rats were either given two weeks of daily practice at reaching through bars for food (C-TRAIN) or were given a diet of soft food in the home cage (C-NO TR). Training increased dendritic branching in the hemisphere contralateral to the trained paw. Rats with motor cortex lesions were given similar experience. The untrained group (F-NO TR) showed an inrease in dendritic branching in the lesioned hemisphere but training produced no additional increase in this hemisphere, although it did lead to an increase in the intact hemisphere (F-TRAIN). (B. Kolb & I.Q. Whishaw, unpublished observations).

UNSOLVED PROBLEMS

Although we have come a considerable way in understanding the brain-behaviour relationships in recovery of function, there are still many significant obstacles that confront us. I shall consider two that I believe to be particularly important for us over the next decade. These are the problems of correlation and behaviour.

The Problem of Correlation

The explanation of behavioural recovery after cerebral injury is by no means solved by correlating post-injury reactions with behaviour. Indeed, the proof of a causal relationship between brain and behaviour requires the results of critical experiments that have only begun to be carried out. For instance, if one is able to show a correlation between a neural or glial reaction to injury and behaviour, at least two critical experiments are necessary before one can seriously entertain causal relationships. First, if there is a causal relationship it should follow that blockade of the brain's reaction will block, or alter, the behavioural recovery. Second, using parallel logic, it should follow that enhancement of the brain's reaction should potentiate behavioural recovery. Such experiments are difficult at best and represent a major challenge for neuropsychological investigations. The experiments are possible, however, as illustrated in some of our recent work.

In view of our intriguing correlation between dendritic branching and behavioural sparing from neonatal frontal lesions, we designed experiments to either block recovery or facilitate recovery and then we examined the dendritic branching[23]. In order to block recovery Sutherland and I took advantage of our earlier finding that neonatal noradrenaline depletion would block sparing of spatial learning after prefrontal lesions at postnatal day seven[34]. We thus replicated the earlier experiment but this time we analyzed dendritic branching. The results showed a significantly greater reduction in dendritic branching in the lesioned animals than in the control animals in response to the NA depletion, a finding which correlated with the behavioural results. Thus, we showed that a treatment that blocked the enhanced dendritic branching also blocked behavioural sparing. Our second experiment aimed to increase dendritic branching by raising animals with postnatal day 1 lesions in an enriched environment. The behavioural analysis revealed a marked decrease in the magnitude of the behavioural deficit in the lesioned animals while the anatomical experiment showed a marked increase in dendritic branching, an increase that was greater in the lesion than in the control animals. In sum, we were able to demonstrate that a treatment that increased dendritic branching improved the behavioural outcome whereas a treatment that decreased dendritic branching led to a worsened behavioural outcome. We are still far from showing a causal relationship between dendritic reaction and behavioural outcome but this is the type of experimentation that will be required if we are to be successful in identifying the neural mechanisms responsible for behavioural recovery.

The Problem of Behaviour

The function of the nervous system is to produce behaviour. Not surprisingly, therefore, behavioural change is undoubtedly the most sensitive measure of injury to much of the CNS, especially the cerebrum. It thus seems paradoxical that whereas much of neuroscience is becoming increasingly molecular in its focus, there is apparently little interest in a parallel development in behavioural analysis. In fact, if reports from journal editors and grant committees can be taken as evidence, there appears to be a growing *disinterest* in basic neuropsychological studies of brain-behavioural relations. An example will illustrate. A couple of years ago I listened to a biochemist lecturing some psychology students at their Society for Neuroscience poster, with his general argument being that behavioural studies were never going to lead anywhere. He clearly believed that molecular biology was going to be the key to understanding brain function. Being unable to resist, I asked him if he really believed that understanding calcium channels was going to explain how he spoke or found his car in the parking lot. His response to me suggested that he most certainly believed me to be crazy and most certainly an exemplar of the point he was trying to make!

The point that I am making is that the analysis of behaviour is every bit as important as the study of other aspects of CNS function (e.g. 43). Furthermore, there needs to be a concerted effort to develop a behavioural methodology that will allow us to make better correlations with increasingly detailed measures of chemistry, anatomy, and physiology of the brain. Equally important, however, there needs to be a recognition that adequate behavioural analysis does not mean reporting the number of errors to criterion on some task. There needs to be a careful determination of how the behaviour has been changed initially by the injury and how it has evolved over time (e.g. 44). Unfortunately it does not follow that if an animal regains the ability to solve some sort of task after cerebral injury, there must be an underlying change in the nervous system. It is incumbent upon the investigator to demonstrate that the apparent recovery does not simply represent the adoption of a different behavioural strategy to solve the task.

DIRECTIONS FOR THE FUTURE

I was asked by the editors of this volume to speculate on the directions that brain-behaviour studies ought to go in the future. I have no crystal ball but I do have some strong biases about the directions that will be most profitable, and unprofitable, in the coming years.

First, I believe that there needs to be more emphasis upon recovery as being merely one example of plasticity in the nervous system. In this way recovery is seen in the same category as learning, memory, long-term potentiation, aging, and so on. Learning and memory, including environmental stimulation, have been the subject of much more intense examination than recovery, and it seems likely to me that we can take advantage of what has been found in such studies. That is, it seems probable that the nervous system is conservative and whatever mechanisms are being used for plasticity in one circumstance are likely to be used in others, such as recovery. There is little reason to believe that the brain has a distinct mechanism for recovery from injury.

Second, I believe that there needs to be more consideration of the parallel between recovery and development. This idea is hardly novel (e.g. 4, 35), but it does not appear to be generally acknowledged. Nonetheless, if we are to repair the nervous system it is likely that it will best be done by repeating what the brain does during development. Furthermore, I do not believe that we have taken advantage of the fact that recovery is exceptional at certain times during development. There must be lessons to be learned here.

Third, I believe that there must be a trend toward studies in which there is not only a detailed analysis of behaviour but also multiple correlating measures in the same animals. Examples include the analysis of behaviour, anatomy, chemistry, and/or physiology in the brains of the same animal. Such studies are necessarily more difficult but in the long run they will provide far richer sources of information than one-shot studies with a single dependent variable.

Fourth, I believe there should be increasing attention paid to the role of various trophic factors in recovery. These include hormones (including sex hormones) growth factors such as NGF, gangliosides, growth associated proteins, etc. Importantly, however, it is essential that studies do not simply administer some factor and report the behaviour of brain-injured animals on a test such as a simple maze. There needs to be a determined effort to understand the nature of the behavioural recovery as well as measures of the brain's reaction to injury with and without the trophic factor.

Finally, I have a strong bias on the direction that we should not be headed. During the 1980s there was a general tendency to hope that administration of a "magic bullet" would lead to recovery from cerebral injury. A good example is the search for a cholinergic agonist that would arrest senile dementias, especially Alzheimer's disease. Another example is the use of cortical grafts to ameliorate the loss of cortical functions. As tantalizing as the initial results of pharmacological and transplant studies might have been, it is naive to think that a system that nature has evolved with multiple inputs and balances can be saved by simply administering a single drug treatment or by grafting in embryonic tissue. Such treatments may prove beneficial in systems where it is known that a single neurochemical component is absent, such as in Parkinson's disease, but I see little reason to believe that recovery from cerebral injury, whether it be vascular, traumatic, or of other origin, is likely to be found in a single treatment. It seems more likely that we will be able to design effective treatment regimes to facilitate recovery from brain injury if we can better identify what mechanisms underlay the recovery process when we see it.

REFERENCES

1. Coleman, P., and Flood, D. G., 1988, Is dendritic proliferation of surviving neurons a compensatory response to loss of neighbors in the aging brain?, in *Brain Injury and Recovery, Controversial and Theoretical Issues,* S. Finger, T.E. LeVere, C.R. Almli, and D.G. Stein, eds., pp. 235-247, Plenum, New York.

2. Cotman, C. W., and Nadler, J. V., 1978, Reactive synaptogenesis in the hippocampus, in *Neuronal Plasticity,* C. W. Cotman, ed., pp. 227-271, Raven Press, New York.

3. Cunningham, T.J., Huddelston, C., and Murray, M., 1979, Modification of neuron numbers in the visual system of the rat, *J. Comp. Neurol.,* **184,** 423-434.

4. Finger, S., and Almli, C. R., 1985, Brain damage and neuroplasticity: mechanisms of recovery or development? *Brain Res. Rev.,* **10,** 177-186.

5. Finger, S., and Almli, C. R., 1988, Margaret Kennard and her 'principle' in historical perspective, in *Brain Injury and Recovery, Controversial and Theoretical Issues,* S. Finger, T.E.LeVere, C.R. Almli, and D. G. Stein eds., pp. 117-132, Plenum, New York.

6. Foerester, A., 1988, Return of function after optic tract lesions in adult rats: Spontaneous axonal regeneration?, in *Post-Lesion Neural Plasticity,* H. Flohr, ed., pp. 473-480, Springer-Verlag, New York.

7. Geschwind, N., 1965, Disconnexion syndromes in animals and man, *Brain,* **88,** 237-294, 585-644.

8. Goldman, P.S., 1974, An alternative to development plasticity: Heterology of CNS structures in infants and adults, in *Plasticity and Recovery of Function in the Central Nervous System,* D. G. Stein, J. J. Rosen, and N. Butters, eds., pp. 149-174, Academic Press, New York.

9. Glassman, R.B., and Smith, A., 1988, Neural spare capacity and the concept of diaschisis: Functional and evolutionary models, in *Brain Injury and Recovery, Controversial and Theoretical Issues,* S. Finger, T.E. LeVere, C. R. ALmli, and D.G. Stein, eds., pp. 45-69, Plenum, New York.

10. Greenough, W.T., Larson, J.R., and Withers, G.S., 1985, Effects of unilateral and bilateral training in a reaching task on dendritic branching of neurons in the rat motor-sensory forelimb cortex, *Behav. and Neural Biol.,* **44,** 301-314.

11. Hicks, S., and D'Amato, C.J., 1970, Motor-sensory and visual behaviour after hemispherectomy in newborn and mature rats, *Exp. Neurol.,* **29,** 416-438.

12. Irle, E., 1987, Lesion size and recovery of function: some new perspectives, *Brain Res. Rev.,* **12,** 307-320.

13. Kawaguchi, S., 1988, Regeneration of cerebellofugal projection in kittens, in *Post-Lesion Neural Plasticity,* H. Flohr, ed., pp. 421-439, Springer-Verlag, New York.

14. Kennard, M.A., 1942, Cortical reorganization and motor function, *Arch. Neurol.,* **48,** 227-240.

15. Kolb, B., and Elliott, W., 1987, Recovery from early cortical damage in rats: **II.** Effects of experiences on anatomy and behaviour following frontal

lesions at 1 or 5 days of age, *Behav. Brain Res.*, **26**, 47-56.

16. Kolb, B., and Gibb, R., 1990, Anatomical correlates of behavioral change after neonatal prefrontal lesions in rats, *Prog. Brain Res.*, **85**, 241-256.

17. Kolb, B., and Gibb, R., 1991, Sparing of function after neonatal frontal lesions correlates with increased cortical dendritic branching: a possible mechanism for the Kennard effect, *Behav. Brain Res.*, **43**, 51-56.

18. Kolb, B., and Gibb, R., 1991, Environmental enrichment and cortical injury: Behavioral and anatomical consequences of frontal cortex lesions, *Cerebral Cortex*, **1**, 189-198.

19. Kolb, B., Gibb, R. and Ladowsky, R., Recovery from early cortical damage in rats: 7. Effects of occipital and temporal lesions at 4 or 10 days of age on cerebral anatomy and behaviour, in submission.

20. Kolb B., Gibb, R., and Muirhead, D., 1991, Anatomical basis of recovery of spatial learning after neonatal prefrontal lesions in rats, *Soc. Neurosci. Abstr.*, **17**, 875.

21.. Kolb, B., Gibb, R., and van der Kooy, D., 1992, Cortical and striatal structure and connectivity are altered by neonatal hemidecortication in rats, *J. Comp. Neurol.*, in press.

22. Kolb, B., Gibb, R., and van der Kooy, D., Frontal cortical lesions in rats at 1 or 10 days have differential effects on cortical structure and connectivity, in submission.

23. Kolb, B., and Sutherland, R.J., 1992, Noradrenaline depletion blocks behavioral sparing and alters cortical morphogenesis after neonatal frontal cortex damage in rats, *J. Neuroscience*, in press.

24. Kolb, B. Sutherland, R.J., & Whishaw, I.Q., 1983, Abnormalities in cortical and subcortical morphology after neocortical lesions in rats, *Exp. Neurol.*, **79**, 223-244.

25. Kolb, B., and Tomie, J., 1988, Recovery from early cortical damage in rats. IV. Effects of hemidecortication at 1, 5, or 10 days of age on cerebral anatomy and behaviour, *Behav. Brain Res.*, **28**, 259-284.

26. Kolb, B., and Whishaw, I.Q., 1981, Decortication in rats in infancy or adulthood produced comparable functional losses on learned and species-typical behaviours, *J. Comp. Physiol. Psychol.*, **95**, 468-483.

27. Kolb, B., and Whishaw, I.Q., 1981, Neonatal frontal lesions in the rat: sparing of learned but not species-typical behaviour in the presence of reduced brain weight and cortical thickness, *J. Comp. Physiol. Psychol.*, **95**, 863-879.

28. Kolb, B., and Whishaw, I.Q., 1989, Plasticity in the neocortex: Mechanisms underlying recovery from early brain damage, *Prog. Neurobiol.*, **32**, 235-276.

29. Kolb, B., and Whishaw, I.Q., 1992, *Fundamentals of Human Neuropsychology*, Third Edition. W.H. Freeman & Co., New York.

30. Kolb, B., and Whishaw, I.Q., 1991, Mechanisms underlying behavioral sparing after neonatal retrosplenial cingulate lesions in rats: Spatial navigation, cortical architecture, and electroencephalographic activity, *Brain Dysfunction*, (in press).

31. Kolb, B., Zaborowski, J., and Whishaw, I.Q., 1989, Recovery from early cortical damage in rats: 5. Unilateral lesions have different behavioral and anatomical effects than bilateral lesions, *Psychobiology*, **17**, 363-369.

32. Lashley, K.S., 1929, *Brain Mechanisms and Intelligence*, University of Chicago, Chicago.

33. LeVere, N.D., Gray-Silva, G., and LeVere, T.E., 1988, Infant brain injury, in

Brain Injury and Recovery, Controversial and Theoretical Issues, S. Finger, T.E LeVere, C.R. Almli, and D.G. Stein, eds., pp. 133-150, Plenum, New York.

34. Marshall, J., 1984, Brain function: neural adaptations and recovery from injury, *Ann Rev. Psych.*, **35**, 277-308.

35. Nieto-Sampedro, M., and Cotman, C.W., 1985, Growth factor induction and temporal order in central nervous system repair, in *Synaptic Plasticity*, C.W. Cotman, ed., pp. 407-456, Guilford Press, New York.

36. Schwartz, M., Cohen, A., Harel, A., Solomon, A, and Belkin, M., 1988, Modulation of glial cell response to injury and CNS regeneration, in *Post-Lesion Neural Plasticity*, H. Flohr, ed., pp. 49-56 , Springer-Verlag, New York.

37. Sohlberg, M.M., and Mateer, C.A., 1989, *Introduction to Cognitive Rehabilitation*, Guilford Press, New York.

38. Sutherland, R.J., Kolb, B., Whishaw, I.Q., and Becker, J.B., 1982, Cortical noradrenaline depletion eliminates sparing of spatial learning after neonatal frontal cortex damage in the rat, *Neurosci. Lett.*, 32, 125-130.

39. Vargha-Khadem, F., Watters, G., and O'Gorman, A.M., 1985, Development of speech and language following bilateral frontal lesions, *Brain Lang.*, **37**, 167-183.

40. Whishaw, I.Q., 1990, The decorticate rat, in *The Cerebral Cortex of the Rat*, B. Kolb and R.C. Tees, eds., pp. 239-267, MIT Press, Cambridge.

41. Whishaw, I.Q., and Kolb, B., 1984, Behavioural and anatomical studies of rats with complete or partial decortication in infancy, in *Early Brain Damage*, Volume 2., S. Finger and C.R. Almli, eds., 117-138, Academic Press, New York.

42. Whishaw, I.Q., and Kolb, B., 1989, Tongue protrusion mediated by spared anterior ventrolateral neocortex in neonatally decorticate rats: behavioural support for the neurogenetic hypothesis, *Behav. Brain. Res.*, **32,** 101-113

43. Whishaw, I.Q., Kolb, B., and Sutherland, R.J., 1983, The annalysis of behaviour in the laboratory rat, in *Behavioral Approaches to Brain Research*, T.E. Robinson ed., pp. 141-210, Oxford Univ. Press, New York.

44.. Whishaw, I.Q., Pellis, S.M., Gorny, B.P., and Pellis, V.C., 1991, The impairments in reaching and the movements of compensation in rats with motor cortex lesions: an endpoint, videorecording, and movement notation analysis, *Behav. Brain Res.*, **42,** 77-91.

RESEARCH ON RECOVERY: ENDS AND MEANS

F D Rose

Department of Psychology
Goldsmiths' College
University of London
London, England

D A Johnson

Department of Clinical Psychology
Astley Ainslie Hospital
Edinburgh, Scotland

INTRODUCTION

The emergence of the study of recovery of function following brain damage as a major research area within the neurosciences dates back less than two decades. During that short period it has developed rapidly and, as Stein and Glasier (this volume) have observed, its growth has been particularly marked in the period since the first European Brain and Behaviour Society meeting on the subject in 1981[45]. Certainly it is an area of neuroscience in which recent developments have captured the imaginations not only of scientists, clinicians and others with an interest in recovery but also, to some extent, the public at large. As we have noted elsewhere:

> "Research on recovery is now a multinational, multidisciplinary and multimillion dollar activity, the progress of which can be charted through numerous conferences, in several major books and, more recently, in the emergence of journals devoted to this area ---" (Rose & Johnson[37]).

That this investment of expertise, enthusiasm and money has paid some dividends is clear: evidence is to be found in the pages of the present volume. Perhaps most notable is the dramatic progress which has occurred in the field of neural implantation (see Hitchcock, Sinden et al., and Stein and Glasier, this volume). Two decades ago the focus of this area of enquiry consisted of just a handful of published reports. Now there are hundreds of publications on the subject and, whilst there are many problems still to resolve, we have a considerable appreciation of the mechanisms underlying successful implantation, the effects of implantation on the host brain and the possible role of such effects in restoring impaired function.

There are many other areas of recovery of function research in which significant, if less news-worthy advances have been made, of course. For example, in a recent review, Zasler [47] concluded:

> "There is now good evidence that many acute, sub-acute and chronic neurological and functional sequelae resulting from brain injury can be lessened and potentially even abated through the thoughtful and appropriate use of pharmacological agents." (p.1)

However, taken overall the picture is uneven and patchy, encompassing both areas of relative neglect such as research on the role of nutrition in recovery (see, for example, Bingham [3] and Dickerson, this volume) but also, we would suggest, areas of apparently disproportionate expenditure of resources. A more general criticism of recovery research is that in all areas there is still insufficient account taken of the complex multifactorial and interactive causation of events during the aftermath of brain damage (for example, Teasdale [43]). An inevitable consequence of this has been to severely limit the extent to which research findings can be generalised across situations. To some considerable degree it is because of this that recovery research has not yielded the much hoped for and much needed guidance for those concerned with the care and rehabilitation of the thousands upon thousands of people whose lives have been blighted by brain damage.

If we reasonably assume that the ultimate objective of research on recovery of function is to counter this "silent epidemic" [23] these shortcomings must surely cause those of us engaged in this type of research to question the efficiency of our activities. How to improve the efficiency and the impact of recovery research was one of the themes of the European Brain and Behaviour Society workshop held at Goldsmiths' College, University of London in April 1991 and one which we wish to take up in this last chapter of the present volume which is based upon that meeting. Here we turn our attention from aspects of the detailed content of recovery research in order to take a more general view of how research in this area is organised and directed: from the content of research we turn to the ends and means of research.

ENDS

Efficiency necessarily is defined in terms of goals. Therefore to increase the efficiency of recovery research we must have clearly defined goals. Crucial to even this elementary level of organisation and direction of our research is a set of agreed definitions pertaining to our subject matter, in terms of which our research goals can be accurately described. Yet a lack of concensus about how recovery and recovery-related processes should be defined persists and continues to form a fundamental hurdle to advancement:

> "The interchangeable use of descriptive words has at times resulted in such high levels of ambiguity that it has impeded progress in the field." (Almli & Finger[1] p.2)

This is an issue which has now been addressed by numerous authors (for example, 1,2,12,20,25,27) and, most recently, has been succinctly summarised by Stein and Glasier in the present volume. We share the concerns of all those who have drawn attention to this problem as, obviously, must all scientists and clinicians working in this field.

There is certainly no shortage of definitions: rather, there are too many alternative definitions of the same terms. In part this reflects the differing professional and disciplinary bases of the clinicians and scientists working in the recovery field but also, it must be said, a regrettable failure of interdisciplinary communication over a period of many years [36]. Related to this is the failure to acknowledge the many differing levels of analysis of recovery and recovery-related phenomena and the ways in which those levels of analysis relate to each other.

In order to overcome the confusion once and for all perhaps what is now required is for a set of definitions of recovery related terms to be drafted and published by an internationally recognised body such as the International Brain Research Organization. In the meantime we offer the following observations on the question of definitions. We believe the way to clarify terminology in this area lies not so much in formulating yet more definitions of existing terms but in applying existing and widely accepted definitions to different levels of analysis of function. This may be aided by viewing recovery research in terms of the sort of matrix shown in the lower part of Figure 1.

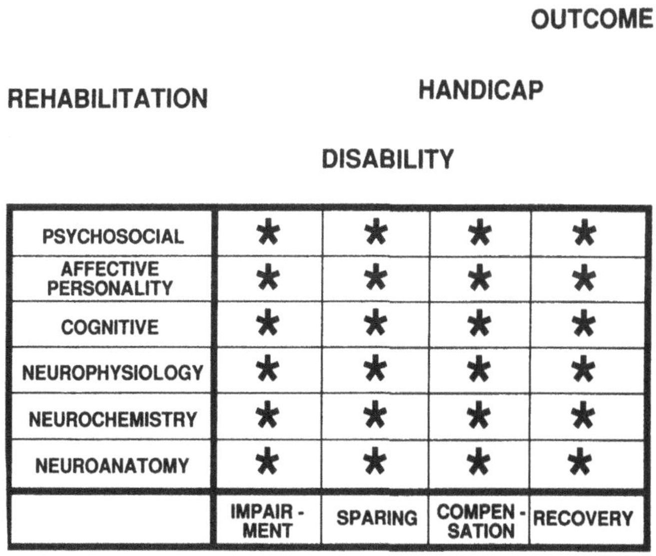

OUTCOME

REHABILITATION   **HANDICAP**

DISABILITY

	IMPAIR-MENT	SPARING	COMPEN-SATION	RECOVERY
PSYCHOSOCIAL	✱	✱	✱	✱
AFFECTIVE PERSONALITY	✱	✱	✱	✱
COGNITIVE	✱	✱	✱	✱
NEUROPHYSIOLOGY	✱	✱	✱	✱
NEUROCHEMISTRY	✱	✱	✱	✱
NEUROANATOMY	✱	✱	✱	✱

Figure 1. Illustration of the relationships between different levels of analysis of recovery and recovery-related processes, and between recovery research and disability, handicap, outcome and rehabilitation. (See text for explanation)

A most important assumption underlying this matrix is that normal function not only may be legitimately defined in terms of different levels of analysis but, to be meaningful, must be defined with reference to a specific level of analysis[12,28]. Here we suggest as the most usual and obvious levels of analysis, neuroanatomical, neurochemical, neurophysiological, cognitive, affective and personality, and psychosocial. Inevitably there is overlap between the levels and additional levels might, arguably, be inserted. However, these six levels adequately encompass descriptions of most studies of brain damage to date. Moving to the horizontal axis of the matrix we come to the terms which have resulted in so much confusion and some of which prompted Almli and Finger's statement quoted above. Yet there need not be confusion as long as in using these terms a level of analysis is also specified. For example, the World Health Organisation definition of impairment[46] is clearly intended to be applicable to all six levels of analysis:

"... any loss or abnormality of psychological, physiological or anatomical structure or function" (WHO[46] p 27)

Equally, the terms sparing (absence of impairment), compensation (achievement of functional objectives by means other than those employed prior to brain damage), and recovery (reinstatement of the impaired function in its original pre brain-damage form) can also occur at all six levels of analysis. Thus the repair of a neural circuit disrupted by brain injury would be just as much an example of recovery of function as would the amnesic patient whose memory was, by some means, restored. However, it is self evident that unless the former were to be referred to as recovery of neural function and the latter as recovery of cognitive function there would indeed be confusion. Similarly, the redirection of a neural message around an area of irreparable damage, and the amnesic overcoming some of the consequences of memory failure by assiduous list making, would both be examples of compensation.

In discussing the terms impairment, sparing, compensation and recovery it is vital to specify the level of analysis, not just in the interests of accuracy and clarity, but also to accommodate the "disengagements" between recovery related processes occurring at different levels of analysis. For example, a *compensatory* neurochemical response to impairment of a neurotransmitter pathway, or the *sparing* of part of that pathway, might be the basis of genuine behavioural *recovery*. Equally it is self evident that *impairment* at the neurochemical level, for example, will not necessarily be accompanied by *impairment* at the psychosocial level. Conversely, *sparing* at the psychosocial level or cognitive level does not necessarily imply *lack of impairment* at the neurochemical level. Although to be expected, these disengagements between levels of functional analysis are frequently the source of confusion about recovery terminology and seen as inconsistencies in the data which can slow or even divert a fruitful line of enquiry.

In summary we suggest the key to resolving our definitional problems, at least in part, lies in a more explicit acknowledgement that the word "function" must be qualified in terms of a particular level of analysis but, that said, the terms impairment, sparing, compensation and recovery can then be applied to whatever level of function is being discussed. As for the generic label "recovery research" or "recovery of function research", we would not advocate attempting any revision. Scientists and clinicians encountering these labels in book or journal titles, or in the descriptions of conference objectives know well enough that the content could embrace everything from neurochemical mechanisms to cognitive or behaviour therapy. To alter the generic labels for the sake of "terminological correctness" is both unneccessary and may even add to the confusion. However, in more detailed discussion of their subject matter we certainly would advocate that scientists and clinicians seek to be specific about the levels of analysis being considered when they use the terms impairment, sparing, compensation and recovery.

In formulating research goals we believe reference to the matrix shown in Figure 1 potentially affords the researcher advantages which go beyond clarification of definitions. Firstly, it provides a context within which a particular piece of research can be viewed and its position relative to other research and other levels of analysis can be readily seen. By the same token it helps in identifying gaps in the overall picture which future research should seek to fill. A second potential advantage of viewing research in terms of the Figure 1 framework lies in providing for the scientist a constant reminder of the relevance of his or her immediate objectives to the ultimate aim of the whole exercise, to maximise outcome for the patient with brain damage.

There are already widely accepted definitions of those terms in Figure 1 which have immediate relevance to clinical objectives:

Disability: " ... any restriction or lack (resulting from an impairment) of ability to perform an activity in the manner or within the range considered normal for a human being." (WHO[46] p 28)

Handicap - "... a disadvantage for a given individual, resulting from an impairment or a disability, that limits or prevents the fulfilment of a role that is normal (depending on age, sex and social and cultural factors) for the individual." (WHO[46] p 29)

Outcome - "... representing the cumulative impact of the individual's entire personal history following onset of the condition." (Fuhrer[14] p 3)

Rehabilitation - " ... the restoration of patients to their fullest physical, mental and social capability." (Mair[29] p 5)

This latter definition has been widely accepted and the objectives of the practice of rehabilitation agreed in general terms[21].

Within this context of defining research goals, the purpose of Figure 1 is to illustrate the relationship between the various levels of analysis of impairment, sparing, compensation and recovery (within which, we have argued, all recovery research to date can be described), and the clinically significant measures of disability, handicap and outcome. More specifically, disability may be seen almost as an algebraic summation of the processes of impairment, sparing, compensation and recovery, occurring at all the various levels of analysis. Pursuing the analogy further, handicap may be seen as the result of this algebraic summation, to which has been applied a weighting factor derived from the pre brain-damage lifestyle expectation for that individual. A series of further weighting factors must then be applied to the equation to represent the effects of whatever rehabilitative interventions may be attempted. These may influence handicap directly (by reducing lifestyle requirements) or disability, by operating on one or more cells of the matrix. The overall result, once this increasingly complex formula has finally been computed, is outcome.

Recovery research, in these terms, can be seen as tackling problems at varying distances from the primary clinical objectives of reducing disability, overcoming handicap and improving outcome. Research in all the cells of the matrix, and at whatever remove from primary clinical practice, is important. However, we believe it can only increase the effectiveness of recovery research if scientists more closely monitor the sequence of moves and the pattern of pathways via which their research might aid primary clinical objectives.

Since resources are limited all our research objectives cannot be pursued with equal vigour. Setting priorities must form part of the exercise of defining goals, therefore. Here also it may help to bear in mind the matrix view of the field of recovery research shown in Figure 1. Ultimately the yardstick against which we measure the value of our research must be that of outcome. This is the measure which is of primary interest to the patient and the patient's family and friends. Of course, contrary to the views of some funding agencies and health authorities, this does not constitute an argument for immediate reallocation of resources to projects thought to have the greatest immediate relevance to direct improvement of outcome. To do this would be to overlook a self evident, if unpalatable truth. A wide variety of factors other than recovery research can influence outcome, for example, improvements in handling compensation claims [6], revisions of legislation regarding discrimination against the disabled[4,7,18] and improved access to public buildings and transport[16]. Moreover, in the immediate future some would argue that these other factors are likely to have so much more impact on outcome than research on brain machanisms of recovery that fine tuning of research priorities in favour of outcome related projects is likely to have very little effect overall. In any case in order to ensure sound theoretical bases of thereapeutic interventions, which in the longer term can be expected to have the most profound and lasting effects on outcome, it is vital that we undertake research to elucidate all aspects of the brain's response to injury. However, to view our research against a wider, outcome-calibrated, reality will certainly help to focus our thinking in ordering our priorities.

For the clinician too this sort of matrix, serving effectively as a "cognitive map" of the recovery research area, should also have value. Being able to see the focus of a piece of research in terms of different levels of analysis of specific recovery related processes will aid assessment of its relevance to the development of therapeutic interventions and to eventual outcome. The matrix also effectively provides a check list for assessing the specific target and theoretical justification for therapies which are in use. What recovery related process is the therapy aimed at and through manipulation of which substrate level (neurochemical, neurophysiological, cognitive etc.) is it intended to have its influence? For example, as yet there is scant empirical support for the efficacy of cognitive rehabilitation (for example, see 15,30,33,34 and Diller, this volume). One likely reason for this is a failure to pay adequate attention to the neurobiological substrates of cognition. An understanding of the neural mechanisms underlying cognition is surely central to explaining both cognitive and psychosocial malfunctioning after brain damage [2,24]. Yet clinical and research reports of cognitive rehabilitation typically make no reference to the neurobiological levels of analysis, preferring to focus exclusively on behavioural and computer-based interventions. That absence of neurobiological analysis therefore impedes the development of an adequate theoretical base for this category of interventions.

In addition to the need for clarification of terms in the recovery of function area there is also a need for a more critical appraisal of the ways in which recovery and related processes are measured. Measures are often too general to be informative: equally they can be too specific. At the cognitive and neuropsychological level complete reliance on traditional global concepts such as memory and intelligence quotients (MQ and IQ) has been roundly criticised by Lezak [26], among others, who has made the point that such an approach:

> "... may obscure specific facets of neuropsychological status or misrepresent it generally." (p 351)

For example, it has been well documented[19,41,42] that patients with severe traumatic brain damage predominantly to the frontal lobes, can perform well on IQ tests and achieve normal scores. Moreover, even when IQ is reduced this may tell us little about the nature of the deficit. After head injury, the Wechsler IQ's may be lowered but the constituent subtests are multifactorial in nature[5] and the performance decrement could be due to any number of problems in visual perception, planning, verbal comprehension, or attention. Of course the Wechsler Intelligence Scales can be meaningful and of great practical benefit in the guidance of the patient's rehabilitation, if they are analysed in terms of their broad factorial structure and used to generate hypotheses for further evaluation.

Potentially just as misleading is adopting too specific a measure of recovery or of recovery-related processes. Given the highly complex inter-relatedness of function at all levels of analysis, which is characteristic of the brain, any conclusions regarding recovery which are couched in terms of a single measure, be it anatomical, biochemical, behavioural or whatever, must be regarded as extremely tentative. This problem is more likely to be found in basic research and has already been the subject of some discussion by Rose et al in the present volume. Clearly there are compelling arguments for greater use of batteries of tests in research on recovery of function in animals.

An additional problem of measurement in recovery of function research is caused by the need to measure the same function repeatedly over a period of time[13]. The point has already been made in this volume and elsewhere[22] that consequences of brain damage are not necessarily immediately apparent but manifest themselves over a period of weeks, months or years. Moreover, it is also clear that the temporal arrangement of the consequences of brain damage are crucially dependent upon the developmental stage of the brain at the time the damage occurs. Therefore, in recovery research it is essential that we have measures of sufficient reliability and validity to be meaningfully applied repeatedly and at different stages of development.

In view of the particular problems of measurement in recovery of function research we would do well to remember Teuber's dictum that absence of evidence is not evidence of absence.

MEANS

A point which has emerged very clearly from recovery of function research over the years, and one which has been further emphasised by Kolb in the present volume, is that the precise functional consequences of brain damage depend upon a multiplicity of factors[8,9,10,11,12,32,40]. Among the most obvious are the causation, location, size and momentum of the lesion, age at the time of the damage, premorbid status in terms of functional capacities, gender, time since the damage occurred, environmental and nutritional conditions during that period and the effects of any therapeutic interventions. Moreover, these factors are frequently interactive. In consequence, investigation of the mechanisms of recovery and identification of the optimal conditions for maximising recovery presents a daunting research challenge. A question which must be addressed is whether the current organisation of our research activities is capable of meeting this challenge.

Scientific research is differently organised in different countries and is obviously subject to change as governments' priorities also change. It is difficult to make general statements, therefore. However, despite occasional international initiatives (for example, the European Science Foundation Network arrangements) and periodic national revisions of the basis of science funding, with consequent minor realignments and regroupings of research workers, for most of us working in the recovery of function area little has changed in recent years. Generally, research has continued within the familiar framework of university, research institute or clinic. To a large extent it continues to be organised in a piecemeal fashion with numerous small research groups pursuing relatively independent lines of enquiry and relying upon conferences, journals and informal contacts to keep in touch with others sharing similar interests. Collaboration between us tends to be patchy and haphazard. When it does occur it tends to be small in scale and, typically, the result of individual and localised initiatives rather than any systematic appraisal of research objectives.

Individuals and research groups working in relative isolation will at best be able to encompass within their experimental designs and resource allocations only a small proportion of the factors known to influence recovery processes. The inevitable consequence will be a continuation of those largely inexplicable failures to replicate results from one laboratory to another and, therefore, continued difficulty in generalising and extrapolating results to new situations. On the other hand if several research groups, organised into a collaborative network, contribute systematically to an agreed research plan using appropriate database systems for handling the much larger volume of results which would ensue, truly multifactorial studies of recovery can be attempted. Moreover, once a central database serving several laboratories has been established it can be interrogated to investigate questions which go beyond the original research plan and which certainly could not be answered by analysis of any one of the contributing data sets. Opponents of such proposals argue that large collaborative networks necessarily engender increased bureaucracy and may stifle individual initiative. The scientist's suspicion of bureaucracy and administration is almost legendary, of course and well illustrated by the following anecdote:

> "...physicists claim to have discovered the heaviest element known to science - "administratium". It has no protons or electrons and its atomic number is zero. What it does have is one neutron, eight assistant neutrons, thirty five vice-neutrons and two hundred and fifty six assistant vice-neutrons. Completely inert, it can be detected chemically because it impedes every action with which it came into contact..." (The Times[44] - Copyright Times Newspapers Ltd. 1991)

A second criticism of centrally organised collaboration is that replication (or not) of the findings of others by truly independent laboratories is an essential element of scientific advance. On both counts we believe the concern to be unfounded. Far from stifling individual initiative we see collaborative networks as providing the levels of resources which will allow new ideas to be taken up. Good ideas, hatched in the context of small, relatively isolated and perhaps relatively poorly resourced research groups, which are not shared and not investigated, will be of little value to those with brain damage. On the question of replication of results we fully accept that this is a vital stage in the scientific process. However, there is surely a greater likelihood of systematic replications being carried out within a multigroup network than within our present system. In any case there is little point in retaining a system which is geared to independent replication of small scale studies (if, indeed, it is) if what is needed to achieve the desired research goals is large scale multifactorial studies.

In addition to facilitating the large scale multifactorial studies which can begin to address the real complexity of recovery from brain damage, we believe there are other advantages in more widespread collaboration between researchers. As Stein and Glasier (this volume) have observed, recovery at the biochemical and neural levels ultimately is only important to the extent that it can be the basis of behavioural and psychological recovery. A vital aspect of recovery research, therefore, is relating empirical findings from the different levels of analysis which are the preserve of different scientific disciplines. Thus a multidisciplinary approach is essential. Since there are few, if any, recovery of function laboratories in which all the relevant disciplines are adequately represented, collaborative networks may provide the best chance of a fostering a truly interdisciplinary approach.

It is not only collaboration between different scientific disciplines which is necessary, of course. If the results of recovery research are to have a real impact on outcome, as we have defined it earlier in this chapter, there must also be communication between scientists and clinicians (neurologists, neurosurgeons, psychologists, psychiatrists, nurses, occupational therapists,physiotherapists, speech therapists) and, through them, with patients, their relatives and patient support groups. This is even more difficult to achieve but to seek to involve clinicians in collaborative research networks is one possible way to proceed. Not only would this help clinicians to make the maximum use of research findings but would also allow scientists to more accurately judge the relevance of their work to the issue of outcome. Additionally such collaboration could considerably increase the pool of raw data. There are many clinicians dealing with brain damage, working outside major research centres, who would like to be involved in some research. Often that wish fails to be translated into action because they have neither the time nor, perhaps, access to a sufficient number or variety of patients to undertake a complete research project. Contributing data to a central database would be entirely feasible, however. Already there are some such networks and databases (see Diller, this volume) but more are needed to avoid unnecessary waste of both data and research ability.

A final aspect of collaboration, which formed a prominent theme of the 1991 EBBS meeting on recovery of function concerns collaboration between those studying humans and those studying animals. Over the last ten to fifteen years reaction against the use of animals in scientific research has grown considerably and, despite some indications that the extremism of the 1980's may now be giving way to a more balanced view[31], the ethics of animal experimentation is still a major issue[39]. Yet for the forseeable future experiments on animals are going to be essential to continued progress in understanding recovery of function following brain damage. The question therefore arises of how scientists working in this area should react to these doubts and misgivings being expressed in society at large. That scientists should adopt the highest standards in carrying out their reseach goes without saying and has certainly been the subject of discussion within the European Brain and Behaviour Society[35]. A greater willingness to publicly defend their particular line of research would also help considerably, although the personal risks involved in doing this can be considerable. However, we also believe that it greatly strengthens the position of scientists if their research is carried out in the context of a collaborative programme involving both scientists and clinicians. As we have already observed such an arrangement allows the relevance of proposed research to immediate clinical problems to be more readily assessed. However, in the public mind there may also a question of credibility. If so one of the most effective defences of animal experimentation in recovery research is that it is being conducted within the framework of an integrated and co-ordinated approach to clinically defined problems.

A FINAL WORD

Recovery of function research is a large, rapidly developing and complex area of science and, out of the whole range of neuroscience, it is an area which has associated with it a particular urgency because of its potential for application to the rehabilitation of those with brain damage. Indeed in this "Decade of the Brain" [17] much is expected:

> "...potential for incalculable reductions in the human and economic costs of brain disease" (Goldstein [17] p. 321)

> "... our basic science colleagues have provided medical science colleagues with a vast background of data and insights that can be readily applied to brain diseases" (Rosenberg and Rowland[38] p, 322)

In addition to the high expectations placed upon it, recovery research has particular requirements in terms of the need for co-ordinated contributions from many scientific disciplines and clinical professions. From an organisational viewpoint, therefore, recovery research is a highly complex activity which merits constant review. The issue can be illustrated by posing two questions. If we were asked to advise on how best to organise research designed to investigate mechanisms of recovery of function would we recommend our existing system? If not, in what ways would we seek to improve it? In the present discussion of the ends and means of recovery research we have sought to stimulate discussion which might help to provide some answers.

REFERENCES

1. Almli, C.R., and Finger, S., 1988, Towards a definition of recovery of function, in S. Finger, T.E. LeVere, C.R. Almli, and D.G. Stein, eds., *Brain Injury. Theoretical and Controversial Issues*, pp 1-14, Plenum, New York.

2. Bach y Rita, P., and Bach y Rita, E. W., 1990, Biological and psychosocial factors in recovery from brain damage in humans, *Canad. J. Psychol.*, **44**, 148-165.

3. Bingham, S., 1991, Dietary aspects of health strategy for England, *Brit. Med. J.*, **303**, 353-355.

4. CORAD, 1982, *Report by the Committee on Restrictions Against Disabled People*, HMSO, London.

5. Crawford, J.R., Johnson, D.A., Mychalkin, B., Cameron, I.M., Allan, K.M., Moole, J.W., Gullion, F., and Moss, A.R. (submitted), Factor structure of the WAIS-R in a clinical sample.

6. Dywan, J., Kaplan, R.D., and Pirozzolo, F.J., eds., 1991, *Neuropsychology and the Law*, Springer, New York.

7. Equal Opportunities Commission, 1982, *Caring for the Elderly and Handicapped*, EOC, London.

8. Finger, S., ed., 1978, *Recovery From Brain Damage, Research and Theory*, Plenum Press, New York.

9. Finger, S., and Almli, C.R., 1984, *Early Brain Damage, Volume 1, Research Orientations and Clinical Observations*, Academic Press, Orlando.

10. Finger, S., and Almli, C.R., 1984, *Early Brain Damage and Recovery. Volume 2. Neurobiology and Behaviour*, Academic Press, Orlando.

11. Finger, S., LeVere, T.E., Almli, C.R., and Stein, D.G., 1988, *Brain Injury and Recovery. Theoretical and Controversial Issues*, Plenum, New York.

12. Finger, S., and Stein, D.G., 1982, *Brain Damage and Recovery. Research and Clinical Perspectives*, Academic Press, New York.

13. Finset, A., 1991, Some methodological problems in assessing neuropsychological recovery of function. A case illustration. Paper presented to the European Brain and Behaviour Society Workshop on Recovery of Function Following Brain Damage, Goldsmiths' College, University of London, April 1991.

14. Fuhrer, M.J., 1987, *Rehabilitation Outcomes: Analysis and Measurement*, Brookes, Baltimore.

15. Fussey, I., 1990, Evaluating the status of cognitive rehabilitation, in R.L. Woods, and I. Fussey, eds., pp. 249-258, *Cognitive Rehabilitation in Perspective*, Taylor and Francis, London.

16. Goldsmith, S., 1976, *Designing for the Disabled*, RIBA, London.

17. Goldstein, M., 1990, The decade of the brain, *Neurology*, **40**, 321.

18. Groves, R., and Gladstone, G., 1982, *Disabled People - A Right to Work?* Bedford Square Press, London.

19. Hebb, D.O., 1949, *Organization of Behaviour. A Neuropsychological Theory*, Wiley, New York.

20. Held, J.M., 1987, Recovery of function after brain damage: theoretical implications for therapeutic intervention, in J.H. Carr, R.B. Shepherd, J. Gordon, A.M. Gentile, and J. M. Held, eds., *Movement Science: Foundations for Physical Therapy in Rehabilitation*, pp 155-177, Aspen, Rockville.

21. Hunter, J., and Walker, J., 1989, *The Role of a Rehabilitation Medicine Service*. Rehabilitation Studies Unit, University of Edinburgh.

22. Johnson, D.A., Uttley, D., and Wyke, M., eds., 1989, *Children's Head Injury. Who Cares?* Taylor and Francis, London.

23. Klein, F.C., 1982, Silent epidemic: head injuries difficult to diagnose, get rising attention, *Wall Street Journal*, 24th November.

24. Kraemer, G.W., 1985, The primate social environment, brain neurochemical changes and psychopathology, *Trends in Neuroscience*, **8**, 339-340.

25. Levin, H.S., Benton, A.L., and Grossman, R.G., 1982, *Neurobehavioural Consequences of Closed Head Injury*, Oxford Unoversity Press, New York

26. Lezak, M.D., 1988, IQ: RIP, *J. Clin. Exp. Neuropsychol.*, **10**, 351-361.

27. Luria, A.R., 1963, *Restoration of Function After Brain Injury*, Pergamon Press, Oxford.

28. Luria, A.R., 1973, *The Working Brain. An Introduction to Neuropsychology*, Penguin Books, London.

29. Mair, A., 1972, *Medical rehabilitation: The pattern for the future,* Report of a sub-committee of the Standing Medical Advisory Committee, Scottish Home and Health Department, HMSO, Edinburgh.

30. Mateer, C.A., and Weber, A.M., 1991, Can competencies be retrained? A critical appraisal of cognitive rehabilitation, in J. Dywan, R.D. Kaplan, and F.J. Pirozzolo, eds., *Neuropsychology and the Law*, Springer, New York.

31. Matfield, M., 1992, Prime time terrorism, *Research Defence Society Newsletter*, April, 1-2.

32. Miller, E., 1984, *Recovery and Management of Neuropsychological Impairments*, John Wiley, Chichester.

33. Robertson, I., 1990, Does computerised cognitive rehabilitation work? A review, *Aphasiology*, **4**, 381-405.

34. Robertson, I., 1992, The rehabilitation of visuo-spatial, visuo-perceptual and apraxic disorders, in R.J.Greenwood, M.P. Barnes, and T.M. McMillan, eds., *Neurological Reahabilitation*, Churchill-Livingstone, Edinburgh (in press).

35. Rose, F.D., 1975, Animal experimentation and animal rights. Time for EBBS to speak out? *European Brain and Behaviour Society Newsletter*, **5**, 9-11.

36. Rose, F.D., and Johnson D.A., 1992, Making the most of what we've got, *THINK*, **2**, 7-8.

37. Rose, F.D., and Johnson, D.A., 1992, Progress in understanding recovery of function after brain damage: the need for collaboration, *Restorative Neurology and Neuroscience,* 4, 241-244.

38. Rosenberg, R.N., and Rowland, L.P., 1990, The 1990's decade of the brain: the need for a national priority, *Neurology*, **40**, 322.

39. Smith, J., and Boyd, K., eds, 1991, *Lives in the Balance. The Ethics of Using Animals in Biomedical Research. The Report of a Study by a Working Party of the Institute of Medical Ethics*, Oxford University Press, London.

40. Stein, D.G., Rosen, J.J, and Butters, N., eds., 1974, *Plasticity and Recovery of Function in the Central Nervous System*, Academic Press, New York.

41. Stuss, D.T., and Benson, D.F., 1984, Neuropsychological studies of the frontal lobes, *Psychol. Bull.*, **95**, 3-28.

42. Stuss, D.T., and Benson, D.F., 1986, *The Frontal Lobes*, Ravens Press, New York.

43. Teasdale, G., 1991, The treatment of head trauma: Implications for the future, *J. Neurotrauma*, **8**, Suppl. 1, S-53-8

44. *The Times*, (London), 15th March, 1991.

45. Van Hof, M.W., and Mohn, G., 1981, *Functional Recovery From Brain Damage*, Elsevier, Amsterdam.
46. World Health Organisation, 1980, *International Classification of Impairments, Disabilities and Handicaps*, World Health Organisation, Geneva.
47. Zasler, N.D., 1992, Advances in neuropharmacological rehabilitation for brain dysfunction, *Brain Injury*, **6**, 1-4.

CONTRIBUTORS

J W T DICKERSON - School of Biological Sciences, University of Surrey, Guildford, Surrey, GU2 5XH, England.

LEONARD DILLER - Rusk Institute, New York University Medical Center, 400 West 34th Street, New York, NY 10016, USA.

MARYLOU M. GLASIER - Brain Research Laboratory, Institute of Animal Behaviour, Rutgers, the State University, Newark, New Jersey 07102, USA.

EDWARD HITCHCOCK - Department of Neurosurgery, University of Birmingham, Midland Centre for Neurosurgery and Neurology, Holly Lane, Smethwick, Warley, West Midlands, B67 7JX, England.

HELEN HODGES - Department of Psychology, Institute of Psychiatry, University of London, De Crespigny Park, London, SE5 8AF, England.

M A JEEVES - Psychological Laboratory, University of St. Andrews, St. Andrews, Fife, KY16 9JU, Scotland.

D A JOHNSON - Department of Clinical Psychology, Astley Ainslie Hospital, Grange Loan, Edinburgh, EH9 2HL, Scotland.

CHRISTIAN KELCHE - Laboratoire de Neurophysiologie et Biologie des Comportements, UPR 419 du CNRS - Centre de Neurochimie, 12 rue Goethe, 67000 Strasbourg, France.

BRYAN KOLB - Department of Psychology, University of Lethbridge, Lethbridge, Alberta, Canada, T1K 3M4.

KATHRYN M MARSDEN - Department of Psychology, Institute of Psychiatry, University of London, De Crespigny Park, London, SE5 8AF, England.

CHARLES E POLKEY - The Neurosurgical Unit, Maudsley Hospital, De Crespigny Park, London, SE5 8AZ, England.

F D ROSE - Department of Psychology, Goldsmiths' College, University of London, London, SE14 6NW, England.

JOHN D SINDEN - Department of Psychology, Institute of Psychiatry, University of London, De Crespigny Park, London, SE5 8AF, England.

DONALD G STEIN - Brain Research Laboratory, Institute of Animal Behaviour, Rutgers, the State University, Newark, New Jersey 07102, USA.

M W VAN HOF - Department of Physiology I, Erasmus University, 3000 DR Rotterdam, The Netherlands.

FARANEH VARGHA-KHADEM - Institute of Child Health, University of London, Neurosciences Unit, The Wolfson Centre, Mecklenburgh Square, London, WC1N 2AP, England.

IAN Q WHISHAW - Department of Psychology, University of Lethbridge, Lethbridge, Alberta, Canada, T1K 3M4.

BRUNO WILL - Laboratoire de Neurophysiologie et Biologie des Comportements, UPR 419 du CNRS - Centre de Neurochimie, 12 rue Goethe, 67000 Strasbourg, France.

AUTHOR INDEX

Black, J. E., 91, 97

Blagowestschenskaja, W., 115, 129, 131

Blakemore, C., 160, 161, 167

Bledsoe, S., 2, 22

Blessed, G., 37, 61, 63

Bloom, F. E., 5, 6, 7, 17

Boast, C. A., 7, 17

Bogdasarian, R. S., 6, 18

Bohn, M. C., 41, 56

Bohne, A., 51, 56

Bolam, J. P., 39, 44, 52, 56, 58, 64

Bond, A., 70, 76

Bond, M., 10, 19, 107, 113

Bornstein, D. L., 27, 33

Bouchon, R., 82, 97

Bowen, D. M., 37, 56

Boyd, K., 195, 197

Bracco, L., 11, 17

Bracken, M. B., 106, 112

Bragin, A. G., 51, 56

Braun, J. J., 10, 17

Breakefield, X. O., 41, 42, 62

Bredesen, D. E., 9, 17

Breedlove, S. M., 91, 103

Breeze, R. E., 70, 76

Bregman, B. S., 12, 18

Bremiller, R., 43, 53, 60

Brenner, E., 89, 93, 98

Brion, J. P., 37, 56

Bromiley, R. B., 115, 129

Brooks, C. M., 126, 129

Brown, D. A., 55, 60

Brown, M., 12, 18

Brundin, P., 9, 19, 45, 46, 48, 50, 57, 59, 64, 68, 69, 75, 77

Brunner, R., 82, 102

Buckingham, J. C., 25, 26, 31

Bucy, P. E., 115, 126, 134

Bunch, S. T., 36, 42, 52, 57, 60, 91, 93, 98

Bures, J., 117, 129

Buresova, O., 117, 129

Burns, R. C., 68, 75

Burright, R. G., 88, 99

Busto, R., 7, 13, 16, 17, 21

Buston, R., 7, 8, 18

Butcher, R., 82, 102

Butler, R. H., 109, 112

Butters, N., 193, 197

Buzsaki, G., 8, 17, 38, 63, 90, 99

Bygdeman, M., 44, 63, 68, 69, 77, 78

C

Cahn, A. P., 70, 75

Calin, L., 43, 53, 60

Camenzuli, L. F., 108, 109, 114

Cameron, I. M., 192, 196

Caminiti, R., 164, 166

Canter, C. J., 68, 71, 75

Card, J. P., 38, 62

Carder, R. K., 43, 57

Carlson, G., A., 39, 64

Carlson, K., 88, 100

Carpenter, K., 93, 98

Carughi, A., 93, 98

Carville, C., 115, 129

Casamenti, F., 11, 17

Cassel, J. C., 50, 51, 57, 64, 90, 91, 98

Castenada, E., 127, 129

Castro, A. J., 39, 51, 63, 125, 127, 130

Cepko, C. L., 55, 62

Cerra, F. B., 27, 31

Chadwick, O., 31, 33

Chambers, J., 89, 102

Chang, F.-L. F., 9, 20

Charlton, H. M., 50, 62

Chen, L. S., 9, 17

Chiarello, C., 162, 163, 165

Choi, D. W., 7, 8, 14, 22

Chong, P. N., 70, 76

Chugani, H. T., 137, 148

Church of Scotland and Social Work, 67, 77

Cicerone, K. D., 111, 112

Clark, C. R., 153, 161, 165

Clark, S. L., 118, 133

Clark, W. E. LeGros, 118, 130

Clarke, A. W., 37, 64

Clarke, D. J., 39, 44, 45, 52, 57, 64

Clarke, J. M., 162, 165

Clifton, G. L., 27, 29, 30, 31

Clough, C. G., 70, 72, 76

Cohen, A., 177, 186

Cohen, D., 26, 32

Cole, D. D., 90, 98

Coleman, P., 177, 184

Colin-Drucker, R., 68, 70, 77

Collerton, D., 37, 57

Collier, J. J., 69, 70, 77

Collier, T., 73, 77

Collier, T. J., 42, 61, 70, 71, 75, 78

Collins, G. H., 38, 64

Collins, W. F., 106, 112

Comella, C. L., 68, 77

Connor, D. J., 37, 57

Contant, C. F., 28, 29, 30, 33

Cooper, J. R., 5, 6, 7, 17

CORAD, 191, 196

Cornbrooks, C. J., 7, 19

Cornwell, P., 81, 83, 98

Cornwell-Jones, C. A., 89, 98

Coscina, D., 89, 102

Cotman, C. W., 7, 8, 16, 17, 20, 21, 39, 41, 42, 43, 52, 53, 58, 60, 61, 90, 101, 171, 176, 177, 183, 184, 186

Cowey, A., 163, 165

Coyle, J. T., 37, 52, 57, 64, 75

Crain, B. J., 7, 21

Crawford, J. R., 192, 196

Crnic, L., 93, 98

Cronin-Golomb, A., 164, 165

Crowder, R. G., 107, 112

Culler, E., 115, 126, 130

Cummins, A. C., 48, 62

Cunningham, M. G., 40, 55, 62

Cunningham, T. J., 175, 184

Cupit, L., 41, 56

Curran, E., 12, 13, 21

Cuthbertson, D. P., 24, 31

D

Dahlstrom, A., 67, 75

D'Alecy, L. G., 28, 32

d'Allest, A. M., 164, 167

Dalrymple-Alford, J. C., 15, 19, 50, 57, 79, 83, 84, 85, 90, 91, 92, 98, 100

Damasio, A. R., 4, 17, 145, 146, 148

Damasio, H., 4, 17, 145, 146, 148

D'Amato, C. J., 125, 127, 130, 175, 184

Dandy, M., 137, 148

Danielsen, E., 39, 51, 63

Das, G. D., 67, 73, 75

Davey, M. J., 96, 101, 102, 115, 116, 120, 122, 123, 125, 126, 127, 130, 133

Davies, C. A., 93, 100

Davis, J. N., 86, 88, 99

Davis, L. G., 38, 62

Davison, A. N., 23, 31, 37, 56

De La Torrer, E., 68, 71, 75

De Voogd, T. J., 79, 99

De Vos Korthals, W. H., 115, 123, 126, 134

Dean, R. L., 37, 56

Deckel, A. W., 52, 57, 73, 75

Deckel, W., 74, 76

Deitcher, D. L., 55, 62

Dekker, A. J. A. M., 37, 57

Del Conte, G., 67, 76

Delay, E. R., 86, 98

Dell, P. A., 96, 101, 102, 115, 116, 120, 122, 123, 125, 126, 127, 130, 133

DeLong, M. R., 37, 45, 46, 55, 64

SUBJECT INDEX

The manufacturer's authorised representative in the EU is Springer
Nature Customer Service Centre GmbH, Europaplatz 3, 69115 Heidelberg,
Germany. If you have any concerns regarding our products, please
contact ProductSafety@springernature.com

Printed and bound by CPI Group (UK) Ltd, Croydon, CR0 4YY
23/04/2026
02095623-0014